Diagnostic Parasitology *for* Veterinary Technicians

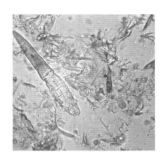

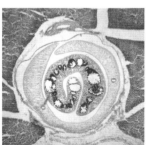

Diagnostic Parasitology
for Veterinary Technicians

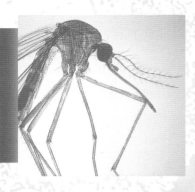

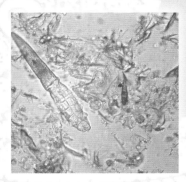

Third Edition

Charles M. Hendrix, DVM, PhD
Professor
Department of Pathobiology
College of Veterinary Medicine
Auburn University, Alabama

Ed Robinson, CVT
Healthy Pet Corporation
DVM Labs
Education Direct

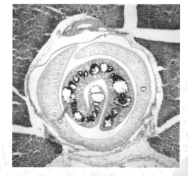

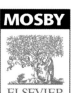
MOSBY

ELSEVIER

with more than 300 color illustrations

MOSBY
ELSEVIER

11830 Westline Industrial Drive
St. Louis, Missouri 63146

Notice

Knowledge and best practice in this field are constantly changing. As new research and experience broaden our knowledge, changes in practice, treatment and drug therapy may become necessary or appropriate. Readers are advised to check the most current information provided (i) on procedures featured or (ii) by the manufacturer of each product to be administered, to verify the recommended dose or formula, the method and duration of administration, and contraindications. It is the responsibility of the practitioner, relying on their own experience and knowledge of the patient, to make diagnoses, to determine dosages and the best treatment for each individual patient, and to take all appropriate safety precautions. To the fullest extent of the law, neither the Publisher nor the Authors assume any liability for any injury and/or damage to persons or property arising out or related to any use of the material contained in this book.

The Publisher

Previous editions copyrighted 1998

ISBN-13: 978-0-323-03614-6
ISBN-10: 0-323-03614-7

Publishing Director: Linda L. Duncan
Managing Editor: Teri Merchant
Publishing Services Manager: Patrician Tannian
Project Manager: Sarah Wunderly
Design Direction: Andrea Lutes

Printed in China

Last digit is the print number: 9   8   7   6   5

To John Schlotthauer, who taught me that the most important part of any veterinary curriculum is the individual student

CMH

To Margi Sirois, who taught me the greatest thing about veterinary technology is helping others learn about the profession

ER

PREFACE

Veterinary clinical parasitology is one of the most important disciplines in any veterinary curriculum, be it a curriculum training veterinary students or one that trains veterinary technicians. This new edition was prepared to follow the educational structure used in parasitology classes in veterinary technology education. Our textbook is intended to inform the reader of the most commonly encountered internal and external parasites of both domesticated and laboratory animals. The text begins with a chapter detailing the language of parasitology, the many terms that describe the intricate host-parasite relationships of veterinary parasitology. These terms are the "framework" of the discipline, the means of communication among veterinarians, veterinary technicians, and their clients. Every veterinary practitioner, veterinarian, veterinary technician, or student, must learn to effectively communicate in this language. Each succeeding chapter describes a different parasite group: protozoans (one-cell organisms), trematodes (flukes), cestodes (tapeworms), nematodes (roundworms), acanthocephalans (thorny-headed worms), arthropods (insects, mites, and ticks), hirudineans (leeches), and pentastomes (tongue worms). As with the last edition, each of these parasite groups is described in detail, with special emphasis placed on morphology, uniqueness of the life cycle, and important parasites within the group. Information on the parasites has been updated and new parasite information has been added to better prepare the technician for the parasites currently seen in the veterinary practice. Treatments and preventive measures have been added to the sections on the major parasites seen in veterinary medicine. A new chapter with a quick reference to the most common parasites has been added, containing pictures of the most common parasite ova seen in diagnostic tests. We have also made a major improvement with this edition with the replacement of black and white photographs with color photographs. We have endeavored to use as many color photographs as possible to assist in the demonstration of key morphologic and diagnostic features needed for proper identification of all classes of parasites. A glossary that defines the terms used in the text and an appendix that provides a quick reference to each parasite in the book, referenced by species, have been added.

This latest edition of *Diagnostic Veterinary Parasitology* was also prepared with the veterinary technician in mind. Parasitology is a large part of the technician's job in any veterinary clinic. Veterinary technicians are responsible for collecting, preparing, and examining fecal tests. In addition, the veterinary technician is responsible for client education in general and parasite education in particular. The information contained within this text will help veterinary technicians become familiar with the parasites seen in veterinary medicine.

Charles M. Hendrix
Ed Robinson

Contents

1

The Language of Veterinary Parasitology

Veterinary medicine continues to be one of the most rapidly evolving health care professions of the twenty-first century. Veterinarians are responsible for many aspects of human health promotion and disease prevention, especially in the areas of food safety, environmental health, prevention and control of zoonotic diseases, and the human-animal bond. To accomplish these important missions, successful veterinarians, along with their professional associates, must learn to communicate effectively with a variety of individuals, ranging from health care professionals in other disciplines, to print and electronic journalists, to the day-to-day clients who walk off the street into the veterinary practice.

One of the most important lines of communication, however, exists between the veterinary practitioner and the members of his or her own veterinary health care team. Veterinary technicians serve as vital members of these health care teams. As such, these technicians must be able to understand and correctly use the nomenclature and terminology for almost every specialty discipline within veterinary medicine. This is especially true for the discipline of *veterinary parasitology*, the study of parasitic relationships affecting domesticated, wild, exotic, and laboratory animals, and, to some extent, those parasites that have the potential to be transmitted directly from animals to humans. If animal parasites are to be effectively treated and controlled, the veterinary technician must become "fluent" in the language of parasitology and be able to communicate effectively, using the specialized terminology associated with these parasites and with the complex interactions between parasites and their animal hosts. This chapter assists the veterinary technician in acquiring fluency with regard to veterinary parasitology.

SYMBIOSIS

Planet Earth is home to millions of species of very diverse, living organisms that include plants, animals, fungi, algae, and unicellular organisms. Likewise, there are millions of complex relationships taking place between and among these differing species of organisms. Many organisms live together in diverse, intricate relationships. The term *symbiosis* (*sym* meaning "together" and *biosis* meaning "living," thus "living together") describes any association, either temporary or permanent, between at least two living organisms of different species. Each member of this association is called a *symbiont.* For example, a lichen growing on the side of a tree (Figure 1-1) is actually a very complex symbiotic relationship between a fungus and an alga. Even the act of

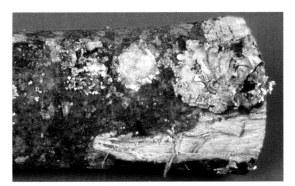

Figure 1-1   Lichen growing on side of tree is symbiotic relationship between fungus and alga.

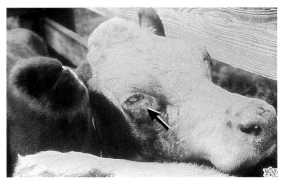

Figure 1-2   *Moraxella bovis*, etiologic agent of infectious bovine keratoconjunctivitis ("pinkeye"), is mechanically carried from eyes of one cow to those of another on sticky foot pads of the face fly *Musca autumnalis.*

a human owning a dog and living with that dog is a type of symbiotic relationship. Two different living species cohabitate; the human "owner" and the "pet" dog are members of a very ancient symbiotic relationship.

There are five types of symbiotic relationships: predator-prey, phoresis, mutualism, commensalism, and parasitism. In a *predator-prey relationship,* there is an extremely short-term relationship in which one symbiont benefits at the expense of the other. For example, the lion (the predator) will kill the zebra (the prey). The prey pays with its life and serves as a food source for the predator.

In *phoresis* (*phore* meaning "to carry") the smaller member of the symbiotic relationship is mechanically carried about by the larger member. The bacterium *Moraxella bovis,* the etiologic agent of infectious bovine keratoconjunctivitis, or "pinkeye" of cattle, is mechanically carried from the eyes of one cow to those of another on the sticky foot pads of the face fly, *Musca autumnalis* (Figure 1-2).

The term *mutualism* describes an association in which both organisms in the symbiotic relationship benefit. For example, within the liquid rumen environment of a cow are millions of microscopic, swimming, unicellular, ciliated protozoans. The cow provides these tiny creatures with a warm, liquid environment in which to live. In return, the rumen ciliates break down

cellulose for the cow and aid in its digestion processes.

The term *commensalism* describes an association in which one symbiont benefits and the other neither benefits nor is harmed. An example is the relationship between the shark and the remora, its "hitchhiker." The remora attaches to the underside of the shark and hitches a ride. The remora also eats the food scraps, or leftovers, after the shark's meal. The remora benefits from this relationship, whereas the shark neither benefits nor is harmed.

In *parasitism* an association exists between two organisms of different species, in which one member (the *parasite*) lives on or within the other member (the *host*), and may cause harm. The parasite has become metabolically dependent on the host.

This book discusses the host-parasite relationships between domesticated and wild animals and their parasites. *Parasitology* is the study of such parasitic relationships.

PARASITISM

Parasitism can occur in differing degrees. In *parasitiasis* the parasite is present on or within the host and is potentially pathogenic (harmful); however, the animal does not exhibit outward

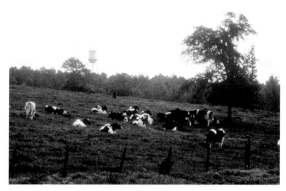

Figure 1-3   Healthy cattle on pasture may harbor bovine trichostrongyles (roundworms) in their gastrointestinal tracts but not exhibit outward clinical signs of parasitism. This condition is known as ***parasitiasis.***

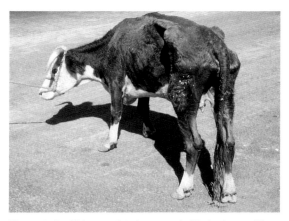

Figure 1-4   This emaciated cow probably harbors millions of bovine trichostrongyles (roundworms) in its gastrointestinal tract. As a result of this parasitism, the cow exhibits obvious outward clinical signs. This condition is referred to as ***parasitosis.***

clinical signs of disease. For example, healthy cattle on pasture may harbor bovine trichostrongyles (roundworms) in their gastrointestinal tracts, but the cattle do not exhibit outward clinical signs of parasitism (Figure 1-3). Parasitiasis describes this type of parasitic relationship.

In *parasitosis* the parasite is present on or within the host and does produce obvious injury or harm to the host animal. The host exhibits obvious outward signs of clinical parasitism (Figure 1-4). For example, an emaciated cow on pasture certainly harbors bovine trichostrongyles (roundworms) in its gastrointestinal tract. Parasitosis describes this type of parasitic relationship.

In any parasitic relationship, the parasite may live on or within the body of the host. If the parasite lives on the body of the host, it is called an *ectoparasite.* Cat fleas (*Ctenocephalides felis*) on a dog are ectoparasites (Figure 1-5). If the parasite lives *within* the body of the host, it is called an *endoparasite.* The dog heartworm (*Dirofilaria immitis*) is an endoparasite (Figure 1-6). *Ectoparasitism* is parasitism by an external parasite. *Endoparasitism* is parasitism by an internal parasite. Similarly, an ectoparasite will produce an *infestation* on the host, and an endoparasite will produce an *infection* within that host.

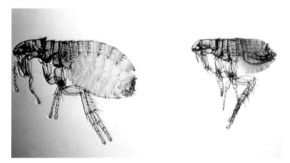

Figure 1-5   These cat fleas *(Ctenocephalides felis)* live within a dog's hair coat. They are ectoparasites and produce **ectoparasitism**. Similarly, these fleas produce infestation in the host's hair coat.

Both endoparasitism and ectoparasitism in domestic animals can be treated by administering *parasiticides,* chemical compounds (both simple and complex) used to treat specific internal and external parasites. The different types of parasiticides include *anthelmintics* (or anthelminthics, compounds developed to kill roundworms, tapeworms, flukes, and thorny-headed worms), *acaricides* (compounds developed to kill mites and ticks), *insecticides* (compounds developed to kill insects), and *antiprotozoals* (compounds developed to kill protozoan organisms).

Sometimes a parasite will wander from its usual site of infection into an organ or location in which it does not ordinarily live. When this

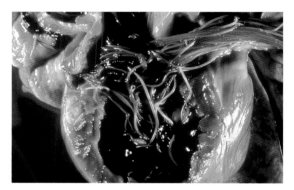

Figure 1-6   These heartworms *(Dirofilaria immitis)* lived in a dog's heart. They are endoparasites and produce **endoparasitism**. Heartworms produce infection within the host's heart. The dog is a definitive host for canine heartworm and harbors adult, sexual, or mature stages of the parasite.

happens, the parasite is called an *erratic parasite,* or *aberrant parasite.* For example, *Cuterebra* species, called "warbles" or "wolves," found in the skin of dogs or cats may accidentally "wander" or migrate into the cranial vault. When this happens, *Cuterebra* becomes an erratic (aberrant) parasite (Figure 1-7).

A parasite can occur in a host in which it does not usually live. When this occurs, the parasite is called an *incidental parasite.* For example, humans can become infected with larval stages of *Dirofilaria immitis,* the canine heartworm (Figure 1-8). Because humans are not the usual host for the heartworm, the canine heartworm is an incidental parasite in humans.

Organisms that are "free living" (nonparasitic) in nature can become parasitic in certain hosts. These organisms are called *facultative parasites.* An example is *Pelodera strongyloides,* a free-living soil nematode (roundworm). This free-living roundworm usually lives in the superficial layers of the soil as a "non-parasite." However, this roundworm is capable of penetrating the skin of many domesticated animals,

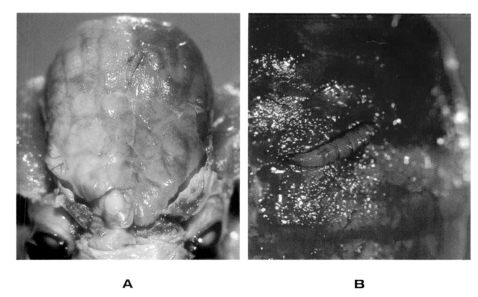

A   **B**

Figure 1-7   A, *Cuterebra* species ("warbles," "wolves") in the skin of dogs or cats may migrate into cranial vault; *Cuterebra* is then an erratic (aberrant) parasite. This parasite has become "lost" on its migration path. **B,** Enlargement of parasite in cranial vault.

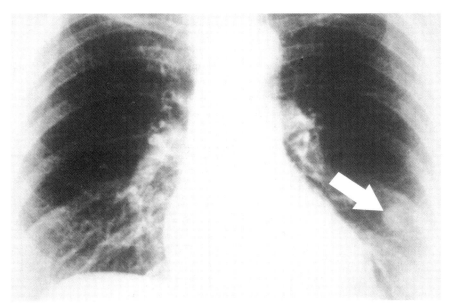

Figure 1-8   Humans can become infected with larval stages of *Dirofilaria immitis*, the canine heartworm. Humans are not the usual host for heartworm, so canine heartworm is an incidental parasite in humans. (Courtesy Ronald E. Bowers, MD.)

particularly dogs lying in moist dirt and "downer cattle," and establishing a parasitic skin infection. *P. strongyloides* is therefore a facultative parasite.

An ***obligatory parasite***, however, is a parasite that must lead a parasitic existence. These are not capable of leading a free-living existence. *D. immitis*, the canine heartworm, is an obligatory parasite; most of the parasites that affect domesticated and wild animals are obligatory parasites.

A parasite does not necessarily have to live on or within a host. It can make frequent short visits to its host to obtain nourishment or other benefits. Such a parasite is called a ***periodic parasite***. The best example of a periodic parasite is the female mosquito, which sucks blood from the vertebrate host; the host's blood is required for her egg development. Without a blood meal, the female mosquito will not have sufficient protein to lay her eggs.

Living creatures or objects that are not parasitic may be mistaken for or erroneously identified as parasites. These are referred to as ***pseudoparasites.*** Sometimes, fecal flotation pro-

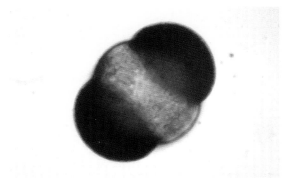

Figure 1-9   Pollen grain from pine tree revealed on fecal flotation. A beginning veterinary student or technician may view this pollen on fecal flotation and erroneously assume the grains are parasites, when they are actually pseudoparasites.

cedures will reveal pollen grains from trees, such as pine pollen (Figure 1-9), or from flowering plants. A novice veterinary student or veterinary technician may view these pollen grains on fecal flotation and erroneously identify them as parasites; they are pseudoparasites.

LIFE CYCLE

Each parasite has its own individual life cycle (Figure 1-10). The life cycle is the development of a parasite through its various life stages. Every parasite has at least one definitive host and may have one or more intermediate hosts. The *definitive host* is the host that harbors the adult, sexual, or mature stages of the parasite. For example, the dog is the definitive host for *D. immitis*; mature male and female heartworms (the sexual stages of the parasite) are found in the right ventricle and pulmonary arteries of the dog's heart (see Figure 1-6). The **intermediate host** is the host that harbors the larval, juvenile, immature, or asexual stages of the parasite. The

female mosquito is the intermediate host for *D. immitis*; larval or immature heartworms (the developing stages of the parasite) are found in the malpighian tubules and proboscis of the mosquito (Figures 1-11 and 1-12). The intermediate host transfers the parasite from one definitive host to another. A parasite may have more than one intermediate host. In the life cycle of *Platynosomum concinum*, the lizard-poisoning fluke of cats, a land snail is the first intermediate host and a lizard is the second intermediate host for the parasite. This liver fluke requires two intermediate hosts to infect the cat.

In a special type of intermediate host, a parasite does not undergo any development, but instead remains arrested, or *encysted* ("in sus-

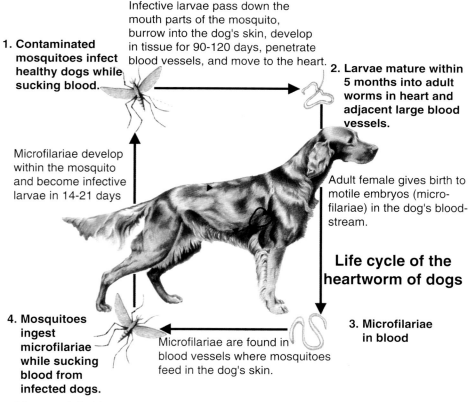

1. Contaminated mosquitoes infect healthy dogs while sucking blood.

Infective larvae pass down the mouth parts of the mosquito, burrow into the dog's skin, develop in tissue for 90-120 days, penetrate blood vessels, and move to the heart.

2. Larvae mature within 5 months into adult worms in heart and adjacent large blood vessels.

Microfilariae develop within the mosquito and become infective larvae in 14-21 days

Adult female gives birth to motile embryos (microfilariae) in the dog's bloodstream.

Life cycle of the heartworm of dogs

4. Mosquitoes ingest microfilariae while sucking blood from infected dogs.

Microfilariae are found in blood vessels where mosquitoes feed in the dog's skin.

3. Microfilariae in blood

Figure 1-10   Life cycle of *Dirofilaria immitis*. In this life cycle the dog is definitive host and the mosquito is intermediate host. Mature male and female heartworms (sexual stages of parasite) are found in right ventricle and pulmonary arteries of dog's heart.

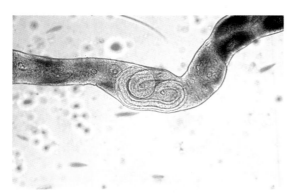

Figure 1-11   The mosquito is intermediate host for *Dirofilaria immitis;* larval or immature heartworms (developing stages of parasite) are found in the mosquito's malpighian tubules.

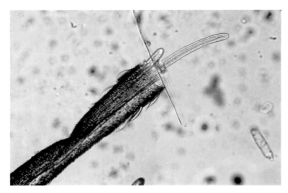

Figure 1-12   Larval or immature heartworms (developing stages of parasite) may also be found in the mosquito's proboscis. The mosquito intermediate host transmits heartworm infection from one dog to another.

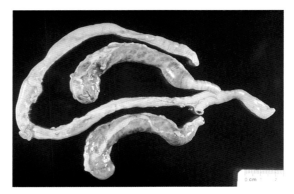

Figure 1-13   *Eimeria tenella* will only infect cecae of chickens; therefore it is a homoxenous or monoxenous parasite.

pended animation"), within the host's tissues. This host is called the **transport host,** or **paratenic host.** The larvae remain in this suspended state until the definitive host eats the transport host. Once within the definitive host, the larvae "wake up," establish an infection, migrate to their predilection site, and grow to adult parasites within the definitive host.

A **reservoir host** is a vertebrate host in which a parasite or disease occurs in nature and is a source of infection for humans and domesticated animals. Heartworms may develop in the right ventricle and pulmonary artery of wild wolves and coyotes. Wolves and coyotes may be reservoir hosts for heartworm; the infection may be spread from the wolf or coyote to the family pet by the mosquito intermediate host.

A **homoxenous** or **monoxenous** parasite is a parasite that will infect only one type of host. For example, *Eimeria tenella,* a coccidian, will only infect chickens. Similarly, a **stenoxenous** parasite is a parasite with a narrow host range. Because *E. tenella* will only infect chickens, it is a stenoxenous parasite. This protozoan parasite only infects the cecae of chickens (Figure 1-13). A **euryxenous** parasite is a parasite with a very broad host range. For example, *Toxoplasma gondii* infects more than 300 species of warm-blooded vertebrates; therefore it is a euryxenous parasite.

A **zoonosis** is any disease or parasite that is transmissible from animals to humans. Examples of parasites that are zoonotic are *T. gondii, Trichinella spiralis, Ancylostoma caninum,* and *Toxocara canis.* Zoonotic parasites are discussed in later chapters.

THE LINNAEAN CLASSIFICATION SCHEME

In beginning biology, students must learn the classification scheme perfected by Linnaeus, an early Swedish biologist. Every organism can be

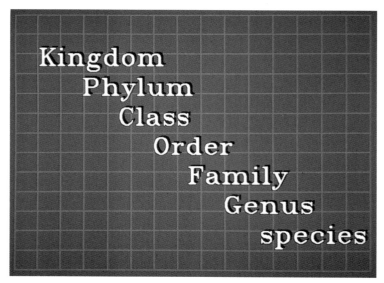

Figure 1-14   All organisms can be classified using the Linnaean classification scheme.

classified using the following classification scheme: kingdom, phylum, class, order, family, genus, and species (Figure 1-14). Students often remember this classification scheme with the simple mnemonic device, "King Philip came over for good spaghetti," in which the first letter of each word in the sentence corresponds to the first letter in the Linnaean classification scheme.

The Linnaean classification scheme works in the following manner. Several million species of animals, plants, fungi, protozoa, and algae live on the earth. These creatures may have different *common names* in different regions of the world. A common name may refer to different organisms in different places. The solution to this problem was to give each organism a *scientific name* composed of two Latin words, which is commonly written in italics. The first word is capitalized and is the *genus name*. The genus indicates the group to which a particular type of animal or plant belongs. The second word is not capitalized; it is the *specific epithet* and indicates the type of animal itself. Examples of common names of animals and their corresponding scien-

tific names are the dog, *Canis familiaris;* the cat, *Felis catus;* the housefly, *Musca domestica;* and a bacterium normally found in the gut, *Escherichia coli.* Similar species are grouped together into the same genus. Similar genera (plural form of genus) are grouped together into the same family. Similar families are grouped together into the same order. Similar orders are grouped together into the same class. Similar classes are grouped together into the same phylum. Similar phyla are grouped together into the same kingdom. Therefore the classification scheme for the dog is as follows:

Kingdom: Animalia
Phylum: Chordata
Subphylum: Vertebrata
Class: Mammalia
Order: Carnivora
Family: Canidae
Genus: *Canis*
Species: *familiaris*

Every living creature has its own unique classification scheme. This text discusses many parasites that affect domesticated animals. It is important to learn the scientific names, the common names, the hosts, and the key identifying features for all these parasites.

The classification scheme contains the following five kingdoms: Planta (plants), Animalia (animals), Protista (unicellular organisms), Monera (algae), and Fungi (fungi). Veterinary parasitology is concerned with only two of these kingdoms as true parasites of domesticated animals. The first is the kingdom *Animalia,* which contains platyhelminths (flatworms— trematodes [flukes] and cestodes [tapeworms]), nematodes (roundworms), acanthocephalans (thorny-headed worms), annelids (leeches), and arthropods (insects, mites, ticks, spiders, pentas- tomes, and other creatures with jointed appendages). The second is the kingdom *Protista,* which contains protozoans (unicellular organisms). The following chapters present parasites from each of these groups and relate their significance in veterinary parasitology.

Any student of veterinary parasitology must use the terms presented in this chapter and their definitions as the "framework" on which to build a greater proficiency in this discipline. As with the veterinarians with whom they work, veterinary technicians must be encouraged to embrace the continual improvement of professional knowledge and competence.

Parasites That Infect and Infest Domestic Animals

2

Chapter 1 describes parasitism as an association between two organisms of different species in which one member (the parasite) lives on or within the other member (the host) and may cause harm. The parasite is metabolically dependent on the host.

In parasitology, the study of parasitic relationships, parasitic groups are classified according to the Linnaean classification system. This chapter presents the parasites that infect and infest domesticated animals, indicating their important characteristics and their place in the Linnaean system.

MONOGENETIC TREMATODES (MONOGENETIC FLUKES)

Kingdom: Animalia (animals)
   Phylum: Platyhelminthes (flatworms)
      Class: Trematoda (flukes)
         Subclass: Monogenea (monogenetic flukes)

Monogenetic flukes are ectoparasites of fish, amphibians, and reptiles. They are rarely parasites of mammals. These flukes are seen most often as ectoparasites of the gills, skin, fins, and mouth of fishes and are rarely observed in a veterinary clinical situation. They might be seen by a veterinarian who specializes in diseases of aquarium fish. Also, some veterinarians may specialize in fish farming or some aspect of aquaculture. Under these conditions, monogenetic flukes frequently may be observed.

DIGENETIC TREMATODES (DIGENETIC FLUKES)

Kingdom: Animalia (animals)
   Phylum: Platyhelminthes (flatworms)
      Class: Trematoda (flukes)
         Subclass: Digenea (digenetic flukes)

Digenetic flukes are important parasites of both large and small animals. These flattened, leaf-shaped flukes are primarily endoparasites of the gastrointestinal tract; however, digenetic flukes can also infect the lungs and blood vasculature. Regardless of the site of infection, the operculated eggs of these flukes can be identified in the feces of domestic animals.

EUCESTODES (TRUE TAPEWORMS)

Kingdom: Animalia (animals)
  Phylum: Platyhelminthes (flatworms)
    Class: Eucestoda (true tapeworms)
Adult true tapeworms are ribbonlike flatworms found in the gastrointestinal tract of their definitive hosts. True tapeworms lack a "gut" or alimentary canal; they absorb nutrients through their tegument (skin). The eggs of these tapeworms are frequently observed on fecal flotation. The larval stages of these true tapeworms may be found in a variety of extraintestinal tissue sites in domestic animals; the animals harboring the larval stages serve as the intermediate hosts. In these extraintestinal sites, the larval stages of these tapeworms may cause more pathology to the intermediate hosts than the adult tapeworm does to the definitive host in its intestinal sites.

COTYLODA (PSEUDOTAPEWORMS)

Kingdom: Animalia (animals)
  Phylum: Platyhelminthes (flatworms)
    Class: Cotyloda (pseudotapeworms)
Similar to true tapeworms, adult pseudotapeworms are flattened and ribbonlike. They resemble true tapeworms and also are found in the gastrointestinal tract of their definitive hosts. Their egg stages may be diagnosed on fecal flotation; they produce operculated eggs. The larval stages of pseudotapeworms are found in microscopic aquatic crustaceans and in the musculature of fish and reptiles. These larval stages seldom produce pathology in domestic animals.

NEMATODES (ROUNDWORMS)

Kingdom: Animalia (animals)
  Phylum: Nematoda (roundworms)
Nematodes, or roundworms, are elongated, unsegmented, cylindric worms. They are called "roundworms" because they are round when observed in cross section on histopathologic examination. Nematodes are the most numerous, complex, and variable among the helminth parasites of domesticated animals. They come in all sizes and shapes and can infect a variety of organs and organ systems. They can produce significant pathology in domesticated animals. On Planet Earth, the nematodes are second only to the arthropods with regard to their numbers and complexity of life cycles. The eggs and larvae of nematodes are most often diagnosed on fecal flotation, so it is important that the veterinary technician become proficient of their identification. Both the adult and the larval stages of nematodes can produce significant pathology in domesticated animals.

ACANTHOCEPHALANS (THORNY-HEADED WORMS)

Kingdom: Animalia (animals)
  Phylum: Acanthocephala (thorny-headed worms)
Acanthocephalans, or thorny-headed worms, are elongated, unsegmented, cylindric worms. They are different, however, from nematodes in that they possess a spiny proboscis on their anterior ends. This spiny proboscis is used as an organ of attachment. Because of this anterior proboscis, acanthocephalans are often referred to as "thorny-headed worms." As with the cestodes (tapeworms), thorny-headed worms lack a gut or alimentary tract; they also absorb nutrients through their tegument (skin). Adult acanthocephalans are very uncommon parasites and are most often found in the gastrointestinal tract. The eggs of these unusual parasites are diagnosed on fecal flotation.

HIRUDINEANS (LEECHES)

Kingdom: Animalia (animals)
  Phylum: Annelida (segmented worms)
    Class: Hirudinea (leeches)
Leeches are blood-feeding ectoparasites of both wild and domesticated animals. These annulated (ringed) worms are typically found in fresh

water, although there may be marine and terrestrial varieties. Leeches may produce significant pathology in both wild and domesticated animals, or they may be beneficial when used after reconstructive surgical procedures in both animals and humans.

ARTHROPODS

Kingdom: Animalia (animals)
  Phylum: Arthropoda (animals with jointed legs)
The phylum Arthropoda is the largest phylum in the animal kingdom. This phylum is quite complex, containing pentastomes, crustaceans, centipedes, millipedes, insects, mites, ticks, scorpions, and spiders.

Arthropods are important in veterinary medicine for the following four reasons:

1. Arthropods may serve as causal agents themselves.
2. They may serve as intermediate hosts for certain helminths and protozoans.
3. They may serve as vectors for bacteria, viruses, spirochetes, and chlamydial agents.
4. They may produce toxins or venomous substances.

Arthropods may parasitize the host as adult or juvenile stages.

PROTISTA (PROTOZOA)

Kingdom: Protista (protozoans—unicellular, or single-cell, organisms)
Trematodes, tapeworms, pseudotapeworms, roundworms, thorny-headed worms, leeches, and arthropods are all members of the animal kingdom. All the parasites described here are *metazoan*, or multicellular, organisms. The remaining parasites belong to the kingdom Protista, which is made up of all of the unicellular organisms. The majority of protozoans on Planet Earth are free living; however, those that are parasitic can cause significant pathology in domesticated animals. Within this kingdom are several phyla, which include flagellates, amoebae, apicomplexans, and ciliates. These protozoans are the primary protozoans that cause significant pathology in domesticated animals. Despite their tiny size, protozoans have complex life cycles and may cause significant pathologic changes in the tissues and organs of domesticated animals.

Each of these groups of parasites and its significance to veterinary parasitology is discussed in detail in the upcoming chapters.

Introduction to the Nematodes

3

Members of the phylum Nematoda, the nematodes, or roundworms, are the most numerous and most diverse group of animals on the Earth. Approximately 10,000 species thrive in very diverse habitats. There are three basic types of nematodes: (1) the free-living nematodes residing in marine water, freshwater, and soil environments; (2) the nematodes that parasitize plants; and (3) the nematodes that parasitize domesticated and wild animals and humans. This chapter discusses the third category, nematodes that parasitize domesticated and wild animals and, to some extent, humans.

NEMATODES OF IMPORTANCE IN VETERINARY MEDICINE

Nematodes in domesticated farm animals in the United States alone cause losses of billions of dollars in animal agriculture resulting from veterinary bills and death. Plant nematodes cause approximately 10% of cultivated crops to be lost each year. It is impossible to determine similar monetary losses in the pet or companion animal "industry."

KEY MORPHOLOGIC FEATURES

Protozoans, discussed in Chapters 10 and 11, are unicellular organisms; nematodes, however, are multicellular organisms. Whereas trematodes (leaflike in form) and cestodes (chainlike or boxcarlike in form) are dorsoventrally flattened in cross section, nematodes are unsegmented, elongate, rounded on both ends, circular in cross section, and bilaterally symmetrical (Figure 3-1); thus they are often referred to as *roundworms*. Nematodes come in a variety of sizes, from *Strongyloides stercoralis* (a tiny parasitic female worm only 2 mm in length and about 35 μm wide (Figure 3-2) to *Dioctophyma renale,* "the giant kidney worm," measuring 100 cm (1 m) in length and 1.2 cm wide (Figure 3-3). As mentioned previously, most nematodes are cylindric and rounded on both ends; however, nematodes do come in a wide variety of shapes, from spherical (definitely not cylindric), such as *Tetrameres* species, which are parasites of the gizzard of domesticated and wild birds (Figure 3-4), to the whiplike *Trichuris* species, which parasitize every domesticated animal except the horse (Figure 3-5).

External Morphologic Features

Nematodes are covered by a thin cuticle (see Figure 3-1). This cuticle covers the exterior body surface of the nematode and extends into all its body openings, that is, the

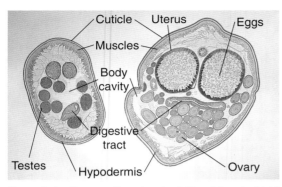

Figure 3-1 Cross section of male *(left)* and female *(right)* *Ascaris suum,* the pig roundworm. Whereas flukes and tapeworms are dorsoventrally flattened, roundworms are usually round in cross section.

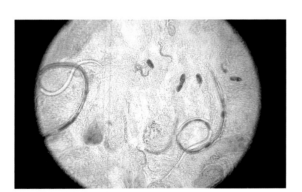

Figure 3-2 Numerous parasitic female *Strongyloides stercoralis* (approximately 2 mm in length and about 35 μm wide) recovered from mucosal scraping from canine small intestine. Also note presence of eggs and first-stage larvae. This is an unusual nematode in that parasitic males do not exist.

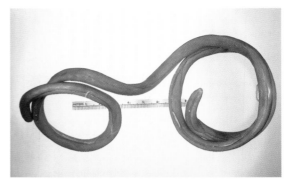

Figure 3-3 Largest nematode known to parasitize domesticated animals, *Dioctophyma renale,* the "giant kidney worm" of dogs. This largest of parasites measures 100 cm (1 m) in length and is approximately 1.2 cm wide.

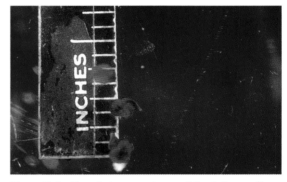

Figure 3-4 Nematodes come in a variety of shapes. Some are spherical, such as *Tetrameres* species, which parasitize the gizzard of domesticated and wild birds.

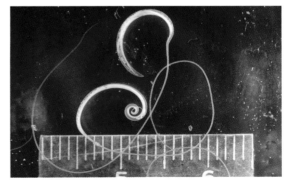

Figure 3-5 Whiplike *Trichuris* species parasitize every domesticated animal except the horse.

mouth, esophagus, and rectal and genital openings. On the external surface the cuticle has a variety of modifications. There may be lateral flattened expansions of the cuticle in the region of the anterior end; these expansions are called *cervical alae* (Figure 3-6). There also may be lateral flattened expansions of the cuticle in the region of the posterior end of some male nematodes; this posterior lateral expansion is called the *copulatory bursa* and serves to hold onto or to grasp the female nematode during the mating

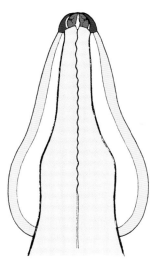

Figure 3-6   Diagrammatic representation of lateral flattened expansion of cuticle on anterior end of *Toxocara cati*, the feline ascarid. These expansions are called cervical alae.

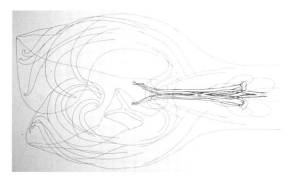

Figure 3-7   Diagrammatic representation of lateral flattened expansion of cuticle on posterior end of male *Haemonchus contortus*, the "barberpole worm" of ruminants. This expansion is called the copulatory bursa and serves to hold onto or grasp the female nematode during the mating process. The copulatory bursa is composed of fingerlike projections called bursal rays. Between each adjacent bursal ray are thin membranes. Male spicules (or intromittent organs) are associated with the copulatory bursa.

process (Figure 3-7). The copulatory bursa is composed of fingerlike projections called **bursal rays**. Between each adjacent bursal ray are thin membranes. The male's highly chitinous and pigmented **spicules** (see Figure 3-7) (the intromittent organs, or "penis") are associated with the copulatory bursa. The cervical alae and the copulatory bursa are only two of the many modifications of the external cuticle of nematodes. The nematode's cuticle is secreted, or formed, by the thin layer directly beneath it, the **hypodermis** (see Figure 3-1).

Just beneath the hypodermis lies the **somatic muscular layer,** the layer of muscles that enables the nematode to move about (see Figure 3-1, muscles). These muscle fibers are spindle shaped and lie along the edge of the hypodermis. Nematodes also possess specialized muscles that aid in feeding and reproductive activities. The muscles line the nematode's **body cavity** (see Figure 3-1). Unlike trematodes (flukes) and cestodes (tapeworms), which lack a body cavity, nematodes (roundworms) do have a body cavity. The body cavity of a typical nematode is not considered a true coelom; it is a **pseudocoelom,** lined by a **pseudocoelomic membrane**.

Internal Morphologic Features

The most important of the nematode's organ systems are the digestive and the reproductive systems.

The digestive tract of the typical nematode is a long, straight tube that extends from the mouth to the anus. On cross section the digestive tract resembles a tube within a tube (see Figure 3-1, *digestive tract*).

The mouth may be surrounded by lips, numbering two up to eight. In some nematodes the lips are replaced by fingerlike projections, or bumps, called **papillae**. Collectively, these papillae may number as many as 40 and are referred to as the **leaf crown** (Figure 3-8). The mouth connects to a buccal cavity, which connects to the esophagus, which connects to a long, winding intestine. The intestine ends with an opening to the outside. Female nematodes have a **rectum**, and male nematodes have a **cloaca**. Remember that the cloaca and the rectum are lined by cuticle and open to the outside through an anus. The

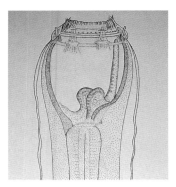

Figure 3-8   Fingerlike projections, or bumps, called papillae on the anterior end of *Strongylus vulgaris.* Collectively, these papillae may number as many as 40 and are referred to as the "leaf crown." The mouth connects to a buccal cavity, which connects to the esophagus, which eventually connects to the long, winding intestine.

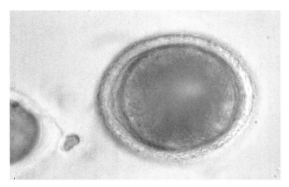

Figure 3-9   Ascaroid, or ascarid, type of nematode egg is best represented by that of *Toxocara canis,* the canine roundworm. Adult female nematode producing this egg type is oviparous. This nematode egg contains a single-cell stage within the eggshell.

part of the nematode's body posterior to the anus is the tail.

Whereas trematodes (flukes) and cestodes (tapeworms) are hermaphroditic (or monoecious), nematodes are **dioecious;** that is, they have separate sexes. There are both male nematodes and female nematodes.

The male reproductive organs consist of one or two **tubular testes** (see Figure 3-1). Usually, a **vas deferens** leads from the testes to the cloaca. There may be a **spicule pouch,** which contains two spicules. Remember that the male nematode's spicules (or intromittent organs) are associated with the copulatory bursa and serve to open the female nematode's vulva during copulation to allow sperm to enter the vagina.

The female reproductive organs consist of one or two **tubular ovaries** (see Figure 3-1, *ovary*). Usually, an **oviduct** leads from the ovary to the uterus. A **seminal receptacle** for sperm storage may be present. The uterus leads to the vagina, which opens to the outside through the vulva. The uterus may contain thousands of eggs or larvae (see Figure 3-1, *uterus* and *eggs*). Parasitic nematodes are very prolific; a single female nematode may produce several thousand eggs (or larvae) each day. The reproductive system is

important because it allows for the production of eggs (and eventually offspring). A veterinary diagnostician confronted with an unrecognized type of nematode can dissect it, and if the nematode is a female, characteristic eggs (or larvae) may be released. When examined microscopically, these eggs or larvae provide a valuable clue as to the type (or species) of nematode.

Female nematodes produce several egg types: (1) the **ascaroid,** or ascarid, type (e.g., *Toxocara canis*) (Figure 3-9); (2) the **trichostrongyle** or strongyle, or hookworm, type (e.g., *Haemonchus contortus* of ruminants, *Strongylus vulgaris* of horses, *Ancylostoma caninum* of dogs) (Figure 3-10); (3) the **spiruroid,** or spirurid, type (e.g., *Spirocerca lupi* of dogs, *Physaloptera* spp. of dogs and cats) (Figure 3-11); and (4) the **trichinelloid** or **trichoroid** type (e.g., *Trichuris vulpis,* the whipworm of dogs, *Capillaria* spp.) (Figure 3-12). In addition, some adult female nematodes produce characteristic larval stages: (1) the microfilariae, or prelarval, stage (e.g., *Dirofilaria immitis* of dogs) (Figure 3-13); (2) the lungworm, or kinkedtail, larvae (e.g., *Aelurostrongylus abstrusus* of cats, *Filaroides osleri* of dogs) (Figure 3-14); and (3) the dracunculoid, or long-tailed, larvae (e.g., *Dracunculus insignis* of dogs) (Figure 3-15). Nematode eggs (and larvae) vary greatly in size

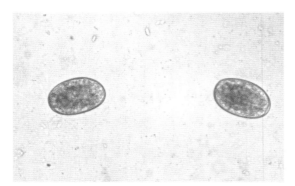

Figure 3-10   Trichostrongyle or strongyle, or hookworm, type of nematode egg is best represented by that of *Ancylostoma caninum*, the hookworm of dogs. Adult female nematode producing this egg type is oviparous. This nematode egg contains a morula stage within the eggshell.

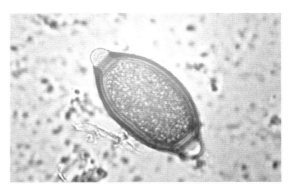

Figure 3-12   Trichinelloid type of nematode egg is best represented by that of *Trichuris vulpis*, the whipworm of dogs. Adult female nematode producing this egg type is oviparous. This nematode egg contains a single-cell stage within the eggshell.

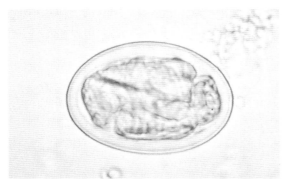

Figure 3-11   Spiruroid, or spirurid, type of nematode egg is best represented by that of *Spirocerca lupi*, the esophageal worm of dogs. Adult female nematode producing this egg type is ovoviviparous. This nematode egg contains a first-stage larva within the eggshell.

and composition. This fact is very important when attempting to render a diagnosis.

Some female nematodes are *oviparous;* that is, the eggs produced by these nematodes contain a single-cell stage (see Figures 3-9 and 3-12) or a *morula stage* within the eggshell (see Figure 3-10). Some female nematodes are *ovoviviparous;* that is, the eggs produced by these nematodes contain a first-stage larva within the eggshell (see Figure 3-11). Finally, some female nematodes are *larviparous;* that is, they retain their eggs within the uterus and incubate them, then give birth to live larvae (see Figures 3-13, 3-14, and 3-15).

LIFE CYCLE OF THE NEMATODE

When compared with the complex life cycles of trematodes (flukes) and cestodes (tapeworms), the typical nematode life cycle is quite simple (Figure 3-16). The adult female nematode produces an egg, which is a single-cell stage within the egg shell. The original cell divides into two cells, two cells divide into four, four cells divide into eight, and so on. The original single-cell stage eventually develops into a morula stage, which in turn develops into a tadpole stage. The tadpole stage develops into a fully formed first-stage larva within the egg shell. This first-stage larva is ready to hatch. The larva emerges from the egg shell, *molts* (sheds its external cuticle), and develops into a second-stage larva. The second-stage larva eventually molts into the third-stage larva. This stage is often referred to as the *infective third-stage larva* because it is infective for the definitive host.

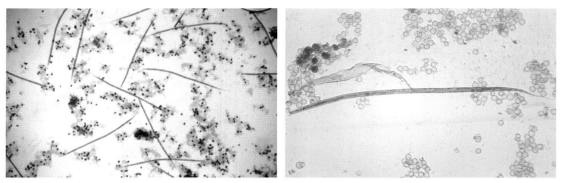

Figure 3-13   Some adult female nematodes produce characteristic larval stages. Microfilariae, or prelarval, stages of *Dirofilaria immitis,* the heartworm of dogs and cats, are characteristic of filarial parasites. Adult female nematode producing this larval type is larviparous. She produces live offspring.

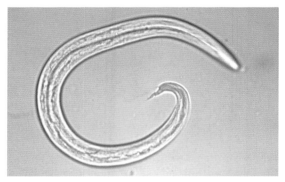

Figure 3-14   The first-stage, kinked-tail larvae of *Aeluro-strongylus abstrusus,* the lungworm of cats, are characteristic of lungworm larvae. Adult female nematode producing this larval type is larviparous. She produces live offspring.

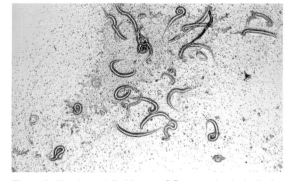

Figure 3-15   Long-tailed larvae of *Dracunculus insignis,* the guinea worm of dogs, are also characteristic larvae. Adult female nematode producing this larval type is larviparous. She produces live offspring.

The first three larval stages can develop in the external environment or within the intermediate host. The intermediate host serves as the means of transmission to the definitive host. Once the infective third larval stage has been reached, it must return to the definitive host to survive. It infects the host either by direct penetration or by intervention of the intermediate host. The intermediate host serves as a means of transmission to the definitive host. Once within the definitive host, the third larval stage molts to the fourth larval stage, which subsequently molts to the fifth larval stage. The fifth larval stage is actually the immature, or preadult, nematode. This stage eventually migrates to its organ or system predilection site and develops into the sexually mature adult stage. The male and female nematodes breed, and the cycle begins again.

Nematodes may or may not use an intermediate host. If there is no intermediate host, the life cycle is said to be a ***direct life cycle***. For example,

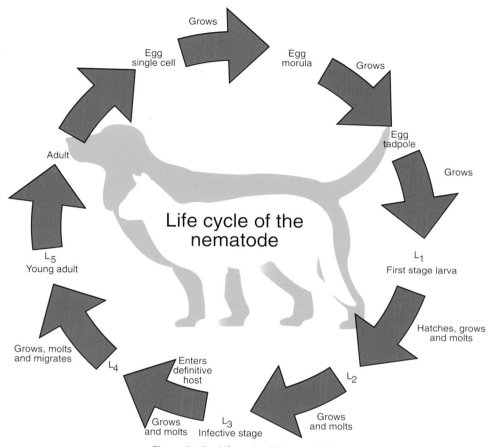

Figure 3-16   Life cycle of the nematode.

canine hookworms (*Ancylostoma* spp.) develop to the infective third stage in the external environment. They penetrate the dog's skin and migrate to the small intestine, where they mature to adults. The canine hookworm's life cycle is said to be "direct."

If the nematode uses an intermediate host, the life cycle is said to be an ***indirect life cycle***. For example, a female mosquito ingests microfilariae of the canine heartworm, *D. immitis,* along with her blood meal. The mosquito incubates the microfilariae, and they eventually develop into infective third-stage larvae within the proboscis

(mouthparts) of the mosquito. When the mosquito takes a blood meal from an uninfected dog, the infective third-stage larvae emerge from the mouthparts and migrate into the puncture wound made by the mosquito. Within the dog, the third-stage larvae molt to fourth-stage larvae and then molt again to fifth-stage larvae (immature, or preadult, heartworms). These larvae migrate to the dog's right ventricle and pulmonary artery, where they mature to adults. The adults breed and the females produce microfilariae. The life cycle begins again. (See Figure 1-10). The canine heartworm's life cycle is said to be "indirect."

A few nematodes produce eggs that do not hatch in the external environment. Within this egg the larva develops to the second stage but does not hatch from the egg. It remains within the egg; the infective stage for these nematodes is the egg containing the second-stage larva.

It is important to remember that there are many variations for this typical nematode life cycle. For every nematode, there is a distinct life cycle; however, the life cycles of most of the nematodes discussed in this book fit those described here.

Nematodes That Infect Domestic Animals

4

This chapter includes brief descriptions of many of the common nematode parasites of domesticated (and wild) animals in the United States. The discussions include information on the tissue, organ, or organ system parasitized in the host. Where appropriate, information is also provided on the *prepatent period* (time from the point of infection until a specific diagnostic stage can be recovered), the diagnostic stage (life cycle stage) most often identified, a morphologic description of this diagnostic stage (e.g., eggs, larvae, or adult), and treatment for the most common parasites.

NEMATODES OF DOGS AND CATS

GASTROINTESTINAL TRACT

Spirocerca lupi, the esophageal worm, is a nematode usually associated with the formation of nodules in the esophageal wall of dogs and cats. Occasionally, this roundworm may be found in granulomas or nodules in the stomach wall of both dogs and cats (Figure 4-1). Adult worms reside in tunnels deep within these nodules and expel their eggs through the fistulous (tract-like) openings in the nodules. Eggs are passed down the esophagus and out in the feces. The thick-shelled eggs of *S. lupi* are 30 to 37 μm by 11 to 15 μm and contain a larva when laid. These eggs have a unique "paper clip" shape (Figure 4-2). Eggs usually can be observed on fecal flotation but may also be recovered from vomitus that has been subjected to standard fecal flotation procedures. Radiographic or endoscopic examination may reveal a characteristic nodule or granuloma within the esophagus or stomach. The prepatent period for this roundworm is 6 months.

Physaloptera species are stomach worms of both the dog and the cat. Although occasionally found in the lumen of the stomach or small intestine, *Physaloptera* species are usually firmly attached to the mucosal surface of the stomach, where they suck blood. With the use of an endoscope, these nematodes can be observed in their attachment sites (Figure 4-3). Their diet consists of blood and tissue derived from the host's gastric mucosa. The feeding habits of these worms may expose their attachment sites, which often continue to bleed after the parasite has detached. Vomiting, anorexia, and dark, tarry stools are often observed in infected animals. The adults are creamy white, sometimes tightly coiled, and 1.3 to 4.8 cm long (Figure 4-4). They may also be recovered in the pet's vomitus; when this happens, *Physaloptera* can easily be confused with

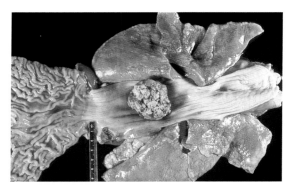

Figure 4-1   *Spirocerca lupi,* the esophageal worm, is a nematode usually associated with formation of nodules in the esophageal wall of dogs and cats.

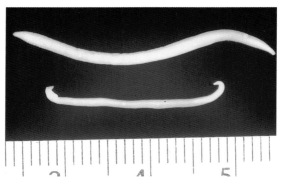

Figure 4-4   Adult of *Physaloptera* is creamy white, sometimes tightly coiled, and 1.3 to 4.8 cm long.

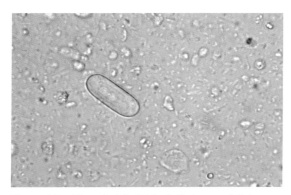

Figure 4-2   Characteristic thick-shelled eggs of *Spirocerca lupi,* with unique "paper clip" shape.

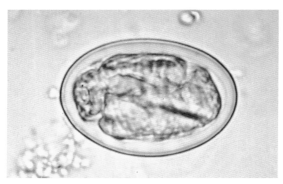

Figure 4-5   Characteristic smooth, thick-shelled, embryonated (larvated) eggs of *Physaloptera* species. Eggs usually can be recovered on standard fecal flotation, using solutions with a specific gravity above 1.25.

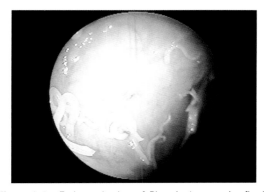

Figure 4-3   Endoscopic view of *Physaloptera* species firmly attached to mucosal surface of stomach.

ascarids. A quick way to differentiate the two parasites is to break open an adult specimen and (if the specimen is female) examine the eggs microscopically.

The eggs of *Physaloptera* species are small, smooth, thick shelled, and embryonated (larvated) when passed in feces. These eggs are quite similar in appearance to the eggs of *S. lupi.* They are 30 to 34 μm by 49 to 59 μm and contain a larva when laid. (See Figure 4-5 for the characteristic egg of *Physaloptera* species.) Eggs can usually be recovered on standard fecal flotation of either feces or vomitus, using solutions with a specific gravity greater than 1.25. The prepatent period for this nematode is 56 to 83 days.

Aonchotheca putorii is commonly referred to as the "gastric capillarid of cats." This nematode was once known by another scientific name, *Capillaria putorii.* This capillarid frequently parasitizes mink but has also been reported in cats. *A. putorii* is rarely reported in North America. The eggs of *A. putorii* are easily confused with other trichuroid nematodes. (See the following section on identification of feline whipworms.) The eggs of *A. putorii* are 53 to 70 μm by 20 to 30 μm and exhibit a netlike surface similar to the eggs of *Eucoleus aerophilus,* another capillarid found in the upper respiratory system. The eggs of *A. putorii* are dense and less delicate than those of *E. aerophilus;* they have flattened sides and contain a one- or two-cell embryo that fills the egg.

Ollulanus tricuspis is the feline trichostrongyle. As a group, the **trichostrongyles** are considered to be parasites of the gastrointestinal tract of ruminants, such as cattle, sheep, and goats; it is quite unusual for the cat to serve as a host for a trichostrongyle. *O. tricuspis* is often diagnosed in cats that exhibit chronic vomiting. These nematodes are usually identified by examining the cat's vomitus under a dissecting or compound microscope. Feline vomitus can also be examined with a standard fecal flotation procedure. The best flotation solution for identification is a modified Sheather's flotation solution. Adult female *O. tricuspis* are tiny, only 0.8 to 1 mm long, and possess three major tail cusps, or toothlike processes, on the tip of the tail (thus the specific epithet *tricuspis*). Adult male nematodes are 0.7 to 0.8 mm long and possess a copulatory bursa. The female worms are larviparous and release infective third-stage larvae (500 × 22 μm), which mature to adults in the cat's stomach. This feline trichostrongyle also is unusual in that these third-stage larvae are immediately infective for any cat that may ingest vomitus containing them. Free-living stages in the external environment are not required for completion of the life cycle.

Toxocara canis, Toxocara cati, and *Toxascaris leonina* are the **ascarids,** or large roundworms, of dogs and cats. These roundworms may be found

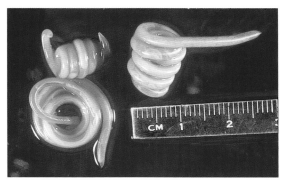

Figure 4-6   Adult ascarids may vary in length from 3 to 18 cm and when passed in feces are usually tightly coiled.

in the small intestine of dogs and cats in most areas of the world. All young puppies and kittens presenting to a veterinary clinic should be examined for the presence of these large, robust nematodes. Adult ascarids may vary in length from 3 to 18 cm and, when passed in the feces, are usually tightly coiled, similar to a coiled bedspring (Figure 4-6). Ascarids in young puppies and kittens may produce vomiting, diarrhea, constipation, and other nonspecific clinical signs. The adult worm does not attach to the host but rather uses an undulating motion to remain in the small intestine. Therefore, adult worms may "swim" into the stomach and cause vomiting. The worm may then be present in the vomitus. Because of the presence of the adult worm in the vomitus, the owner may describe the vomitus as having "spaghetti" in it.

The eggs of *Toxocara* species are unembryonated, spherical, and have a deeply pigmented center and rough, pitted outer shell. Eggs of *Toxocara canis* are 75 by 90 μm in diameter (Figure 4-7), whereas those of *Toxocara cati* are smaller, 65 to 75 μm in diameter (Figure 4-8). The eggs of *Toxascaris leonina* are spherical to ovoid, with dimensions of 75 by 85 μm. In contrast to the eggs of *Toxocara* species, the eggs of *T. leonina* have a smooth outer shell and a hyaline, or "ground glass," central portion (Figure 4-9). The prepatent period for *T. canis* is 21 to 35 days, whereas that of *T. leonina* is 74 days. Ascarids are

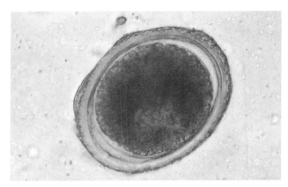

Figure 4-7 Egg of *Toxocara canis* with unembryonated, spherical form with deeply pigmented center and rough, pitted outer shell.

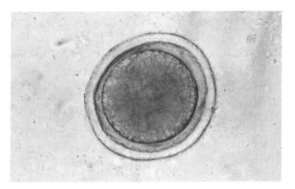

Figure 4-8 Characteristic egg of *Toxocara cati* is similar in structure to that of *T. canis* but smaller in diameter.

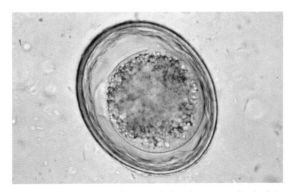

Figure 4-9 Eggs of *Toxascaris leonina* are spherical to ovoid, with dimensions of 75 by 85 μm. In contrast to eggs of *Toxocara* species, these eggs have a smooth outer shell and hyaline, or "ground glass," central portion.

among the most frequently diagnosed nematodes in young puppies and kittens.

The adult "roundworms" are present in the small intestine, where they mate. The female produces umembryonated eggs that are passed in the host's feces. The eggs embryonate to the point that they contain **L2 larvae** on the ground, where they are ingested by a host and the L2 larvae are released from the egg. The L2 larvae may go into dormancy in an adult host, but they grow and migrate to various tissues in the young host. Finally, the L2 larvae migrate to the young host's lungs, where they are coughed up and swallowed by the host. They grow to adulthood in the host's small intestine and begin a new life cycle (Figure 4-10).

In the adult female host, the infective larvae remain dormant until the female host mates and produces hormones during pregnancy. At this time the larvae become active once more and migrate through the female host's body. The larvae (with the exception of *T. cati*) can cross the placental barrier to infect the host's offspring. The most common symptoms of a "roundworm" infection are diarrhea, vomiting, and a pot-bellied appearance.

The most common way of identifying an infection by *Toxocara canis, Toxocara cati,* or *Toxascaris leonina* is through the fecal flotation technique. Usually the pregnant female will have feces tested for these parasites to determine the chances of her puppies or kittens becoming infected with the parasites. Puppies and kittens are routinely dewormed during their first few visits to the veterinary office.

Several types of anthelmintics can be used to treat a "roundworm" infection. A *vermifuge* (anthelmintic that paralyzes the parasite so it passes out in the feces) such as piperazine or pyrantel is often used to treat this type of parasite. A *vermicide* (anthelmintic that kills the parasite and allows the parasite to be broken down by the body) such as thiabendazole or mebendazole can also be used to treat a roundworm infection.

T. canis, although primarily a parasite of the dog, can also infect humans *(visceral larva*

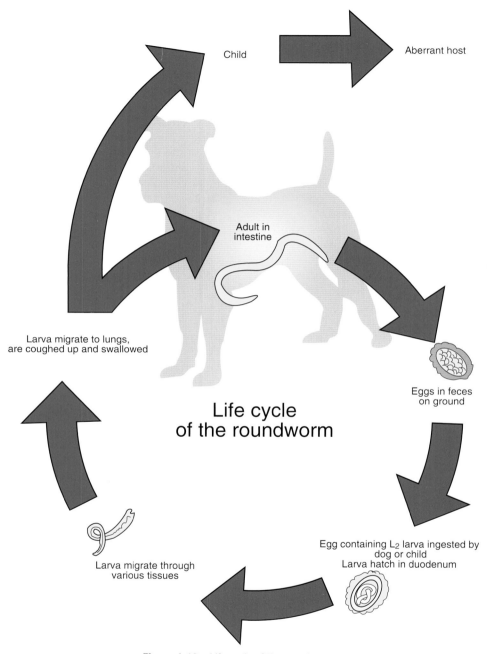

Child

Aberrant host

Adult in intestine

Larva migrate to lungs, are coughed up and swallowed

Eggs in feces on ground

Life cycle of the roundworm

Egg containing L_2 larva ingested by dog or child
Larva hatch in duodenum

Larva migrate through various tissues

Figure 4-10   Life cycle of the roundworm.

migrans), as discussed in Chapter 17. The best way to prevent infection to humans and other animals is cleaning up the feces in the yard at least once a week. Also, prevent children from playing in the yard and placing their contaminated hands to their mouths.

Ancylostoma caninum, the canine hookworm; *Ancylostoma tubaeforme,* the feline hookworm; *Ancylostoma braziliense,* the canine and feline hookworm; and *Uncinaria stenocephala*, the northern canine hookworm, are nematodes that infect the small intestine. Hookworms are found throughout the world but are most often found in tropical and subtropical areas of North America. Hookworms attach to the small intestinal mucosa and suck blood. *A. caninum* demonstrates a frightful buccal cavity—it has three pairs of ventral teeth with which it attaches to the mucosa of the small intestine (Figure 4-11). These parasites may change feeding sites and reattach elsewhere in the small intestine. Because this hookworm feeds on blood, it secretes an anticoagulant from its mouth, which causes the former attachment sites to continue to bleed. Thus the hookworm's voracious feeding activity and the secondary hemorrhage produced can cause significant anemia. Because this bleeding occurs within the small intestine, the blood is digested

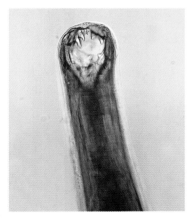

Figure 4-11 *Ancylostoma caninum* demonstrates a frightful buccal cavity, with three pairs of ventral teeth with which it attaches to mucosa of the small intestine of dogs.

by the host and often appears as a black, tarry stool. The resulting anemia can be quite severe in young kittens and puppies. Hookworms often produce serious problems in kennels and catteries. The prepatent period depends on the species of hookworm. Animals are usually infected through percutaneous, prenatal, and transmammary routes.

The male and female worms attach to adjacent villi of the intestinal wall. The male and female mate continuously, and therefore the female continually produces eggs that are laid in the feces. The egg contains the morula stage as it is passed out of the host's body in the feces. These eggs embryonate into L1 larvae in the external environment. The L1 larvae hatch, feed, grow, and molt to L2 larvae. The L2 larvae feed, grow, and molt to L3 larvae, but do not release the cuticle of the L2 larva. They are ensheathed L3 larvae that do not feed. They are the infective stage larvae. The L3 larvae can be ingested, or they can penetrate the host's intact skin and migrate through the tissues of the body until they reach the lungs. Once in the lungs, the larvae are coughed up and swallowed by the host (Figure 4-12).

The larvae of this parasite are able to cross the placenta and also can be passed from mother to offspring through the colostrum. Therefore the pregnant host should be checked several times during pregnancy for the presence of these parasites. Since these parasites can penetrate intact skin, they can also enter the skin of humans (cutaneous larval migrans), as discussed in Chapter 17.

Eggs of all hookworm species are oval or ellipsoidal, thin walled, and contain an 8- to 16-cell morula when passed in feces. Because these eggs embryonate, or larvate, rapidly in the external environment (as early as 48 hours), fresh feces are needed for diagnosing hookworm infections. Eggs of *A. caninum* are 56 to 75 μm by 34 to 47 μm; those of *A. tubaeforme,* 55 to 75 μm by 34.4 to 44.7 μm; those of *A. braziliense,* 75 by 45 μm; and those of *U. stenocephala,* 65 to 80 μm by 40 to 50 μm. These eggs can be easily recovered on standard fecal flotation (Figure 4-13).

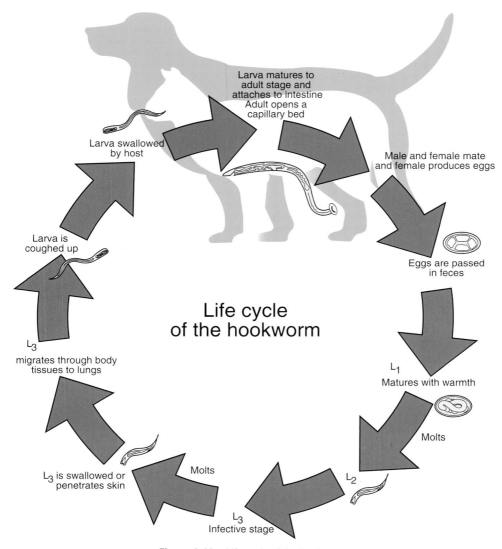

Larva matures to
adult stage and
attaches to intestine
Adult opens a
capillary bed

Larva swallowed
by host

Male and female mate
and female produces eggs

Larva is
coughed up

Eggs are passed
in feces

Life cycle
of the hookworm

L_3
migrates through body
tissues to lungs

L_1
Matures with warmth

Molts

L_3 is swallowed or
penetrates skin

Molts

L_2

L_3
Infective stage

Figure 4-12 Life cycle of the hookworm.

Treatment for the hookworm species can take two forms. The first is prevention with the use of once-a-month heartworm preventive agents; Interceptor and Heartgard are the most common brands. Many of these preventive medications are also labeled for the prevention of hookworms. If the parasite eggs are found on fecal flotation or other techniques, the veterinarian may choose a vermicide such as mebendazole or fenbendazole.

The best way to prevent hookworm species from infecting animals or humans is removing the feces after defecation by the host. Removal during warm weather should take place immediately after defecation, whereas removal during cold months may take place every other day.

Strongyloides stercoralis and *S. tumiefaciens* are often referred to as intestinal threadworms. These nematodes are unique in that only a parthenogenetic female is parasitic in the host.

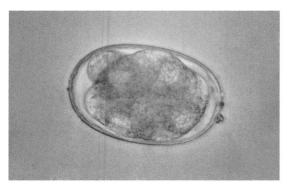

Figure 4-13 Eggs of all hookworm species are oval or ellipsoidal, thin walled, and contain an 8- to 16-cell morula when passed in feces. These eggs may represent one of several genera that parasitize dogs and cats: *Ancylostoma caninum, A. tubaeforme, A. braziliense,* and *Uncinaria stenocephala.*

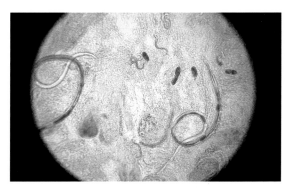

Figure 4-14 Parasitic adult females, eggs, and first-stage larvae of *Strongyloides stercoralis,* intestinal threadworms.

Parasitic males do not exist. These females produce embryonated or larvated eggs, but in dogs the eggs hatch in the intestine, releasing first-stage larvae that may be observed in fresh feces. (See Figure 4-14 for the parasitic adult females, eggs, and first-stage larvae of *Strongyloides* species.) The larval *Strongyloides* species are 280 to 310 μm long and possess a rhabditiform esophagus, with a club-shaped anterior corpus, a narrow median isthmus, and caudal bulb. The prepatent period is 8 to 14 days. These nematodes frequently are associated with a moderate-to-severe diarrhea in young puppies,

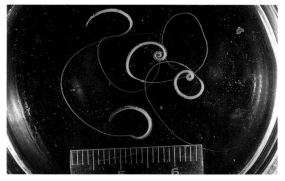

Figure 4-15 *Trichuris vulpis,* the canine whipworm, derives its common name from the fact that adults possess a thin, filamentous anterior end ("lash" of the whip) and thick posterior end ("handle" of the whip).

particularly in kennel environments during the summer months.

Trichuris vulpis, the canine whipworm, and *Trichuris campanula* and *Trichuris serrata,* the feline whipworms, reside in the cecum and colon of their respective definitive hosts. Whipworms are a common clinical occurrence in dogs; however, it is important to remember that feline whipworms are quite rare in North America and have been diagnosed only sporadically throughout the world. Whipworms derive their name from the fact that the adults have a thin, filamentous anterior end (the "lash" of the whip) and a thick posterior end (the "handle" of the whip (Figure 4-15). The egg of the whipworm is described as *trichuroid* or *trichinelloid;* it has a thick, yellow-brown, symmetric shell with polar plugs at both ends. The eggs are unembryonated (not larvated) when laid. Eggs of *T. vulpis* are 70 to 89 μm by 37 to 40 μm. (See Figure 4-16 for the characteristic egg of *T. vulpis.*) The prepatent period for *T. vulpis* is 70 to 90 days.

The adult *Trichuris* species are attached to the wall of the cecum or colon and produce eggs. The eggs are passed out in the feces of the host. Once in the environment, the eggs will go through a period of development to become an L1 (infective) larva within the egg. Unlike the hookworm species, the whipworm species must be ingested

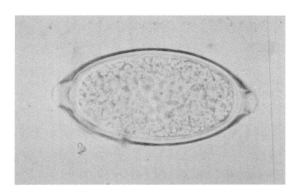

Figure 4-16 Characteristic egg of *Trichuris vulpis* is described as *trichinelloid* or *trichuroid;* it has a thick, yellow-brown, symmetric shell with polar plugs at both ends. Eggs are unembryonated (not larvated) when laid.

by the host. The L1 larva will hatch from the egg once in the host's small intestine. The larva will molt several times in the small and large intestine before becoming an adult. The new adult will migrate back through the colon to the cecum and attach to the intestinal wall (Figure 4-17). The most common symptoms seen in infected animals are diarrhea, anemia, and mucus-coated stool.

The eggs of *T. campanula* and *T. serrata,* the feline whipworms, may be easily confused with *Aonchotheca putorii, Eucoleus aerophilus,* and *Personema feliscati,* parasites of the feline stomach, respiratory tract, and urinary system, respectively. The eggs of *T. campanula* average 63 to 85 µm by 34 to 39 µm (Figure 4-18). When examining a cat's feces for trichurids, it is important that the diagnostician remember that pseudoparasites, that is, the eggs of trichurids or capillarids, may parasitize nonfeline hosts, such as mice, rabbits, or birds (an outdoor cat's prey). The eggs of trichurids or capillarids from a cat's prey may pass undigested and unaltered through the cat's gastrointestinal system, remaining intact and unembryonated.

Fecal flotation is the most common way of identifying the eggs of this parasite; however, the whipworm eggs do not float well in most common fecal flotation mediums. Therefore, it is

imperative that the eggs be allowed to float for a minimum of 15 minutes before viewing under the microscope. Once identified, the veterinarian will most often use the vermicides mebendazole or fenbendazole for treatment of these worms. Prevention involves daily feces removal to remove the uninfective eggs from the host's environment.

Dogs and cats may often be blamed as serving as host for certain parasites of humans. *Enterobius vermicularis* is the pinworm found in humans and is often found in young children. This pinworm *does not* parasitize dogs or cats. Nevertheless, the family pet is often falsely incriminated by physicians, family practitioners, and pediatricians as a source of pinworm infection in young children. The veterinary diagnostician should remember this rule: Pinworms are parasites of omnivores (mice, rats, monkeys, and humans) and herbivores (rabbits and horses) but *never* carnivores (dogs and cats).

CIRCULATORY SYSTEM

Dirofilaria immitis is often referred to as the canine heartworm (Figure 4-19); however, this nematode has been known to parasitize cats and ferrets as well (Figure 4-20). The definitive host for *D. immitis* is the canine. Although cats and ferrets have been parasitized by this parasite, they rarely serve as a source for transmission. Heartworms are long, slender parasites (Figure 4-21). As adults, these parasites are found within the right ventricle and the pulmonary artery and its fine branches. The offspring of filarial worms such as *D. immitis* are known as **microfilariae.** Among the nematodes of small animals, *D. immitis* is perhaps the one nematode that may be found in sites other than its normal predilection sites. This parasite is often recovered in a variety of aberrant sites, such as the brain, anterior chamber of the eye (Figure 4-22), and subcutaneous sites. The prepatent period in dogs is approximately 6 months.

The life cycle of *D. immitis* requires an intermediate host to be transmitted from animal to animal. The adults live in the right ventricle and

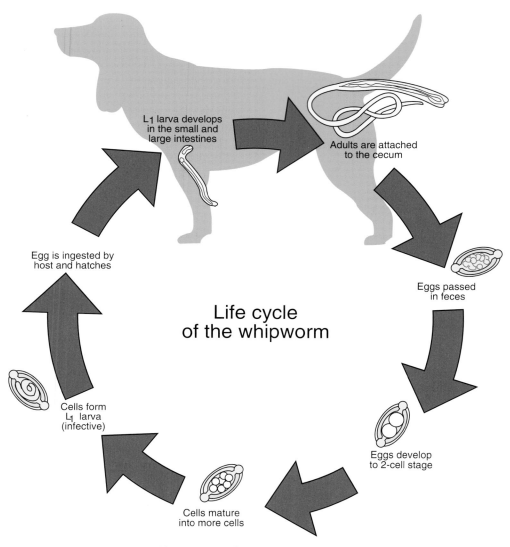

Figure 4-17   Life cycle of the whipworm.

pulmonary artery. The male and female adults mate, and the female produces microfilariae. The microfilariae are released into the host's bloodstream, where they are ingested by feeding female mosquitoes. The microfilariae grow and molt in the mosquito until they reach the infective stage. Once they become infective, they enter a new host the next time the mosquito feeds (Figure 4-23). Once in the new host, the larvae migrate and molt through various body tissues on their way to the heart. It is at this time that the larve may grow and molt to become adults in sites other than the heart.

In microfilaremic dogs, diagnosis is made by observing microfilariae in blood samples, using one of several concentration techniques, such as the modified Knott's test (Figures 4-24 and 4-25) or commercially available filter techniques

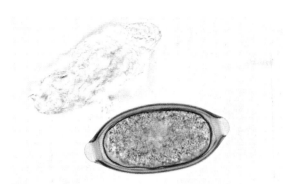

Figure 4-18 Egg of *Trichuris campanula* (pictured) and *T. serrata,* the feline whipworms, may be easily confused with *Aonchotheca putorii, Eucoleus aerophilus*, and *Personema feliscati,* parasites of the feline stomach, respiratory tract, and urinary system, respectively. Eggs of *T. campanula* average 63 to 85 μm by 34 to 39 μm.

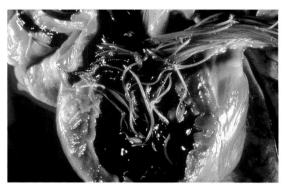

Figure 4-19 Adults of *Dirofilaria immitis,* the canine heartworm, are found within right ventricle and pulmonary artery and its fine branches.

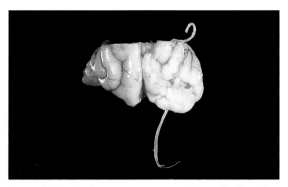

Figure 4-20 Canine heartworms may be found in sites other than the heart and in hosts other than the dog. These heartworms have been recovered from the brain of a ferret.

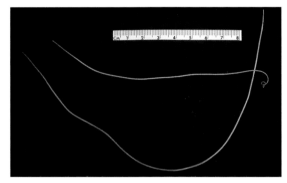

Figure 4-21 Heartworms are long, slender parasites, evolved for fitting into the fine branches of pulmonary arteries.

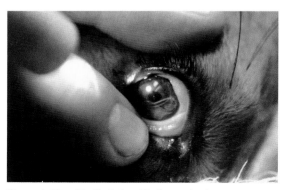

Figure 4-22 *Dirofilaria immitis,* the canine heartworm, may also be recovered from a variety of aberrant sites, such as the anterior chamber of the eye.

(Figure 4-26). For dogs (amicrofilaremic or microfilaremic), infection can also be diagnosed using one of the commercially available *e*nzyme-linked *i*mmuno*s*orbent *a*ssay (ELISA) tests (Figure 4-27). It is important to remember that a subcutaneous filariid of dogs, *Acanthocheilonema* (formerly known as *Dipetalonema*) *reconditum,* also produces microfilariae in the peripheral blood (Figures 4-28 and 4-29). The microfilariae of this nonpathogenic nematode must be differ-

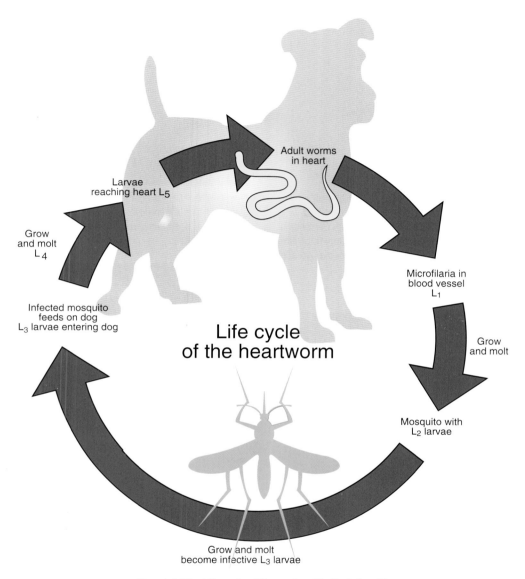

Adult worms
in heart

Larvae
reaching heart L_5

Grow
and molt
L_4

Microfilaria in
blood vessel
L_1

Infected mosquito
feeds on dog
L_3 larvae entering dog

Life cycle
of the heartworm

Grow
and molt

Mosquito with
L_2 larvae

Grow and molt
become infective L_3 larvae

Figure 4-23 Life cycle of the canine *Dirofilaria immitis.*

entiated from those of *D. immitis* (see Figures 4-24 and 4-25).

The damage that *D. immitis* causes to the heart will cause the hallmark symptoms of heartworm disease in dogs. The symptoms are a decrease in exercise tolerance, right-sided heart enlarge-ment, and abdominal ascites (fluid accumulation in the abdomen). These symptoms are caused by the parasite's location in the heart and pulmonary arteries, which reduces blood flow on the right side of the heart and causes inflammation to the lining of the blood vessels.

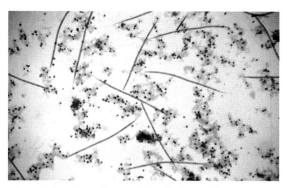

Figure 4-24   Microfilariae of *Dirofilaria immitis* subjected to modified Knott's test. Microfilariae of this pathogenic nematode must be differentiated from those of *A. reconditum*.

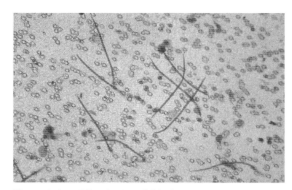

Figure 4-26   Microfilariae of *Dirofilaria immitis* subjected to commercially available filter technique.

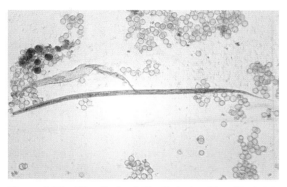

Figure 4-25   Microfilaria of *Dirofilaria immitis* subjected to modified Knott's test. Note tapering anterior end and straight tail. This microfilaria measures approximately 310 μm in length.

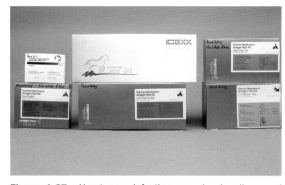

Figure 4-27   Heartworm infection can also be diagnosed using commercially available enzyme-linked immunosorbent assay (ELISA) tests.

The treatment for heartworm disease involves pretreatment testing, treatment, and posttreatment rest. The first step in treatment involves determining the canine's ability to withstand the treatment by performing blood work; this determines the status of the internal organs. Radiographs are taken to determine the status of the heart and the stage of the disease. After testing, the canine is treated for the adult heartworms. *Adulticides* (drugs that will kill the adult stages of the parasite) such as Immiticide (Merial Limited, 888-637-4251) are used to kill the adult heartworms. As the adults die, they will move with the flow of blood toward the lungs. This could cause problems for the canine if it is allowed to exercise after the adulticide treatment. The canine must be kept quiet for several weeks after treatment while the body resorbs the dead adults. Once the adults have been treated and resorbed by the body, the canine is treated with a *microfilaricide* (usually ivermectin) to clear the blood of any microfilariae. The final part of the treatment is the heartworm testing. This usually involves a microfilariae test and an ELISA test to confirm the microfilariae and adults have been cleared from the canine's body.

The treatment for canine heartworm disease can be very stressful on the dog's body. There-

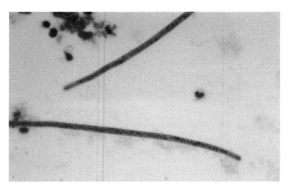

Figure 4-28 Microfilariae of *Acanthocheilonema reconditum* subjected to modified Knott's test. Note "broom handle" anterior end. This microfilaria measures approximately 280 μm in length. Microfilariae of this nonpathogenic nematode must be differentiated from those of *D. immitis.*

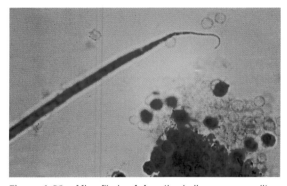

Figure 4-29 Microfilaria of *Acanthocheilonema reconditum* subjected to modified Knott's test. Note "buttonhook" posterior end, which is an artifact of formalin fixation used in modified Knott's procedure.

fore, prevention is recommended so that the dog does not contract the parasite. Preventive regimens include daily preventive medications, monthly medications, and an injection every 6 months.

Feline hosts for *Dirofilaria immitis* occur in the same areas that canines are infected. Cats are susceptible to the parasite but tend to be very resistant. Therefore, it takes a greater exposure to the microfilariae from the mosquito to infect a cat than it does a dog. Whereas *D. immitis* causes enough damage to produce hallmark symptoms in dogs, cats do not show specific symptoms of the infection. Cats tend to show signs similar to those seen with respiratory disease.

The life cycle of *D. immitis* in cats begins as it does in dogs. The adults live in the right ventricle and pulmonary arteries of the dog. The adults mate, and the female produces microfilariae, which are present in the vessels of the dog. Mosquitoes feed on the infected canine and ingest the microfilariae. The microfilariae grow and molt to the infective L3 larvae. Once infective, the mosquito feeds on a cat, and the larvae are transferred to the cat. The larvae grow, molt, and migrate in the cat on their way to the heart (Figure 4-30).

Identification of the parasite in the cat is difficult. The adults do not produce many microfilariae in the cat, so the microfilariae tests will produce negative results in most cases. Tests developed for dogs are not sensitive enough for the infection in cats, so ELISA tests have been developed for detection of *Dirofilaria immitis* in cats. Two types of tests are available for in-clinic use: antigen tests and antibody tests. The antigen test is the definitive test, although a negative result does not rule out a heartworm infection. The antibody test can detect a reaction by the cat's body to the microfilariae, but the microfilariae may die before becoming adults. Therefore the positive antibody test does not positively detect an active infection. A positive antigen or antibody test in the presence of clinical respiratory symptoms indicates an active infection (www.heartwormsociety.org/felineheartworminfo).

At this time there are no approved treatments for feline heartworm disease. Therefore the best treatment is prevention. Preventive options available for cats include once-a-month pills and a single topical monthly application for the prevention of feline heartworm disease.

RESPIRATORY SYSTEM

Aelurostrongylus abstrusus is the feline lungworm. The adults live in the terminal respiratory

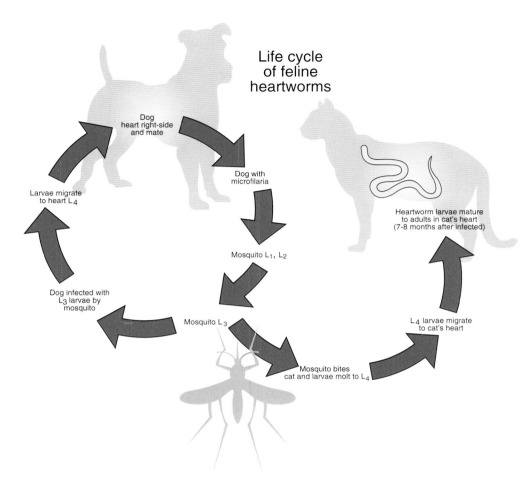

Figure 4-30 Life cycle of the feline *Dirofilaria immitis*.

bronchioles and alveolar ducts, where they form small egg nests or nodules. Initially, this parasite lays embryonated (larvated) eggs. The eggs of this parasite are forced into the lung tissue, where they hatch to form characteristic first-stage larvae, approximately 360 μm long. These larvae are quite distinct; each has a tail with a unique, S-shaped bend with a dorsal spine (Figure 4-31). These larvae are coughed up by the cat, swallowed, and passed out in the feces. Diagnosis is by finding these characteristic larvae on fecal flotation or by the Baermann tech-

nique (see Chapter 17). It is also possible to recover the larvae using a tracheal wash (Figure 4-32). The prepatent period for the feline lung-worm is approximately 30 days.

Filaroides osleri, *F. hirthi*, and *F. milksi*, the canine lungworms, are found in the trachea, lung parenchyma, and bronchioles, respectively. The larva is 232 to 266 μm in length and has a tail with a short, S-shaped appendage. *Filaroides* species are unique among nematodes in that their first-stage larvae are immediately infective for the canine definitive host. No period of devel-

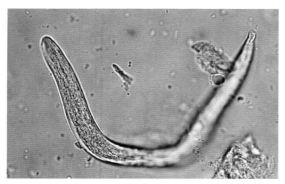

Figure 4-31 First-stage larva of *Aelurostrongylus abstrusus*, the feline lungworm. Each larva has a tail with an S-shaped bend and dorsal spine. Diagnosis is by finding these characteristic larvae on fecal flotation or by the Baermann technique.

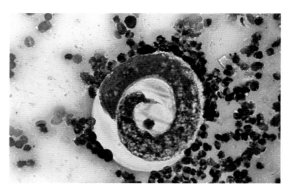

Figure 4-33 Tracheal wash revealing characteristic first-stage larva of *Filaroides osleri*, the canine lungworm, which has a tail with a short, S-shaped appendage. *Filaroides* species are unique among nematodes in that their first-stage larvae are immediately infective for the canine definitive host. No period of development is required outside the host.

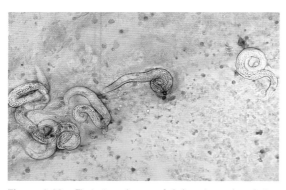

Figure 4-32 First-stage larvae of *Aelurostrongylus abstrusus* recovered on tracheal wash.

opment is required outside the host. These parasites are transmitted from the dam to her offspring as she licks and cleans her puppies. Diagnosis is by finding these characteristic larvae on fecal flotation or by the Baermann technique. (See Figure 4-33 for the unique infective larvae of *F. osleri*.) Nodules of *F. osleri* are usually found at the bifurcation of the trachea, where they can be easily observed at necropsy (Figure 4-34). The prepatent period for *F. osleri* is approximately 10 weeks.

Eucoleus aerophilus (Capillaria aerophila) is a capillarid nematode found in the trachea and bronchi of both dogs and cats. The prepatent period is approximately 40 days. During standard fecal flotation, eggs of *Eucoleus* species are often confused with those of *Trichuris* species (whipworms). Eggs of *E. aerophilus* are smaller than whipworm eggs (59-80 μm × 30-40 μm), more broadly barrel-shaped, and lighter in color. The egg has a rough outer surface with a netted appearance (Figure 4-35). *Eucoleus böehmi* is found in the nasal cavity and frontal sinuses of dogs. Its eggs are smaller and have a smoother outer surface than those of *E. aerophilus*. Its shell has a pitted appearance. *E. böehmi* can be diagnosed by standard fecal flotation.

URINARY TRACT

Dioctophyma renale is the giant kidney worm of dogs. This largest of the parasitic nematodes that affect domestic animals (Figure 4-36) frequently infects the right kidney of dogs and ingests the parenchyma, leaving only the capsule of the kidney (Figure 4-37). Eggs may be recovered by

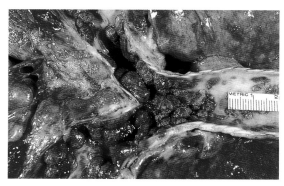

Figure 4-34 Nodules of *Filaroides osleri* are usually found at the bifurcation of the trachea, where they can be easily observed at necropsy.

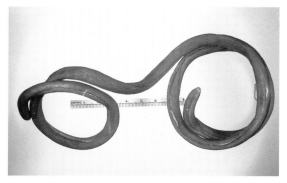

Figure 4-36 *Dioctophyma renale,* the giant kidney worm of dogs, is the largest of parasitic nematodes that affect domestic animals.

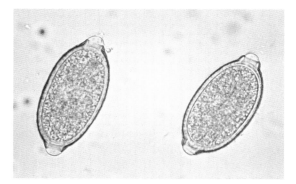

Figure 4-35 Egg of *Eucoleus aerophilus (Capillaria aerophila),* a capillarid nematode found in trachea and bronchi of dogs and cats. Eggs are smaller than whipworm eggs and more broadly barrel-shaped and lighter in color. Eggs have rough outer surface with netted appearance.

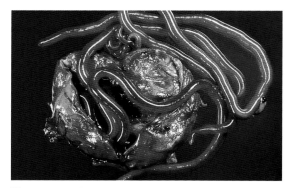

Figure 4-37 *Dioctophyma renale* frequently infects the right kidney of dogs and ingests the entire parenchyma, leaving only the capsule of the kidney.

centrifugation and examination of the urine sediment. They are characteristically barrel-shaped, bipolar, and yellow-brown. The shell has a pitted appearance. Eggs measure 71 to 84 µm by 46 to 52 µm. (See Figure 4-38 for the characteristic egg of *D. renale.*) *D. renale* is also known for its wandering activity; it often "gets off course" during its migration to the kidney. This nematode also may occur freely within the peritoneal cavity. When the kidney worm is in an aberrant site, its

eggs cannot be passed to the external environment. The prepatent period for this largest of nematodes is approximately 18 weeks.

Capillaria plica and *Capillaria feliscati* are nematodes of the urinary bladder of dogs and cats, respectively. Their eggs may be found in urine or in feces contaminated with urine. Eggs are clear to yellow, measure 63 to 68 µm by 24 to 27 µm, and have flattened, bipolar end plugs. The outer surface of the shell is roughened (Figure 4-39). These eggs may be confused with eggs of the respiratory and gastric capillarids and eggs of the whipworms.

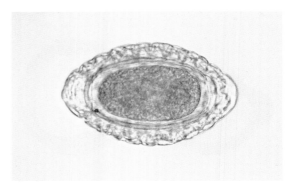

Figure 4-38   Egg of *Dioctophyma renale* with its characteristic barrel-shaped, bipolar, yellow-brown appearance. Shell has a pitted appearance.

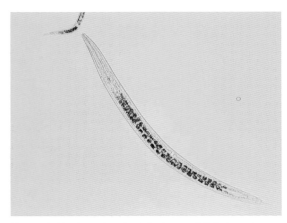

Figure 4-40   Larval and adult stages of *Pelodera strongyloides* can be identified following superficial skin scrapings of affected areas that have come in contact with infected soil.

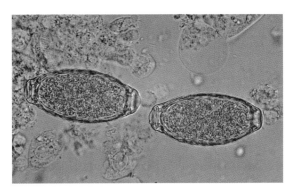

Figure 4-39   Egg of *Capillaria plica*, the urinary capillarid. Eggs are clear to yellow and have flattened bipolar end plugs and a rough outer surface. Eggs may be confused with those of respiratory and gastric capillarids and whipworms.

SKIN

Pelodera strongyloides are free-living saprophytic nematodes that normally live in moist soil. These roundworms are facultative parasites; that is, they are normally free-living, but under certain circumstances they invade mammalian skin and develop to a parasitic mode of existence. Male and female adult *P. strongyloides* are found in soil mixed with moist organic debris, such as straw or hay. The females produce eggs that hatch into first-stage larvae. These larvae invade the super-

ficial layers of damaged or scarified skin, producing a mild dermatitis. The skin may become reddened, denuded, and covered with a crusty material. Occasionally, a pustular dermatitis develops. Because dogs acquire the infection by lying on contaminated bedding or soil, these lesions are usually observed on the ventral, or inner, surface of the limbs. Larvae of *P. strongyloides* also can be recovered from the skin of almost any domesticated animal, particularly downer cattle when these cows come in direct contact with soil containing larval *P. strongyloides.*

Larval (and adult) stages can be identified following superficial skin scrapings of the affected areas on the ventral, or inner, surface of the thighs (Figure 4-40). Larvae of *P. strongyloides* are 596 to 600 μm long. These larvae must be differentiated from the microfilariae of the canine heartworm, *Dirofilaria immitis* (see Figures 4-24 and 4-25), the microfilariae of *A. reconditum* (see Figures 4-28 and 4-29), and the first-stage larvae of *Dracunculus insignis* (Figure 4-41).

As discussed earlier, *Dirofilaria immitis*, the canine heartworm, normally resides in the right ventricle and pulmonary arteries of the canine

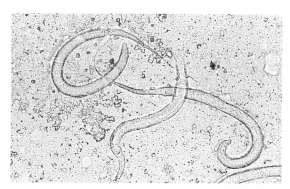

Figure 4-41 Unique first-stage larva of *Dracunculus insignis* with characteristic long, pointed tail.

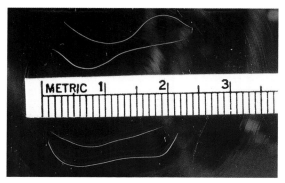

Figure 4-43 Adults of *Acanthocheilonema reconditum,* the subcutaneous filarial worm, are nonpathogenic. They reside in subcutaneous tissues of the dog and are seldom recovered at necropsy.

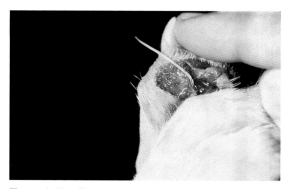

Figure 4-42 Aberrant adult *Dirofilaria immitis* in subcutaneous interdigital cyst. Heartworms found aberrantly are usually single, immature, isolated worms "lost" en route to the heart.

definite host. This parasite tends to wander aberrantly and may be found in a variety of extravascular sites, including cystic spaces in subcutaneous sites. Figure 4-42 shows an aberrant adult *D. immitis* in a subcutaneous interdigital cyst. When heartworms are found aberrantly, they are usually single, immature, isolated worms that have become "lost" en route to the heart. If the worm within the cyst is female, she will not have been fertilized by a male heartworm. Therefore she will not be gravid and will not produce microfilariae.

However, other adult male and female heartworms may be in their predilection sites, the right ventricles and pulmonary arteries. It is possible for these adult females to produce microfilariae. These microfilariae occasionally may be recovered in deep skin scrapings that draw blood.

Aberrant *D. immitis* within cystic spaces in the skin can be removed surgically. When subjected to the modified Knott's procedure, the microfilariae of *D. immitis* are 310 to 320 μm long, with straight tails and tapering anterior ends. They must be differentiated from microfilariae of *A. reconditum* (see Figures 4-28 and 4-29), the first-stage larvae of *P. strongyloides* (see Figure 4-40), and first-stage larvae of *D. insignis* (see Figure 4-41).

Adult *Acanthocheilonema reconditum,* the subcutaneous filarial worm, is a nonpathogenic nematode residing in the subcutaneous tissues of the dog. The adult filarial parasites are seldom found (Figure 4-43). (See Figures 4-28 and 4-29 for the frequently seen microfilariae.) These parasites may also be found within the body cavity. Occasionally, subcutaneous abscesses and ulcerated areas have been associated with *A. reconditum.* The intermediate host for this parasite is the cat flea, *Ctenocephalides felis.* Because this parasite is found in enzootic areas where *D. immitis* is present, it is necessary to differentiate the microfilariae of these two filarial parasites.

Adult *A. reconditum* are rarely recovered from subcutaneous sites. More often, their microfilariae are recovered in peripheral blood samples. These microfilariae may be rarely recovered in deep skin scrapings that draw blood. On examination of microfilaremic peripheral blood subjected to the modified Knott's procedure, the microfilariae of *A. reconditum* average about 285 µm in length and have "buttonhook" tails and blunt (broom handle–shaped) anterior ends (see Figures 4-28 and 4-29). It is important to differentiate these microfilariae from the microfilariae of *D. immitis* (see Figures 4-24 and 4-25), the first-stage larvae of *P. strongyloides* (see Figure 4-40), and first-stage larvae of *D. insignis* (see Figure 4-41).

Dracunculus insignis, the guinea worm, is a nematode found in the subcutaneous tissues of the dog. The adult female nematode may be extremely long, up to 120 cm in length. In comparison, the male is quite short, only 2 to 3 cm in length; however, it is rarely seen. The female resides subcutaneously and produces a draining, ulcerous lesion in the skin, usually on the dog's limb (Figure 4-44). The anterior end of the female worm extends from this ulcer. If the female worm within the lesion comes in contact with water, her uterus will prolapse through her anterior end and rupture, releasing a mass of first-stage larvae into the water. These larvae are 500 to 750 µm in length and have long tails that are quite distinct. (See Figure 4-41 for the first-stage larvae of *D. insignis*.) Larvae are ingested by tiny crustaceans in the water; within the crustaceans, the larvae develop to the infective third stage. Dogs become infected with *D. insignis* by drinking water containing these infected crustaceans.

If *D. insignis* is observed in the ulcerous lesion, the ulcer with its associated worm should be dipped in cool water. The cool water is a stimulus for the female worm to expel her larvae. The water containing expelled larvae should be collected and centrifuged; the sediment must then be examined for the presence of the characteristic first-stage larvae. Larvae of *D. insignis* must be differentiated from the microfilariae of *D. immitis* (see Figures 4-24 and 4-25), the microfilariae of *A. reconditum* (see Figures 4-28 and 4-29), and the first-stage larvae of *P. strongyloides* (see Figure 4-40). Once diagnosed, the adult female worm must be surgically removed.

EYE AND ADNEXA

Thelazia californiensis is the eyeworm of dogs and cats. Adult parasites can be recovered from the conjunctival sac and lacrimal duct (Figure 4-45). Examination of the lacrimal secretions may also reveal eggs or first-stage larvae.

As mentioned previously, *Dirofilaria immitis* can be recovered from a variety of aberrant sites, including the anterior chamber of the eye (see Figure 4-42). As with aberrant parasites that occur in the skin, those found in the eye are usually single, immature, isolated worms that have become lost en route to the heart. If the worm within the anterior chamber is female, she will not have been fertilized by a male heartworm. Therefore she will not be gravid and will not produce microfilariae. This nematode can be surgically removed from the eye.

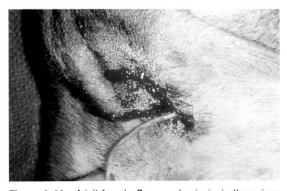

Figure 4-44 Adult female *Dracunculus insignis*, the guinea worm, is often found in subcutaneous tissues of the dog. She causes a draining, ulcerous lesion in the skin, usually on the limb.

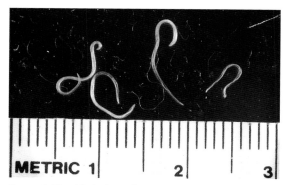

Figure 4-45 *Thelazia californiensis* is the eyeworm of dogs and cats. Adult parasites can be recovered from the conjunctival sac and lacrimal duct. Examination of lacrimal secretions may also reveal eggs or first-stage larvae.

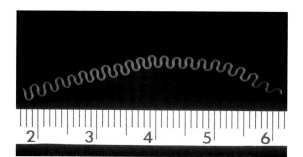

Figure 4-46 *Gongylonema pulchrum* inhabits the esophagus of sheep, goats, cattle, and occasionally pigs and horses. Parasite lies embedded within submucosa or mucosa of esophagus; it has a unique appearance in that it lies in a zigzag fashion.

NEMATODES OF RUMINANTS

GASTROINTESTINAL TRACT

Gongylonema pulchrum inhabits the esophagus of sheep, goats, cattle, and occasionally pigs and horses. This parasite lies embedded within the submucosa or mucosa of the esophagus; it has a unique appearance in that it lies in a zigzag fashion (Figure 4-46). Its eggs are 50 to 70 μm by 25 to 37 μm.

The *bovine trichostrongyles* comprise several genera of nematodes within the abomasum and

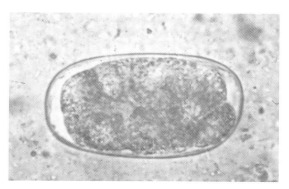

Figure 4-47 Oval, thin-shelled eggs that typify eggs of ruminant trichostrongyles. Eggs contain a morula with four or more cells. Some eggs can be identified to their respective genera; however, identification is usually difficult because mixed infections are common. Identification of these should be recorded as "trichostrongyle types of eggs," and no attempt should be made to identify them to individual genus names.

the small and large intestines of cattle and other ruminants. The genera that can be classified as producing the trichostrongyle type of eggs are *Bunostomum, Chabertia, Cooperia, Haemonchus, Oesophagostomum, Ostertagia,* and *Trichostrongylus* species. These seven genera (there are many others) produce oval, thin-shelled eggs. The bovine trichostrongyles have a similar life cycle. The adults live in the abomasum and intestines. The female passes eggs in the feces. The eggs have a morula that contains four or more cells and are 70 to 120 μm in length (Figure 4-47). Some of these eggs can be identified to their respective genera; however, identification is usually difficult because mixed infections are quite common. On identification of the characteristic eggs, the veterinary diagnostician should record the identification as "trichostrongyle type of egg" and should not attempt to identify them to the individual genus names. Identification to genus and species is usually performed by fecal culture and larval identification. (See Figure 4-48 for representative examples of trichostrongyle type of eggs.) The trichostrongyles are perhaps the most common nematodes diagnosed on fecal flotation of ruminants.

The most common dewormers used for the trichostrongyles are fenbendazole, levamisole, and ivermectin.

Nematodirus species and *Marshallagia* species are also ruminant trichostrongyles; however, the eggs of these nematodes are much larger than those of the genera just mentioned and are the largest in the trichostrongyle family. Figure 4-49 shows the eggs of *Nematodirus* species. In standard fecal flotation, the eggs of *Nematodirus* species are large, 150 to 230 μm by 80 to 100 μm, and have tapering ends and a four- to eight-cell morula. The eggs of *Marshallagia* species are also large, 160 to 200 μm by 75 to 100 μm, and have parallel sides, a rounded end, and contain a 16- to 32-cell morula.

Strongyloides papillosus is the intestinal threadworm of cattle. These nematodes are unique in that only a parthenogenetic female is parasitic in the bovine host. Parasitic male *Strongyloides* do not exist. The female worms produce larvated eggs measuring 40 to 60 μm by 20 to 25 μm. Eggs are usually recovered in flotation of fresh feces. (See Figure 4-14 for the parasitic adult females, eggs, and first-stage larvae of *Strongyloides* species.) The eggs grow and molt as they pass through the feces to the environment. Once the eggs hatch, the larvae become free-living adults or infective-stage female larvae. The infective-stage larvae can enter the host by penetration of the skin (usually between the hooves) or by ingestion. The larval *Strongyloides* species are 280 to 310 μm long and possess a rhabditiform esophagus, with a club-shaped anterior corpus, narrow median isthmus, and caudal bulb. The larvae migrate to the lungs through the circulatory system, are coughed up, and swallowed. Once in the intestines, they mature to adults. The larvae can be passed to the ruminant neonate through the colostrum. The prepatent period is 5 to 7 days. Light infections may be asymptomatic, but heavy infections will produce diarrhea, anorexia, blood and mucus in the feces, and weight loss.

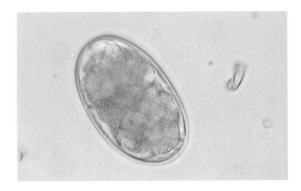

A

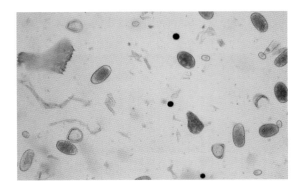

B

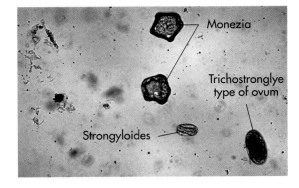

C

Figure 4-48 Representative examples of trichostrongyle type of eggs. Trichostrongyles are perhaps the most common nematodes diagnosed on fecal flotation of ruminants.

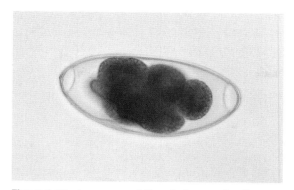

Figure 4-49   Large eggs of *Nematodirus* species. Eggs are largest of the ruminant trichostrongyle eggs and have tapering ends and a morula with four to eight cells.

The most common anthelmintics for *S. papillosus* are the **benzimidazoles** (e.g., fenbendazole, oxfendazole, albendazole), the **probenzimidazoles** (e.g., thiophanate, febantel, netobimin), and ivermectin. Since most ruminants spend part or all of their lives in pasture, the animals are subject to constant reinfection. Treatment with dewormers is only part of the treatment for ruminant parasites. Prevention plays a major role in the treatment procedure. Pasture rotation with nonruminant animals, such as horses, mules, and donkeys, will reduce the infective larvae in the pasture.

Trichuris ovis parasites are commonly called "whipworms" and infect the cecum and colon of ruminants. (See discussion of nematode parasites of gastrointestinal tract of dogs and cats for details of gross morphology of adult whipworms.) The egg of the whipworm is described as trichinelloid or trichuroid; it has a thick, yellow-brown, symmetric shell with polar plugs at both ends. The eggs are unembryonated (not larvated) when laid. Eggs of bovine whipworms measure 50 to 60 μm by 21 to 25 μm. (See Figure 4-16 for the characteristic egg.) Symptoms are usually not apparent with *Trichuris ovis* but can include dark feces, anorexia, and anemia. The most common anthelmintics are the benzimidazoles, probenzimidazoles, and ivermectin.

CIRCULATORY SYSTEM

Elaeophora schneideri, the arterial worm, is found in the common carotid arteries of sheep in the western and southwestern United States. Although the adults are found in these predilection sites, their microfilariae are restricted to the skin. Microfilariae are 270 μm in length by 17 μm in thickness, bluntly rounded anteriorly, and tapering posteriorly. In the skin the microfilariae usually reside in the capillaries of the forehead and face. In sheep, filarial dermatitis is seen on the face, poll region, and feet.

Diagnosis of *E. schneideri* is by observation of characteristic lesions and identification of microfilariae in the skin. The most satisfactory means of diagnosis is to macerate a piece of skin in warm saline and examine the fluid for microfilariae after about 2 hours. In sheep, microfilariae are rare and may not be found in the skin of affected animals. Postmortem examination may be necessary to confirm the diagnosis of adult parasites within the common carotid arteries. The prepatent period for *E. schneideri* is $4\frac{1}{2}$ months or longer.

RESPIRATORY SYSTEM

Dictyocaulus species are the lungworms of cattle (*D. viviparus*), sheep, and goats (*D. filaria*). Adult parasites are found in the bronchi of infected hosts. The prepatent period varies between the species but is approximately 28 days. The female worm lays her eggs in the lungs. The eggs are usually coughed up, swallowed, and hatch in the intestine, producing larvae that may be recovered in the feces. Larvae of *D. filaria* have brown food granules in their intestinal cells, a blunt tail, and an anterior cuticular knob. These larvae are from 550 to 580 μm in length. Larvae of *D. viviparus* also have brown food granules in their intestinal cells, but they have a straight tail. They are from 300 to 360 μm in length but lack the anterior cuticular knob. (See Figure 4-50 for representative examples of eggs and larvae of *D. viviparus*.) The larvae pass out of the host through the feces to grow and molt from L2 to

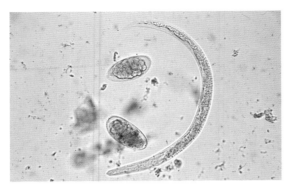

Figure 4-50   Representative examples of eggs and larvae of *Dictyocaulus viviparus* species, the lungworms of cattle. Eggs are usually coughed up, swallowed, and hatch in the intestine, producing larvae that may be recovered in feces. Larvae of *D. viviparus* have brown food granules in their intestinal cells, a straight tail, and an anterior cuticular knob.

L3 larvae in the environment. The L3 infective larvae are ingested by the host and migrate through the tissues to the lymph vessels. The larvae grow and molt to **L4 larvae** and follow the lymph vessels to the heart. From the heart, the larvae follow the circulatory system to the lungs, where they mature into adults (Figure 4-51). The most common symptom is coughing. The eggs can be found in mucous discharge or coughed-up sputum. Benzimidazoles, probenzimidazoles, and ivermectin are the most common anthelmintics used in ruminants.

Muellerius capillaris is often called the "hair lungworm" of sheep and goats. Adults are found within the bronchioles, mostly in nodules in the lung parenchyma. The eggs develop in the lungs of the definitive host, and first-stage larvae are coughed up, swallowed, and passed out with the feces. The larvae are from 230 to 300 μm long. The larval tail has an undulating tip and a dorsal spine. Figure 4-52 shows representative examples of eggs and larvae of *M. capillaris*.

Adult *Protostrongylus* species occur in the small bronchioles of sheep and goats. The eggs develop in the lungs of the definitive host. First-

stage larvae are coughed up, swallowed, and passed out with the feces. These larvae are 250 to 320 μm long. This nematode's larval tail has an undulating tip but lacks the dorsal spine.

The Baermann technique is used to diagnose lungworm infection in ruminants (see Chapter 17).

SKIN

Stephanofilaria stilesi parasites are small nematodes found in the skin of cattle and goats and buffalo and other wild ruminants. In the United States they typically produce a dermatitis along the ventral midline of cattle (Figure 4-53). The infective larvae are transmitted by the bite of the horn fly, *Haematobia irritans*. The skin lesions are thought to be caused by both adult and microfilarial stages of this parasite.

The lesions caused by *S. stilesi* are located at or near the umbilicus and consist initially of small, red papules. Later, the lesions develop into large pruritic areas (up to 25 cm) of alopecia, with thick, moist crusts. Both the adults (6 mm) and microfilariae may be found in deep skin scrapings after the crusts have been removed from the lesions.

Although *Elaeophora schneideri*, the arterial worm, is found in the common carotid arteries of sheep in the western and southwestern United States, the microfilariae are restricted to the skin (see earlier discussion under Circulatory System).

It is important that the veterinary diagnostician remember that larvae of *Pelodera strongyloides* also can be recovered from the skin of almost any domesticated animal, particularly downer cattle that come in contact with moist soil containing larvae of the genus *Pelodera*. The larvae actively penetrate the skin and can produce a severe dermatitis (see Figure 4-40).

EYE AND ADNEXA

Thelazia rhodesii and *Thelazia gulosa* are the eyeworms of cattle, sheep, and goats. Adult parasites can be recovered from the conjunctival sac

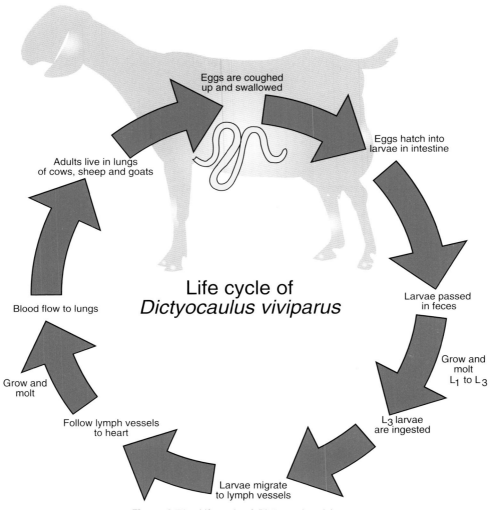

Eggs are coughed
up and swallowed

Eggs hatch into
larvae in intestine

Adults live in lungs
of cows, sheep and goats

Larvae passed
in feces

Life cycle of
Dictyocaulus viviparus

Blood flow to lungs

Grow and
molt
L_1 to L_3

Grow and
molt

L_3 larvae
are ingested

Follow lymph vessels
to heart

Larvae migrate
to lymph vessels

Figure 4-51   Life cycle of *Dictyocaulus viviparus.*

and lacrimal duct. Examination of lacrimal secretions may reveal eggs or first-stage larvae.

ABDOMINAL CAVITY

Setaria cervi is the abdominal worm of cattle. Adults are usually observed on postmortem examination and are found free within the peritoneal cavity (Figure 4-54). The sheathed microfilariae are approximately 250 by 7 μm.

Antemortem diagnosis is by demonstration of microfilariae in peripheral blood smears.

NEMATODES OF EQUIDS

GASTROINTESTINAL TRACT

Habronema microstoma, Habronema muscae, and *Draschia megastoma* are nematodes found in the stomach of horses. *H. microstoma* and *H. muscae*

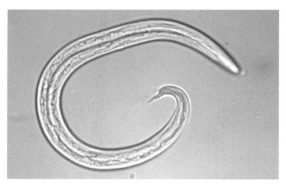

Figure 4-52 Representative examples of eggs and larvae of *Muellerius capillaris,* the hair lungworm of sheep and goats. Eggs develop in lungs of definitive host, and first-stage larvae are coughed up, swallowed, and passed out with feces. Larval tail has undulating tip and dorsal spine.

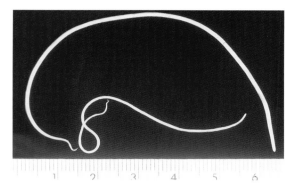

Figure 4-54 *Setaria cervi* is the abdominal worm of cattle. Adults are usually observed on postmortem examination and found free within the peritoneal cavity.

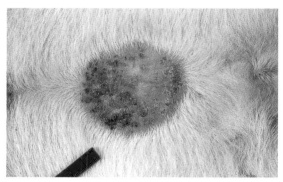

Figure 4-53 *Stephanofilaria stilesi* are small nematodes found in skin of cattle, goats, buffalo, and other wild ruminants. They typically produce dermatitis along ventral midline of cattle in the United States.

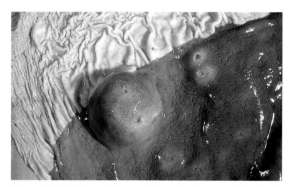

Figure 4-55 *Draschia megastoma* is often associated with formation of large, thickened fibrous nodules within stomach mucosa of horses.

reside on the mucosa of the stomach, just beneath a thick layer of mucus. *D. megastoma* is often associated with the formation of large, thickened fibrous nodules within the stomach mucosa (Figure 4-55). Larvae of both *Habronema* and *Draschia* species may parasitize skin lesions, causing a skin condition of horses known as "summer sores" (see Figure 4-65 and later discussion under Skin).

Larvated eggs or larvae may be recovered on standard fecal flotation. The eggs of both genera are elongate, thin-walled, and measure 40 to 50 μm by 10 to 12 μm (Figure 4-56). These eggs (or the hatched larvae) pass to the outside environment and are ingested by flies belonging to the family Muscidae. The larvae develop to the infective third-stage within the fly, and if a horse accidentally ingests the fly, the larvae develop to the adult stage within the stomach of the horse. The prepatent period is approximately 60 days. Antemortem diagnosis of gastric habronemiasis is based on observation of eggs or larvae on fecal flotation. Symptoms for *H. microstoma, H. muscae,* and *D. megastoma* occur with heavy infections and include gastritis, colic, and diarrhea.

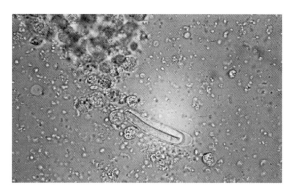

Figure 4-56 Larvated eggs or larvae of *Habronema* and *Draschia* species may be recovered on standard fecal flotation. Eggs of both genera are elongate, thin-walled, and often contain first-stage larvae.

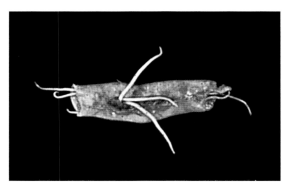

Figure 4-57 *Parascaris equorum* nematodes are often called "equine ascarids" or "equine roundworms." These nematodes are found in the small intestine of young foals.

Benzimidazoles and ivermectin are the most common anthelmintics used for these species in horses. As with ruminants, equines are pasture animals, so pasture management plays an important role in treatment and prevention. In addition, a good fly control program will help reduce the infected flies in the horse's environment.

Trichostrongylus axei is another species of nematode that may reside in the stomach of horses. These unusual nematodes can cross species lines and can also infect cattle, sheep, and swine. The egg of *T. axei* is classified as a strongyle type of egg and measures 79 to 92 µm by 31 to 41 µm (see following discussion on strongyles).

Parascaris equorum is often called the "equine ascarid" or "equine roundworm." These nematodes are found in the small intestine of young foals (Figure 4-57). These large, robust nematodes are the largest of the equine nematodes. Sometimes, young foals will pass these nematodes in their feces (Figure 4-58). The eggs are passed in the feces, which tends to be sticky, and the larvae grow and molt within the egg. The infective egg is ingested by the young foal and hatches in the intestines. The larvae migrate to the liver through the hepatic portal vein, where they grow and molt to the next stage of larvae. The larvae are carried to the lungs through the circulatory system, where they are coughed up

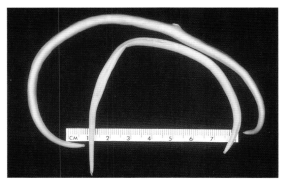

Figure 4-58 *Parascaris equorum* is the largest of the equine nematodes. Young foals may pass these large parasites in feces.

and swallowed. Once back in the intestines, the larvae mature into adults (Figure 4-59). The prepatent period for these ascarids is 75 to 80 days. The eggs are recovered from the feces of young horses and are round to oval and deeply pigmented. The shell is thickened, with a finely granular surface. These eggs measure 90 to 100 µm in diameter. The center of the egg contains one or two cells (Figure 4-60). Eggs can be easily recovered on standard fecal flotation.

The adult worms of *P. equorum* also may be passed in the feces of the young foal. This is one of the largest nematodes to infect horses and

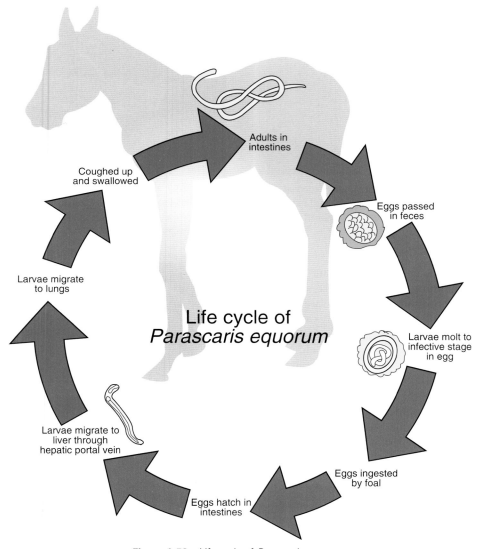

Life cycle of
Parascaris equorum

Adults in
intestines

Eggs passed
in feces

Larvae molt to
infective stage
in egg

Eggs ingested
by foal

Eggs hatch in
intestines

Larvae migrate to
liver through
hepatic portal vein

Larvae migrate
to lungs

Coughed up
and swallowed

Figure 4-59 Life cycle of *Parascaris equorum*.

may grow to a length of 50 cm; however, such large specimens are the exception rather than the rule.

Mild infections of *P. equorum* are usually asymptomatic, but heavy infections can cause unthriftiness, depression, a pot-bellied appearance, anorexia, colic, and a cough with nasal discharge. Treatment involves pasture management to reduce chances of reinfection and a sound deworming program with benzimidoles, ivermectin, piperazine, moxidectin, or pyrantel. Prevention includes thoroughly washing the feeders and waterers to remove the contaminating eggs. In addition, pasture management

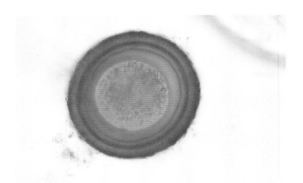

Figure 4-60 Egg of *Parascaris equorum*. Eggs are recovered from feces of young horses and are round to oval and deeply pigmented. Shell is thickened, with a finely granular surface.

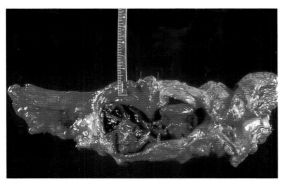

Figure 4-61 *Strongylus vulgaris* is often associated with thrombi in anterior mesenteric artery of horses.

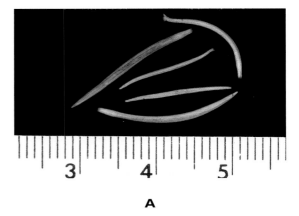

A

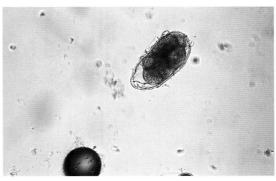

B

Figure 4-62 Strongyles are nematodes that parasitize the large intestine of horses and are typically divided into two types, large strongyles and small strongyles. **A,** Small strongyles comprise several genera that vary in pathogenicity. **B,** Large strongyles are the most pathogenic strongyles. Both large and small strongyles produce the typical strongyle type of egg.

involves rotating the pastures where the weanlings and foals graze.

Strongyles are nematodes that parasitize the large intestine of horses and are typically divided into two types, large strongyles and small strongyles. The small strongyles comprise several genera that vary in pathogenicity. The large strongyles are the most pathogenic of the strongyles. *Strongylus vulgaris* is often associated with thrombi within the anterior mesenteric artery of horses (Figure 4-61). *Strongylus vulgaris, S. edentatus,* and *S. equinus* are the large strongyles (Figure 4-62).

Regardless of whether these endoparasites are a small strongyle or a large strongyle, their eggs are virtually identical. Identification to the species level is accomplished by fecal culture and identification of larvae. Strongyle eggs are most often observed during standard fecal flotation of horse feces. The eggs contain an 8- to 16-cell morula and measure approximately 70 to 90 μm by 40 to 50 μm. In addition, the life cycles of the strongyles are very similar. The eggs are passed

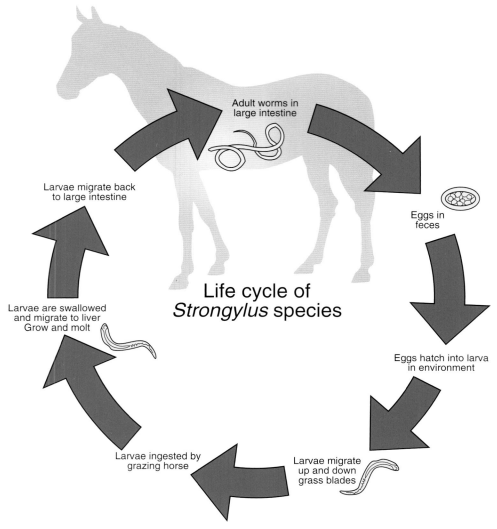

Life cycle of
Strongylus species

Adult worms in
large intestine

Eggs in
feces

Larvae migrate back
to large intestine

Larvae are swallowed
and migrate to liver
Grow and molt

Larvae ingested by
grazing horse

Larvae migrate
up and down
grass blades

Eggs hatch into larva
in environment

Figure 4-63 Life cycle of the *Strongylus* species.

in the feces and hatch in the environment. The infective-stage larvae migrate up and down blades of grass until the equine host ingests the larvae. The larvae are swallowed and migrate through the intestines to the mesenteric arteries and the liver, where they grow and molt to the next larval stage. The larvae migrate back toward the large intestine and grow and molt on their way. Once in the large intestine, the larvae enter the mucosa of the large intestine and mature to adults (Figure 4-63). When these characteristic eggs are found on fecal flotation, the veterinary diagnostician should record their presence as a "strongyle type of egg," rather than trying to identify a particular species of large or small strongyles.

Clinical signs of a strongyle infection include colic, weight loss, lethargy, fever, and poor appetite. Most of the signs are related to the migration of the larvae through the mesenteric arteries and liver. The most common anthelmintics include fenbendazole, oxfendazole, thiabendazole, and ivermectin. Preventive measures include pasture management, a good deworming program, and routine fecal examinations.

Strongyloides westeri is the intestinal threadworm of horses. These nematodes are unique in that only a parthenogenetic female is parasitic in the host. Parasitic males do not exist. *S. westeri* produces larvated eggs measuring 40 to 52 μm by 32 to 40 μm. The mare can transmit the parasite to the foal through the colostrum. Eggs are usually recovered on flotation of fresh feces. The prepatent period is 5 to 7 days (see Figure 4-14). The clinical symptoms include diarrhea, weight loss, anemia, and poor appetite. A good deworming program for the mare and foal with oxibendazole, thiabendazole, or ivermectin will help control the parasite.

Oxyuris equi is a pinworm of horses. The adult worms are found in the cecum, colon, and rectum. Adult worms are often observed protruding from the anus. Adult female worms attach their eggs to the exterior of the anus with a gelatinous, sticky material that produces anal pruritus in infected horses. The eggs can be rubbed off the anus onto waterers, feeders, and fences, where the eggs can be ingested by the same host or a new host. Pinworm eggs can also be recovered from the feces; eggs are 90 by 40 μm and have a smooth, thick shell. They are operculate and slightly flattened on one side. Pinworm eggs may be larvated (Figure 4-64). The prepatent period is approximately 4 to 5 months.

Diagnosis of pinworms in horses is made by finding the characteristic eggs on microscopic examination of cellophane tape impressions or by scraping the surface of the anus. The pruritus produced will often cause the horse to rub its rump against solid objects to relieve the itching. As a result, hairs in the region of the tail head are often broken. A good deworming program with oxibendazole, thiabendazole, or ivermectin and

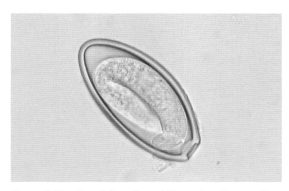

Figure 4-64   Egg of *Oxyuris equi*, the equine pinworm. Eggs are operculate and slightly flattened on one side. Pinworm eggs may be larvated.

thoroughly washing the anus of infected horses will help control the spread of *Oxyuris equi*.

RESPIRATORY SYSTEM

Dictyocaulus arnfieldi, the equine lungworm, is found in the bronchi and bronchioles of horses, mules, and donkeys. Its eggs are ellipsoidal, embryonated, and measure approximately 80 to 100 μm by 50 to 60 μm. Eggs can be recovered on fecal flotation of fresh feces (<24 hours old). Larvae hatch from the eggs within a few hours after feces are passed to the outside. The lungworm larvae become infective in the external environment; horses become infected by ingesting the larvae. The larvae migrate to the bronchi through lymphatic vessels. The prepatent period for the equine lungworm is 42 to 56 days. The common anthelmintics (thiabendazole, fenbendazole, ivermectin) used in a good deworming program will also treat *Dictyocaulus arnfieldi*.

SKIN

Adult *Habronema* species that occur in horses are gastrointestinal nematodes (see earlier discussion). The adults never parasitize the skin; however, the larval stages can be deposited by flies (*Musca domestica* and *Stomoxys calcitrans*) into the skin wounds of horses. Here the larvae are aberrant, or "off course," and produce a condition known as ***cutaneous habronemiasis,***

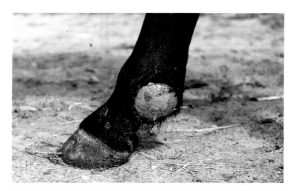

Figure 4-65 Lesions of cutaneous habronemiasis (cutaneous draschiasis, or summer sores) vary in size and have uneven surface that consists of soft, reddish-brown material and covers a mass of firmer granulation tissue. Lesions are seen on body parts that are likely to be injured, such as legs, withers, male genitalia, and medial canthus of the eye.

cutaneous draschiasis, or *summer sores.* The lesions vary in size and have an uneven surface that consists of a soft, reddish-brown material and covers a mass of firmer granulation tissue. These lesions are seen on the parts of the body likely to be injured, such as the legs, withers, male genitalia, and medial canthus of the eye (Figure 4-65). These wounds tend to increase in size and do not respond to usual treatment until the following winter, when they spontaneously heal.

Diagnosis of cutaneous habronemiasis is based on clinical signs and skin biopsies, which may reveal cross sections or longitudinal sections of these aberrant larvae.

The microfilariae of *Onchocerca cervicalis,* the equine filarial parasite, produce recurrent dermatitis and periodic ophthalmia in horses. The adults live in the ligamentum nuchae of horses. The female worms produce microfilariae that migrate to the dermis through connective tissue. This parasite is spread by the biting midges of *Culicoides* species. The flies feed on host blood and ingest the microfilariae, which develop to the infective third stage within the fly. When the fly bites another horse, larvae are injected into the connective tissue and develop to adults during migration to the ligamentum nuchae.

The microfilariae produce the characteristic lesions of **cutaneous onchocerciasis:** patchy alopecia and scaling on the head, neck, shoulders, and ventral midline that may be accompanied by intense pruritus.

Many infected horses are asymptomatic. Microfilariae of *Onchocerca* concentrate in certain areas, most often the ventral midline. Because more than 90% of normal hosts are probably infected with *O. cervicalis,* detection of microfilariae in the skin of the ventral midline is not diagnostic for cutaneous onchocerciasis. However, the presence of microfilariae in diseased skin is highly indicative of, although not diagnostic of, cutaneous onchocerciasis.

Onchocerca microfilariae may be demonstrated by the following procedure. After clipping and a surgical scrub, a 6-mm punch biopsy is obtained (see Chapter 17). With a single-edged razor blade or scalpel blade, half the tissue is minced in a small amount of preservative-free physiologic saline on a glass slide and allowed to stand for 5 to 10 minutes. Drying of the specimen is prevented by placing the slide in a covered chamber with a small amount of saline. The slide is then examined under a low-power (10×) objective. Because the translucent microfilariae are difficult to observe, low-intensity light and high contrast (achieved by lowering the condenser) are essential. Live microfilariae are identified by the vigorous swimming activity at the edge of the tissue. *O. cervicalis* microfilariae are slender and 207 to 240 μm long. The other half of the biopsy should be submitted for routine histopathologic examination.

EYE AND ADNEXA

Thelazia lacrymalis is the eyeworm of horses throughout the world. Adult parasites can be recovered from the conjunctival sac and lacrimal duct. Examination of the lacrimal secretions may reveal eggs or first-stage larvae.

The unsheathed microfilariae of *Onchocerca cervicalis* have been incriminated as causing periodic ophthalmia and blindness in the eyes of horses. These may be detected by ophthalmic examination.

ABDOMINAL CAVITY

Setaria equina is the abdominal worm of horses. Adults are found free within the peritoneal cavity. The sheathed microfilariae are 240 to 256 μm long. Antemortem diagnosis is by demonstration of microfilariae in peripheral blood smears. Adults may be observed freely within the peritoneal cavity during postmortem examination.

NEMATODES OF SWINE

GASTROINTESTINAL TRACT

Ascarops strongylina and *Physocephalus sexalatus* are the thick stomach worms of the porcine stomach. Both these nematodes produce thick-walled, larvated eggs that can be recovered on fecal flotation. The eggs of both species are similar in appearance. The egg of *A. strongylina* is 34 to 39 μm by 20 μm and has a thick shell surrounded by a thin membrane, producing an irregular outline (Figure 4-66). The egg of *P. sexalatus* is 34 to 39 μm by 15 to 17 μm. The prepatent period for both species is approximately 42 days. Diagnosis is by observation of typical eggs on routine fecal flotation. Clinical

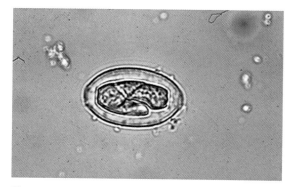

Figure 4-66   Egg of *Ascarops strongylina* is 34 to 39 μm by 20 μm and has a thick shell surrounded by a thin membrane that produces an irregular outline.

signs include anemia, diarrhea, and weight loss. Anthelmintics used for treating *A. strongylina* and *P. sexalatus* are ivermectin, fenbendazole, thiabendazole, and oxfendazole.

Hyostrongylus rubidus is the red stomach worm of swine. The egg is a trichostrongyle type of egg, that is, an oval, thin-shelled egg. It contains a morula with four or more cells and measures 71 to 78 μm by 35 to 42 μm. These eggs can be recovered on fecal flotation. As with the bovine trichostrongyles, definitive diagnosis can only be made by fecal culture and larval identification. The prepatent period is approximately 20 days. Clinical signs include dehydration, weight loss, diarrhea, and anemia. Deworming with benzimidazoles (fenbendazole, thiabendazole, oxibendazole) and ivermectin will control the parasite.

Trichostrongylus axei is another species of nematode that may reside in the stomach of pigs. It is important to remember that *T. axei* can cross species lines and also parasitize cattle, sheep, and horses. The eggs of *T. axei* are classified as the trichostrongyle type and measure 79 to 92 μm by 31 to 41 μm. As with bovine trichostrongyles, definitive diagnosis can be made only by fecal culture and larval identification. Benzimidazoles are the anthelmintics of choice.

Ascaris suum, the swine ascarid, or large intestinal roundworm, is the largest nematode found in the small intestine of pigs (Figure 4-67). It may attain a length of up to 41 cm and can be as wide as 5 mm. These large, robust nematodes may be passed in feces. They produce eggs that are passed in the feces and hatch in the environment. The larvae grow to infective larvae within the eggs, which are ingested by the pig. The larvae hatch and migrate to the liver, where they grow to the next larval stage. The larvae migrate through the circulatory system to the lungs and the bronchial tree, where they are swallowed. Once in the intestines, the larvae mature into adults.

Eggs of *A. suum* can be recovered on standard fecal flotation. They are oval and golden brown with a thick, albuminous shell bearing pro-

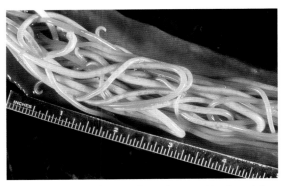

Figure 4-67 *Ascaris suum,* the swine ascarid or large intestinal roundworm, is largest nematode found within small intestine of pigs.

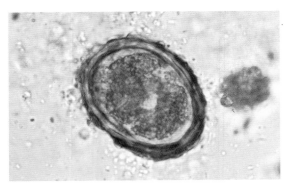

Figure 4-68 Eggs of *Ascaris suum* can be recovered on standard fecal flotation. Eggs are oval and golden brown, with a thick, albuminous shell bearing prominent projections that give a lumpy, bumpy appearance.

minent projections that give a lumpy, bumpy appearance. The eggs measure 70 to 89 μm by 37 to 40 μm (Figure 4-68). *A. suum* can cause a reduced growth rate, weight loss, unthriftiness, respiratory symptoms (coughing, abdominal breathing, or *thumps*). Benzimidazoles, levamisole, ivermectin, pyrantel, piperazine, and hydromycin (a feed-additive dewormer) are the anthelmintics of choice.

Strongyloides ransomi, the intestinal threadworm of pigs, is unique in that only a parthenogenetic female is parasitic in the host. Parasitic males do not exist. These females produce lar-

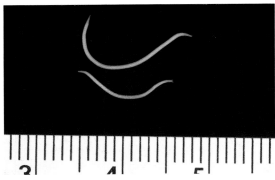

Figure 4-69 *Oesophagostomum dentatum,* the nodular worm of swine, is found in large intestine of swine.

vated eggs measuring 45 to 55 μm by 26 to 35 μm. Eggs are usually recovered in flotation of fresh feces. The life cycle of *S. ransomi* closely resembles that of *Strongyloides papillosus* (see Figure 4-63). Transmission can occur through the colostrum. The prepatent period is 3 to 7 days. (see Figure 4-14). *S. ransomi* can produce diarrhea, anemia, and weight loss in the host. Anthelmintics of choice are the benzimidazoles and ivermectin.

Oesophagostomum dentatum, the nodular worm of swine, is found in the large intestine of swine (Figure 4-69). It is called the "nodular worm" because its larval stages induce the formation of large nodules within the wall of the large intestine (Figure 4-70). The prepatent period is 50 days. The eggs of *O. dentatum* are of the trichostrongyle type, that is, oval, thin-shelled eggs. They contain 4 to 16 cells and measure 40 by 70 μm. These eggs can be recovered on standard fecal flotation. As with the bovine trichostrongyles, definitive diagnosis can be made only by fecal culture and larval identification. The parasite can cause anorexia, diarrhea, weight loss, and gastrointestinal disturbances in the host. Benzimidazoles, ivermectin, levamisole, piperazine, and pyrantel are the anthelmintics of choice.

Trichuris suis, commonly called "whipworms," infect the cecum and colon of swine. (See previous discussion of nematodes of dogs

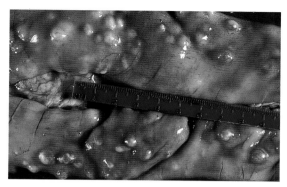

Figure 4-70 *Oesophagostomum dentatum* is called the "nodular worm" of swine because its larval stages induce formation of large nodules within the wall of the large intestine.

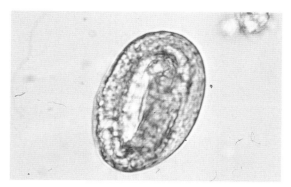

Figure 4-71 *Metastrongylus elongatus (apri)*, the swine lungworm, is found in bronchi and bronchioles of pigs. Oval, thick-walled eggs measure 60 by 40 μm and contain larvae.

and cats for gross morphology of adult worms and life cycle.) The egg of the whipworm is trichuroid or trichinelloid and has a thick, brown, barrel-shaped shell with polar plugs at both ends (see Figure 4-16). The eggs are unembryonated (not larvated) when laid. Eggs of porcine whipworms measure 50 to 60 μm by 21 to 25 μm. The prepatent period is 42 to 49 days. Common symptoms seen in the host are anemia, bloody diarrhea, anorexia, and stunted growth. Levamisole, dichlorvos, and fenbendazole are the anthelmintics of choice.

The adult *Trichinella spiralis,* the "trichina worm," is found in the small intestine of the porcine definitive host. The adult worm is very fine and slender. The female is very tiny, only 4 mm in length; the male is even smaller. This stage is seldom recovered by the veterinarian. The egg is larvated and measures 30 by 40 μm. (See discussion under Musculoskeletal System for larval stage in porcine intermediate host.) *T. spiralis* is a very unusual parasite because the definitive host and the intermediate host may be the same animal. *T. spiralis* can be passed to humans in undercooked pork (see Chapter 16). Most animal hosts are *asymptomatic* (showing no symptoms).

RESPIRATORY TRACT

Metastrongylus elongatus, the swine lungworm, is found within the bronchi and bronchioles of pigs. The oval, thick-walled eggs measure 60 by 40 μm and contain larvae (Figure 4-71). Eggs can be recovered on fecal flotation using flotation medium with a specific gravity greater than 1.25 or by using the fecal sedimentation technique. The prepatent period is approximately 24 days. *M. elongatus* uses the earthworm as an intermediate host. Therefore, control of earthworms in the pigs' environment will help eliminate this parasite. Control may include keeping pigs on concrete rather than pasture or dirt. Infected pigs may have a persistent cough, reduced growth rate, and unthriftiness. Infected pigs can be treated with fenbendazole, ivermectin, or levamisole.

URINARY TRACT

Stephanurus dentatus, the swine kidney worm, is found in cystic spaces that connect to the kidney, ureters, and perirenal tissues of pigs (Figure 4-72). The eggs are the oval, thin-shelled strongyle type of eggs, containing 4 to 16 cells and measuring 90 to 120 μm by 43 to 70 μm. Eggs can be recovered from the urine using sedimentation (Figure 4-73). The prepatent period is extremely long, approximately 9 to 24 months. Infected pigs may show signs of anorexia, decreased growth rate, and weight loss. Anthelmintics of choice include fenbendazole, levamisole, and ivermectin.

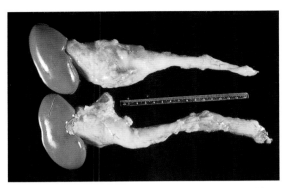

Figure 4-72 *Stephanurus dentatus,* the swine kidney worm, is found in cystic spaces that connect to kidney, ureters, and perirenal tissues of pigs.

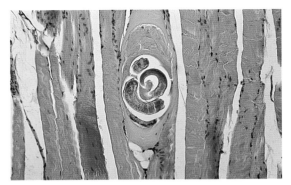

Figure 4-74 Muscle biopsy revealing larval form of *Trichinella spiralis,* the trichina worm, found in musculature of porcine intermediate host. Larvae measure approximately 1 mm in length and are found in cystic spaces in musculature.

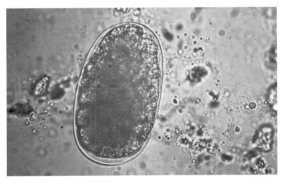

Figure 4-73 Eggs of *Stephanurus dentatus* are of the strongyle type, that is, oval, thin-shelled eggs. They contain 4 to 16 cells and measure 90 to 120 μm by 43 to 70 μm. Eggs can be recovered from urine using sedimentation.

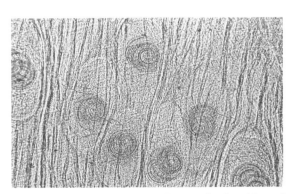

Figure 4-75 Histopathologic section revealing larval form of *Trichinella spiralis,* the trichina worm found in musculature of porcine intermediate host.

MUSCULOSKELETAL SYSTEM

The larval form of *Trichinella spiralis,* the "trichina worm," is found in the musculature of the porcine intermediate host. The adult worm is very fine and slender and is found within the small intestine. The larval *T. spiralis* is found in striated muscle fibers. It measures approximately 1 mm in length and is found in cystic spaces within the musculature (Figures 4-74 and 4-75). The cyst measures 0.4 to 0.6 mm by 0.25 mm. In chronic cases the cyst may become calcified. (See discussion under Gastrointestinal Tract for adult stage of this parasite in the definitive host.) Humans may become infected with *T. spiralis.*

Diagnosis of the larval stage of *T. spiralis* is made by performing a biopsy of muscle tissue and demonstrating encysted larvae within skeletal musculature. As a result of the zoonotic potential for this parasite, pork should *always* be cooked thoroughly.

NEMATODES OF MICE

GASTROINTESTINAL TRACT

Oxyurids, or pinworms, of mice include *Syphacia obvelata, Aspiculuris tetraptera,* and to a lesser extent, *Syphacia muris,* the common pinworm of rats. Patent *Syphacia* infections can be detected both antemortem and postmortem with the perianal cellophane test. The adults of *Syphacia* reside in the cecum of the mouse until the gravid female migrates the length of the colon to deposit a large batch of eggs in the perianal region, at which time the female dies.

Eggs of *A. tetraptera* cannot be detected with the perianal cellophane tape test. *A. tetraptera* adults reside mainly in the proximal loop of the colon of the mouse and do not migrate to deposit eggs on the perianal area, as do *Syphacia* species. Eggs of *A. tetraptera* can be detected antemortem by fecal flotation and occasionally by direct smear examination of feces.

The banana-shaped eggs of *S. obvelata* are elongated with pointed ends (Figure 4-76). They are flat on one side and convex on the other, measuring 118 to 153 μm by 33 to 55 μm. *S. muris* is found less frequently and in smaller numbers in mice than *S. obvelata.* The more symmetric,

football-shaped eggs of *S. muris* are smaller than those of *S. obvelata,* measuring only 72 to 82 μm by 25 to 36 μm, and are blunted or rounded on the ends (Figure 4-77). When observed on fecal flotation, the eggs of *A. tetraptera* are seen to have a thinner shell than the eggs of the *Syphacia* species and do not have a flattened side. *A. tetraptera* eggs are 89 to 93 μm by 33 to 42 μm, symmetrically ellipsoid, and midway in size between eggs of the two *Syphacia* species.

On postmortem examination, pinworms of mice may be detected by placing a small piece of the cecum and proximal loop of the colon in a Petri dish with a small amount of normal saline. Within a few minutes, pinworms may be observed in the saline grossly or with the aid of a hand-held magnifying lens or a dissecting microscope (Figure 4-78). The adult pinworms can be collected with a bulb and pipette, applied to a glass slide with a coverslip, and examined microscopically at low magnification (4× objective). *A. tetraptera* is usually recovered from the proximal colon and is easily distinguished from *Syphacia* species by its oval esophageal bulb and prominent cervical ala (Figure 4-79, *A*). *S. obvelata* and *S. muris* are usually recovered from the cecum. *Syphacia* species have a rounded

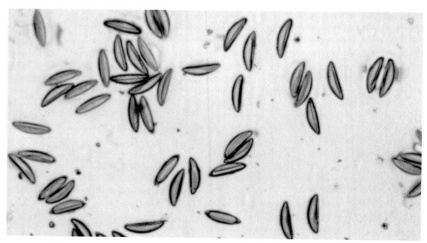

Figure 4-76 Eggs of *Syphacia obvelata,* the mouse cecal pinworm, as they appear on cellophane tape presentation.

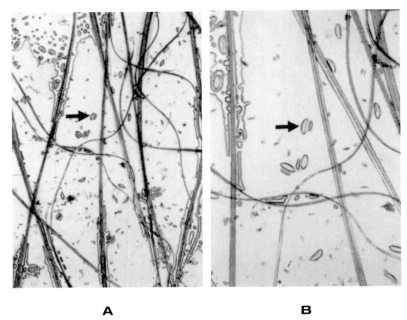

A   **B**

Figure 4-77 Cellophane tape presentation of *Syphacia muris* eggs viewed at **A**, low and **B**, medium magnification. Arrow points to same egg at each magnification. Smaller object right of egg is an artifact.

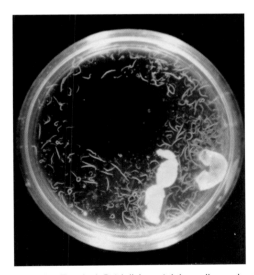

Figure 4-78 Two-inch Petri dish containing saline and proximal loops of colon from three mice. White, hairlike objects are *Aspiculuris tetraptera* roundworms that have moved into saline from colon sections.

esophageal bulb and a small cervical ala (Figure 4-79, *B*). Additionally, the vulva is in the cranial one sixth of the body of *S. obvelata* females (Figure 4-79, *C*), whereas the vulva of *S. muris* is in the cranial one fourth of the body (Figure 4-79, *B*). Adult males of the two *Syphacia* species can be differentiated by the position of the three ventral mamelons. In males of *S. obvelata*, the middle mamelon is located centrally on the length of the body (see Figure 4-83, *A*). The first mamelon is at the center of the male in *S. muris* (see Figure 4-83, *B*). Although differentiation of the adults of the two *Syphacia* species may be difficult and time-consuming for veterinary technicians, experienced diagnosticians can easily differentiate the eggs on the cellophane tape preparations by size and shape (see Figures 4-76 and 4-77).

In general, mice carry light-to-medium loads of pinworms without demonstrating clinical signs of infection. However, large numbers of

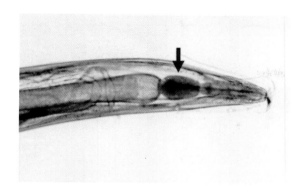

A

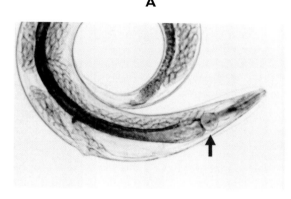

B

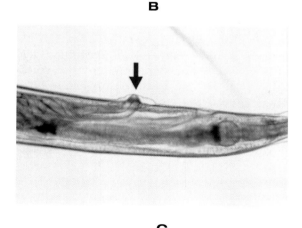

C

Figure 4-79 **A,** Cranial end of *Aspiculurus tetraptera* female, showing oval esophageal bulb *(arrow)*. **B,** *Syphacia muris,* showing round esophageal bulb *(arrow)*. **C,** Cranial end of *Syphacia obvelata* female *(arrow* indicates vulva).

pinworms may lead to rectal prolapse, enteritis, sticky stools, and pruritus, which results in biting at the base of the tail.

Pinworms are transmitted by the ingestion of the eggs. The eggs are hardy, resistant to environmental extremes, and light enough to aerosolize, making control difficult. Retrograde infection is also possible with *Syphacia* species. The multispecies owner should be instructed that *Syphacia* species can be easily transmitted among mice, rats, hamsters, and gerbils. *A. tetraptera* has also been diagnosed in rats. Rodent pinworms are not of zoonotic significance.

NEMATODES OF RATS

GASTROINTESTINAL TRACT

The three oxyurids, or pinworms, discussed in the previous section, *Syphacia muris, S. obvelata,* and *Aspiculuris tetraptera,* may also infect rats. *S. muris* is by far the most common pinworm and is often referred to as the "rat pinworm."

Trichosomoides crassicauda is a nematode found in the urinary bladder of rats. The adult female *T. crassicauda* is approximately 10 mm long; it is a thin worm and is grossly visible in the wall of the urinary bladder. This parasite is unique in that the male is **neotenic.** This means that he is very small and resides in the vagina of the immature female and the uterus of the mature female *T. crassicauda.* The eggs are double operculate, approximately 65 by 33 μm, and resemble whipworm eggs, especially those of *Trichuris vulpis.* The main difference between the eggs is that the eggs of *T. crassicauda* are lighter in color and slightly smaller. This parasite has been associated with bladder tumors in rats; however, few clinical signs are associated with infection by *T. crassicauda.* Transmission is by the urinary-oral route. This parasite can be a significant problem in rat colonies but can be eliminated by cesarean delivery of neonates. This is a species-specific nematode and is not of zoonotic significance.

Infections with *T. crassicauda* may be diagnosed in three ways: antemortem or postmortem

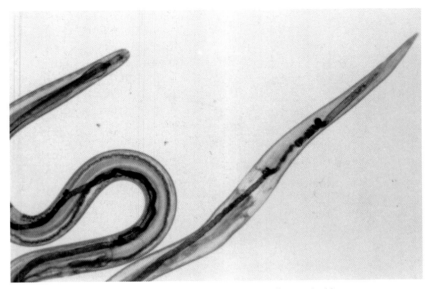

Figure 4-80 Adult female *Dentostomella translucida.*

observation of eggs in the urine, gross observation at postmortem of adult worms in the wall or lumen of the urinary bladder, and microscopic observation of the adult worms in histopathologic sections of the urinary bladder, ureters, or renal pelvis.

NEMATODES OF HAMSTERS

GASTROINTESTINAL TRACT

Hamsters are susceptible to infection with the mouse and rat pinworm, *Syphacia obvelata* and *S. muris,* although it is unlikely that hamsters will develop clinically apparent infections (see previous discussion of nematodes of mice).

NEMATODES OF GERBILS

GASTROINTESTINAL TRACT

Dentostomella translucida, the gerbil pinworm, is not reported as frequently as other rodent pinworms (*Syphacia* species and *Aspiculuris tetraptera*). This may be the result of the lack of information on its life cycle. Adult male and female nematodes have a short, muscular esophagus. The vulva of the female is located just cranial to the midbody (Figure 4-80). Males are distinguished by a cuticular inflation just cranial to the cloaca (Figure 4-81). Adults are 6 to 31 mm long, with the female generally larger than the male, as is true of other rodent pinworms. Eggs of *D. translucida* are asymmetric and oval, measuring 120 to 140 µm by 30 to 60 µm (Figure 4-82). They resemble those of *A. tetraptera,* which are smaller, measuring 89 to 93 µm by 36 to 42 µm.

Fecal flotation may be used to detect eggs of *D. translucida,* but this method is unreliable because of the poorly understood life cycle (intermittent shedding of eggs). On postmortem examination, *D. translucida* may be found in the stomach and the proximal one third of the small intestine.

D. translucida has a direct life cycle and is transmitted by ingestion of infective eggs from feces of infected animals. The parasite has been found in the golden hamster, as well as the gerbil. This parasite has no zoonotic significance.

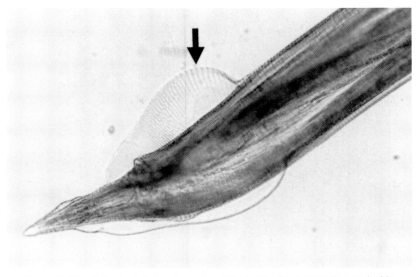

Figure 4-81   Cuticular inflation *(arrow)* on tail of male *Dentostomella translucida.*

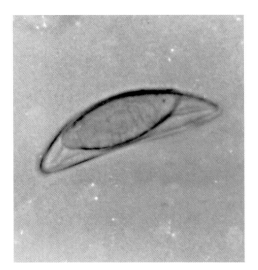

Figure 4-82   Egg of *Dentostomella translucida* in fecal flotation.

As with hamsters, gerbils are susceptible to infection with the mouse and rat pinworm, *S. obvelata* and *S. muris* (Figure 4-83; see also Figures 4-76, 4-77, and 4-79 and previous discussion of nematodes of mice).

NEMATODES OF GUINEA PIGS

GASTROINTESTINAL TRACT

Paraspidodera uncinata is generally a nonpathogenic nematode of guinea pigs that can be found in cecal contents or in the mucosa of the cecum and colon. Adult worms are 11 to 28 mm by 0.3 to 0.4 mm. The male of *P. uncinata* has a sucker and two spicules of equal length immediately cranial to the anus. The eggs are oval and have a characteristic thick ascarid shell (Figure 4-84). Eggs are 40 to 50 μm by 30 to 40 μm. Antemortem eggs may be detected by fecal flotation or direct fecal smear. Occasionally, extremely heavy infections may cause diarrhea and weight loss.

The life cycle of *P. uncinata* is direct, and transmission occurs through feed and water contaminated with infective eggs. *P. uncinata* has not been found in other species of animals and is not considered a public heath hazard.

NEMATODES OF RABBITS

GASTROINTESTINAL TRACT

Passalurus ambiguus is a nonpathogenic pinworm found in the cecum and colon of domestic and

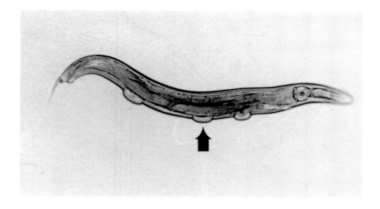

A

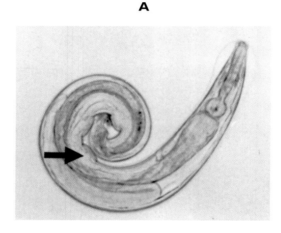

B

Figure 4-83 **A,** *Syphacia obvelata* male, showing middle mamelon *(arrow)* at center of body. **B,** *Syphacia muris* male, showing first mamelon at midbody *(arrow).*

cottontail rabbits and hares. It is a pinworm that has an obvious round esophageal bulb. Adult females are approximately 10 mm long (Figure 4-85), and males are 4 to 5 mm long (Figure 4-86). Females have a long, finely pointed tail. Eggs are oval and slightly flattened on one side, measuring approximately 43 by 103 μm (Figure 4-87). Eggs are deposited in the feces and resemble morulated hookworm eggs of dogs.

Infection with *P. ambiguus* can be detected antemortem by observing typical eggs in fecal flotation preparations. On postmortem examination, the white, hairlike adult worms can be found in the cecum and the proximal colon. Rabbits can tolerate heavy infections with no apparent clinical signs. It is believed that these pinworms feed on bacteria in the intestinal contents without disturbing the mucosal lining of the cecum.

Eggs passed in the feces are immediately infective, so control of this parasite is quite difficult. Transmission is by ingestion of infective eggs. Clients should be advised to use feeders elevated off of the floor of the rabbit hutch and to prevent access of wild hares and cottontail rabbits to pet rabbits and to the feed and bedding. *P. ambiguus* is species specific and has no zoonotic potential.

Trichostrongyles are primarily parasites of ruminants and other large animals. However, these nematodes are also common in wild rabbits, although uncommon in domestic rabbits. Diagnosticians must be aware of the possibility of

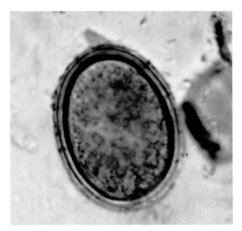

Figure 4-84 Egg of *Paraspidodera uncinata*, the cecal pinworm of guinea pigs.

infection with one or more rabbit trichostrongyles. Adult *Obeliscoides cuniculi* are found in the stomach of rabbits, and adult *Trichostrongylus calcaratus* are found in the small intestine. The males of these species are distinguished by the copulatory bursa on the posterior end. *O. cuniculi* females are 16 mm long and 0.5 mm wide, and males are 12 by 0.2 mm. Male and female adults may be found in the stomach on postmortem examination. Eggs are 80 by 45 μm and are thin shelled and oval. They may be easily observed on fecal flotation procedures. This nematode can produce a hemorrhagic gastritis. Transmission is by ingestion of the larval form after eggs are passed in the feces.

Adults of *T. calcaratus* are found in the small intestine and generally are smaller than those of *O. cuniculi*. Females of *T. calcaratus* are 6.4 mm by 100 μm, and males are 5.7 mm by 115 μm. The thin-shelled eggs are 65 by 33 μm and may be observed on fecal flotation. Rabbits infected with *T. calcaratus* may develop anemia. The life cycle of this trichostrongyle is direct, and transmission is by ingestion of infective larvae. As with other parasites that infect wild rabbits, prevention and

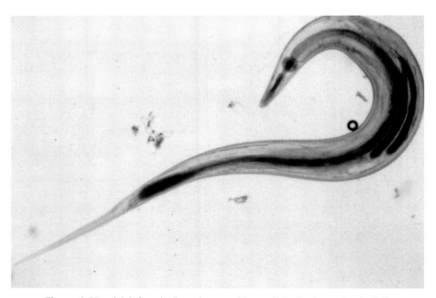

Figure 4-85 Adult female *Passalurus ambiguus*. Note the long, slender tail.

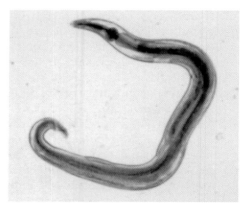

Figure 4-86　Adult male *Passalurus ambiguus.*

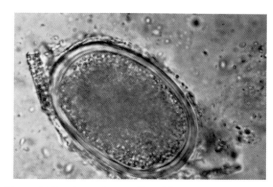

Figure 4-88　A roundworm *(Ascaridia)* egg in a fecal smear from a cockatiel.

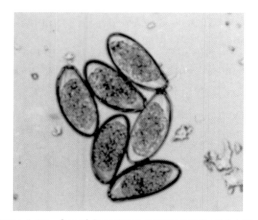

Figure 4-87　Ova of *Passalurus ambiguus* in fecal flotation.

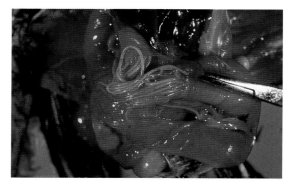

Figure 4-89　Nematodes occur infrequently in pet and aviary birds. *Ascaridia* is occasionally seen in small intestine of lovebirds, cockatiels, and macaws.

control depend on storing feed and bedding safely from wild hares and cottontail rabbits.

NEMATODES OF PET AND AVIARY BIRDS

GASTROINTESTINAL TRACT

Nematodes occur infrequently in pet and aviary birds. *Ascaridia* is occasionally seen in lovebirds, cockatiels, and macaws (Figures 4-88 and 4-89). Ascarids are very common in grass parakeets and can be demonstrated on both direct smear examination and fecal flotation. These roundworms are also common in backyard poultry and

in waterfowl. In turkeys and peafowl, *Heterakis gallinarum* serves as an intermediate host for *Histomonas meleagridis,* the protozoan that produces infectious enterohepatitis.

Spirurids can infect a variety of avian species but are generally uncommon in pet birds. *Spiroptera incesta* can infect Australian finches; *Dyspharynx nasuta* infects other finches. Infection by spirurids can be difficult to detect in finches. When spirurids are suspected, histologic examination of the ventriculus is recommended. The eggs of the spirurids are characterized by a thick wall and the presence of an embryonating larva within each egg. *Tetrameres,* a globose (spherical) spirurid, is typically found in the wall of the proventriculus of pigeons (see Figure 4-4).

Capillaria species may be found in the crop and upper alimentary tract of pheasants, peafowl, and other poultry. These hairlike nematodes have been reported in a variety of imported psittacine birds. The tiny adult worms often can be recovered from the wall of the esophagus or the crop. A direct smear of a sample from this area or a fecal flotation often reveals the characteristic thick-walled bipolar eggs, which are similar to whipworms, the *Trichuris* species.

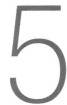

The Phylum Platyhelminthes, Class Cestoda

The phylum Platyhelminthes, the flatworms, includes the *trematodes* (or flukes), discussed in Chapters 7 and 8, and the *cestodes* (or tapeworms) detailed in this chapter and Chapter 6. Remember that the morphologic feature shared by these two classes is that they are both dorsoventrally flattened. However, whereas the flukes are flattened and leaf shaped, the tapeworms are ribbonlike and segmented into identical compartments called *proglottids* (Figure 5-1).

Members of the phylum Platyhelminthes, class Cestoda, are often referred to as cestodes or "tapeworms." Their bodies are usually long, segmented, and flattened, almost ribbonlike in appearance. Within the class Cestoda are two subclasses, the subclass Eucestoda (true tapeworms) and the subclass Cotyloda (pseudotapeworms). Members of both of these classes are important parasites of domesticated and wild animals and of humans.

EUCESTODA (TRUE TAPEWORMS)

Phylum: Platyhelminthes
    Class: Cestoda

KEY MORPHOLOGIC FEATURES

As mentioned, tapeworms are long, segmented, flattened, almost ribbonlike parasites. On the extreme anterior end of the typical true tapeworm is the holdfast organelle, the *scolex,* or head (Figure 5-2). The scolex of the adult true tapeworm has four suckers called *acetabula,* with which the tapeworm holds on to the lining of the small intestine, the predilection site, or "home," of most adult tapeworms. Unlike the oral sucker of the digenetic trematode, the suckers of the true tapeworm are *not* associated with intake of food but rather serve as organs of attachment. True tapeworms do not have a mouth; instead, they absorb the nutrients acquired from the host's intestine through their *tegument,* or body wall. In addition to the suckers, some true tapeworms may possess an anchorlike organelle called the *rostellum* (Figure 5-3). The rostellum usually has backward-facing hooks. With these hooks, the tapeworm further anchors itself in the mucosa of the small intestine. If the tapeworm has a rostellum, it is said to be an

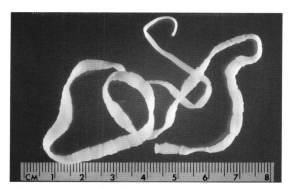

Figure 5-1 Example of typical tapeworm with dorsoventrally flattened, ribbonlike appearance. Every tapeworm is segmented into identical compartments called proglottids.

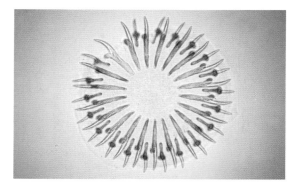

Figure 5-3 Anchorlike organelle, the rostellum, on anterior end of tapeworm. The rostellum usually has backward-facing hooks used to anchor the tapeworm further in the mucosa of the small intestine. If the tapeworm has a rostellum, it is said to be an "armed" tapeworm; if the tapeworm lacks the rostellum, it is said to be an "unarmed" tapeworm.

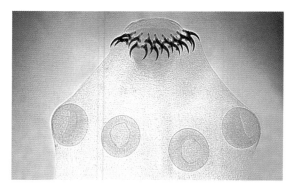

Figure 5-2 Located on the anterior end of the true tapeworm is the holdfast organelle, the scolex, or head. The scolex of the adult true tapeworm has four suckers called acetabula, with which the tapeworm holds on to the lining of the small intestine, the predilection site of most adult tapeworms.

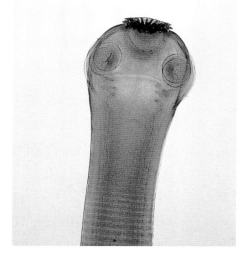

Figure 5-4 Proglottids closest to scolex and neck of the true tapeworm are immature, or "youngest," proglottids. Immature proglottids contain immature, nonfunctional male and female reproductive organs.

armed tapeworm; if the tapeworm lacks the rostellum, it is said to be an *unarmed tapeworm.*

Just posterior to the scolex of the true tapeworm is a germinal, or growth, region called the *neck.* It is from the neck that the rest of the true tapeworm's body, the *strobila,* arises. The strobila is composed of individual proglottids that are arranged similar to the boxcars in a railroad train. The proglottids closest to the scolex and the neck of the true tapeworm are the *immature,* or youngest, proglottids (Figure 5-4); those that are intermediate in distance from the scolex and

the neck are the *mature* proglottids (Figure 5-5); and those farthest from the scolex and the neck are the *gravid,* or oldest, proglottids (Figure 5-6).

As with the hermaphroditic digenetic trematodes, each proglottid of a true tapeworm

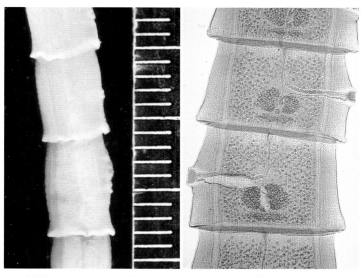

Figure 5-5   Tapeworm proglottids intermediate in distance to scolex and neck of the true tapeworm are mature, or "adolescent," proglottids. Mature proglottids contain mature, functional male and female reproductive organs.

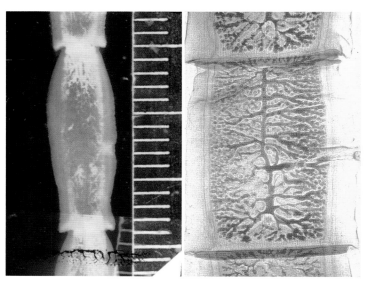

Figure 5-6   Tapeworm proglottids farthest from the scolex and the neck of the true tapeworm are gravid, or "aged," proglottids. Gravid proglottids contain male and female reproductive organs that have grown old and degenerated so that only the uterus filled with eggs remains.

contains complete sets of both male and female reproductive organs. As with the flukes, tapeworms are hermaphroditic. The sex organs of these tapeworms are usually located along the lateral aspects of the proglottid. Cross-fertilization and self-fertilization take place between and among individual proglottids. Immature proglottids contain male and female reproductive organs that are sexually immature; these are "prepuberty" proglottids. Mature proglottids contain male and female reproductive organs that are sexually mature and completely functional, or capable of reproduction. Gravid proglottids contain male and female reproductive organs that have grown old or are "spent," having degenerated to the point that the only portion remaining is the uterus filled with tapeworm eggs. Tapeworm proglottids can usually be observed with the naked eye in the feces of the definitive host (Figure 5-7). Other organ systems (nervous, excretory) are represented; however, they are not as important as the reproductive system. As with the digenetic trematodes, or flukes, tapeworms are "designed" to reproduce and produce offspring.

The eggs found in the gravid proglottids contain the larval stage, or *hexacanth,* with six hooks. The hexacanths can be contained within one of three egg types: pseudophyllidia, dipylidium, and taenia. The *pseudophyllidian egg* resembles on the *Ancylostoma* egg, however, it

has an operculum (Figure 5-8, *A*). It has an oval shape with the operculum at one end. The *Dipylidium egg* packet contains multiple hexacanths within one egg (Figure 5-8, *B*). Each hexacanth contains six hooks. The *Taenia egg* has a wide outer shell with a thicker outer covering and a six-hooked hexacanth within the egg (Figure 5-8, *C*).

LIFE CYCLE OF THE TRUE TAPEWORM

The life cycle of a typical true tapeworm is more complicated than that of a digenetic trematode. In most cases the gravid proglottids of the true tapeworm pass to the outside environment, sometimes singly and sometimes in chains, one behind the other. These proglottids rupture in the external environment and release thousands of *hexacanth embryos,* or eggs, to the outside environment (Figure 5-9). To continue the life cycle, the egg must be ingested by a suitable intermediate host, either an invertebrate or a vertebrate. Within this host, the egg develops into a *metacestode,* or larval tapeworm. The metacestode may take one of several forms: *cysticercoid, cysticercus, coenurus, hydatid cyst,* or *tetrathyridium.* These larval stages differ in their choice of host, their structure, their predilection site, and their pathogenicity to the intermediate host. Sometimes the metacestode, or larval, stage of the tapeworm is more pathogenic to the intermediate host than the adult or mature tapeworm is to the definitive host. The definitive host becomes infected by ingesting the intermediate host containing the metacestode stage. The "juvenile," or developing, tapeworm emerges from the metacestode stage, attaches to the lining of the small intestine, and begins to produce the strobila, which is composed of proglottids.

Tapeworm proglottids have muscles that enable them to move about. Owners of infected animals often observe these tapeworms as "little white worms" crawling on the animal's feces, hair coat, or bedding. Tapeworm proglottids often contain eggs when they are passed into the feces. These hexacanth embryos are eggs with

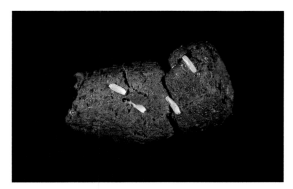

Figure 5-7 Tapeworm proglottids *(Dipylidium caninum)* observed in feces of definitive host.

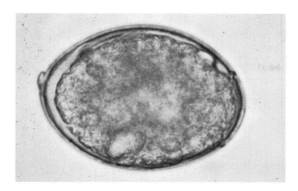

A

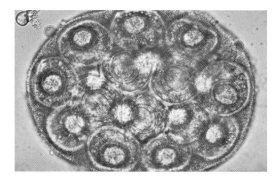

B

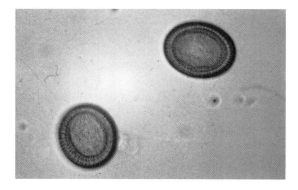

C

Figure 5-8 Tapeworm eggs can be seen in three basic types. **A,** Pseudophyllidia egg, as seen in *Diphyllobothrium latum.* **B,** Dipylidium eggs, as seen in *Dipylidium caninum.* **C,** Taenia egg, as seen in *Taenia pisiformis.*

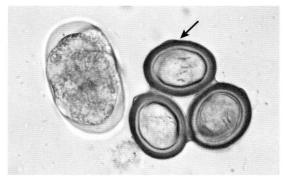

Figure 5-9 Tapeworm egg, or hexacanth embryo. Tapeworm eggs are released to outside environment. Each tapeworm egg is infective for the intermediate host and produces one metacestode stage.

embryos that have an internal structure and six hooks (see Figure 5-9). The hexacanth embryos are ingested by the intermediate host in which the tapeworm develops.

The intermediate host may be an arthropod, such as a flea or a grain mite. In this host the hexacanth embryo develops into a microscopic larval stage known as a *cysticercoid* (Figure 5-10). The cysticercoid is tiny and contains a small, fluid-filled space. The definitive host becomes infected by ingesting the intermediate host containing the cysticercoid larval stage. Examples of tapeworms that develop into a cysticercoid stage in an intermediate host are the fringed tapeworms of cattle *(Thysanosoma actinioides)* and the double-pored tapeworm of dogs and cats *(Dipylidium caninum).*

Sometimes the intermediate host is a mammalian host, such as a rabbit, in which the hexacanth embryo develops into a *cysticercus,* or "bladder worm," stage (Figure 5-11). The bladder worm is a fluid-filled larval stage within the tissues of the vertebrate intermediate host. The definitive host becomes infected by ingesting the intermediate host containing the bladder worm larval stage (Figure 5-12). Examples of tapeworms that have a bladder worm stage (or a variation of the bladder worm stage) in an

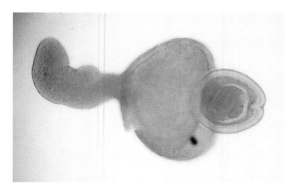

Figure 5-10 Microscopic larval (metacestode) stage known as a **cysticercoid.** The cysticercoid is tiny (microscopic) and contains a small, fluid-filled space; the cysticercoid develops within the intermediate host. Definitive host becomes infected by ingesting the intermediate host containing cysticercoid larval stage. Examples of tapeworms that develop into cysticercoid stage in the intermediate host are *Thysanosoma actinoides* of cattle, *Anoplocephala* species of horses, and *Dipylidium caninum* of dogs and cats.

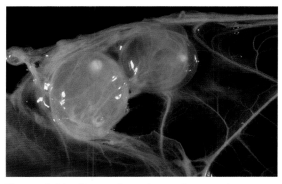

Figure 5-11 Hexacanth embryo of some tapeworms develops into a **cysticercus,** or "bladder worm," stage. Bladder worm is a fluid-filled larval stage within tissues of vertebrate intermediate host. Definitive host becomes infected by ingesting the intermediate host containing bladder worm larval stage. Examples of tapeworms that develop into cysticercus stage in an intermediate host are *Taenia* species.

intermediate host are the canine Taeniid tapeworm *(Taenia pisiformis)* and the *Coenurus* tapeworm *(Multiceps multiceps).* Other tapeworms that use a variation of the bladder worm stage are *Echinococcus granulosus* and *E. multilocularis,*

the hydatid cyst tapeworms. Chapter 6 covers these tapeworms and their larval stages in greater detail.

COTYLODA (PSEUDOTAPEWORMS)

Phylum: Platyhelminthes
  Class: Cestoda

KEY MORPHOLOGIC FEATURES

Members of the subclass Cotyloda, the pseudotapeworms, are tapeworms; they are long, segmented, flattened, almost ribbonlike parasites. These tapeworms resemble true tapeworms in that on the extreme anterior end of the typical pseudotapeworm is the holdfast organelle, the scolex, or head. Instead of possessing four holdfast suckers, or acetabula, the typical pseudotapeworm has two slitlike organelles called *bothria* (Figure 5-13). Bothria are longitudinal grooves along the length of the scolex. The pseudotapeworm attaches to the lining of the small intestine by means of the bothria. As with true tapeworms, pseudotapeworms do not have a mouth; instead, they absorb the nutrients acquired from the host's intestine through their tegument, or body wall.

The strobila of the pseudotapeworm is similar to that of the true tapeworm. The neck, or growth region, is just posterior to the scolex, and the pseudotapeworm's body arises from this. The strobila of the pseudotapeworm also is composed of immature, mature, and gravid proglottids. As with true tapeworms, pseudotapeworms are hermaphroditic, and each proglottid of a pseudotapeworm contains complete sets of both male and female reproductive organs. The sex organs of these tapeworms are usually located along the central region of each proglottid. There is a centrally located uterine pore through which eggs are voided to the external environment. The eggs of the pseudotapeworm do not resemble those of the true tapeworm. Oddly, they resemble the eggs of a digenetic trematode—they are operculated. In most cases the spent proglottids

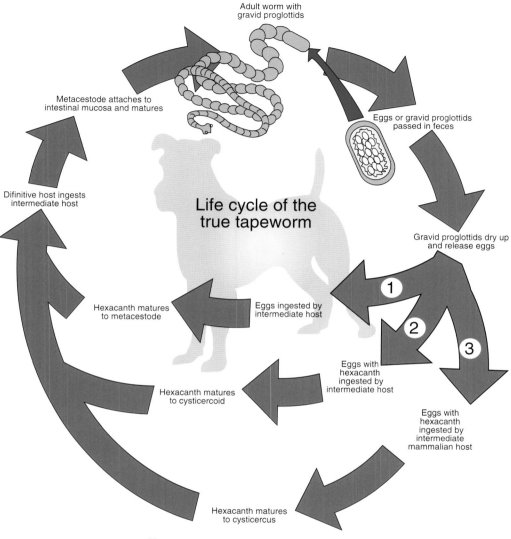

Figure 5-12 Life cycle of the true tapeworm.

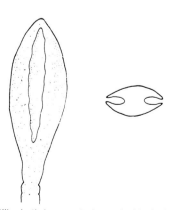

Figure 5-13 Slitlike bothria on anterior end of typical pseudotapeworm.

of the pseudotapeworm pass to the outside environment in long chains.

LIFE CYCLE OF THE PSEUDOTAPEWORM

The life cycle of the pseudotapeworm is slightly more complicated than that of a true tapeworm. The operculated eggs are passed singly to the external environment. If these eggs make contact with water, they hatch, releasing a ciliated hexa-canth embryo out of the operculum. This ciliated hexacanth embryo is called a *coracidium.* The coracidium must be ingested by a suitable first intermediate host, an aquatic Crustacean called a *copepod.* Within the copepod, the coracidium develops to a stage called a *procercoid.* If the copepod containing the procercoid is ingested by the second intermediate host, usually a fish of some type, the procercoid develops into the

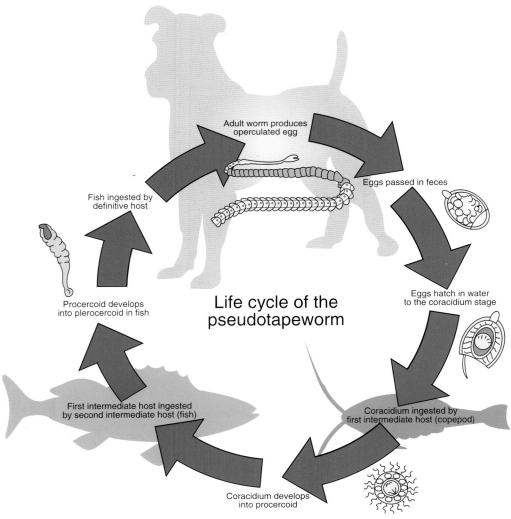

Figure 5-14   Life cycle of the pseudotapeworm.

second stage, which is infective for the definitive host. This stage is called the *plerocercoid* stage. The definitive host becomes infected by ingesting the second intermediate host containing the plerocercoid stage. This plerocercoid stage is the "juvenile," or developing, tapeworm; it possesses slitlike bothria. When the plerocercoid stage is ingested by the definitive host, it emerges from the metacestode stage, attaches to the lining of the small intestine, and begins to produce the strobila (Figure 5-14).

There are two important species of pseudotapeworms: *Diphyllobothrium latum,* the "broad fish tapeworm," and *Spirometra mansonoides,* the "zipper tapeworm."

Chapter 6 details the major true tapeworms and pseudotapeworms that infect domesticated animals.

Tapeworms That Parasitize Domestic Animals and Humans

EUCESTODA (TRUE TAPEWORMS)

Phylum: Platyhelminthes (flatworms)
   Class: Cestoda (tapeworms)
      Subclass: Eucestoda (true tapeworms)

MICE, RATS, GERBILS, AND HAMSTERS
Intestinal Tract

Hymenolepis nana and *Hymenolepis diminuta* parasitize mice, rats, gerbils, and hamsters. These tapeworms are small and slender. Adults of *H. nana* are 1 mm wide and 25 to 40 mm in length, and adults of *H. diminuta* are 3 to 4 mm wide and 20 to 60 mm in length. These true tapeworms reside in the small intestine of the rodent definitive host and are usually detected on postmortem examination of the small intestine. The scolex of *H. nana* has a ring of hooks on its anterior end; it has an armed rostellum (Figure 6-1). The scolex of *H. diminuta* has no hooks; it is unarmed (Figure 6-2).

The life cycle of *H. nana* is a direct life cycle, whereas *H. diminuta* requires an intermediate host for infection. The eggs of *H. nana* are passed in the feces and are swallowed by a host. The hexacanth enters the villus of the small intestine and matures into a nontailed cysticercoid. The cysticercoid returns to the lumen of the small intestine, attaches to the lining, and matures to adulthood. *H. diminuta* also passes its eggs in the feces, which are ingested by an intermediate arthropod host. The **hexacanth embryo** (embryo containing three pairs of hooks) matures into a tailed cysticercoid. The arthropod is ingested by a definitive host, and the cysticercoid attaches to the lining of the small intestine and matures into an adult.

The eggs of *Hymenolepis* species may be detected on fecal flotation. Veterinary technicians should be aware that the eggs of this tapeworm are shed intermittently in the feces. Sometimes, individual proglottids may also be recovered, but these do not float. Figure 6-3 shows stained proglottids of *H. diminuta.* The oval egg of *H. nana* measures 44 to 62 μm by 30 to 55 μm (Figure 6-4). The egg of *H. diminuta* is more spherical and measures 62 to 88 μm by 30 to 55 μm. The embryo within the egg of both species measures 24 to 30 μm by 16 to 25 μm and contains three pairs of hooks

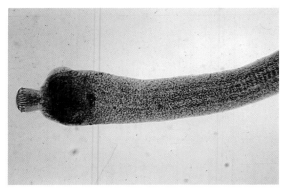

Figure 6-1 Scolex of *Hymenolepis nana*, showing armed rostellum on scolex.

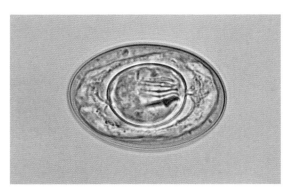

Figure 6-4 Oval egg of *Hymenolepis nana* measures 44 to 62 µm by 30 to 55 µm.

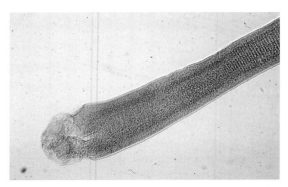

Figure 6-2 Scolex of *Hymenolepis diminuta*, showing unarmed scolex.

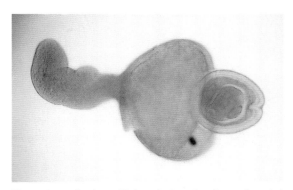

Figure 6-5 Cysticercoid (larval) stage has been dissected from insect intermediate host.

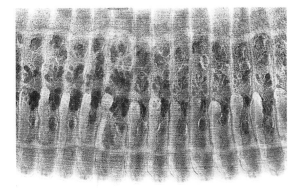

Figure 6-3 Stained proglottids of *Hymenolepis diminuta*.

(hexacanth embryo). Infected animals may be treated with niclosamide or praziquantel.

Both of these tapeworms have zoonotic potential. *H. nana* is unique in that it does not require an intermediate host; therefore it is directly infective to other rodents and to humans. Autoinfection by *H. nana* can occur when its eggs hatch in the small intestine of the host and subsequently infect that host. *H. diminuta* uses an insect (flea, grain beetle, or cockroach) as an intermediate host to complete its life cycle. The cysticercoid develops within the insect intermediate host (Figure 6-5).

RUMINANTS

Intestinal Tract

Moniezia species and *Thysanosoma actinoides* are true tapeworms that infect the intestinal tract of ruminants.

MONIEZIA SPECIES. *Moniezia* species are long (up to 6 m) tapeworms found in the small intestine of cattle, sheep, and goats. *Moniezia* species are large tapeworms and can be up to 1.6 cm at the widest margins (Figure 6-6). The scolex of *Moniezia* is unarmed; it lacks an armed rostellum (Figure 6-7). Individual proglottids are very short and wide. Each proglottid contains two sets of laterally located genital organs and associated pores (Figure 6-8). These tapeworms produce eggs with a characteristic square or triangular shape. The eggs of both species possess a *pyriform* (pear-shaped) *apparatus.* Two species are common among ruminants: *Moniezia benedini* in cattle and *Moniezia expansa* in cattle, sheep, and goats. The eggs of both species can be easily differentiated using standard fecal flotation procedures. The eggs of *M. expansa* are triangular or pyramidal in shape and 56 to 67 μm in diameter. The eggs of *M. benedini* are square or cuboidal in shape and approximately 75 μm in diameter (Figure 6-9). The prepatent period for these tapeworms is approximately 40 days.

The *metacestode,* or larval, stage of *Moniezia* is the cysticercoid stage, which may be found within the intermediate hosts, *oribatid* grain mites. Intact proglottids and eggs are found in the feces of the ruminant definitive host. Mites become infected by ingesting the hexacanth embryo, which develops into the cysticercoid stage within the body of the grain mite. Ruminants become infected by ingesting cysticercoid-infected mites that infest the grain. The cysticercoid is a tiny, microscopic stage and probably will not be observed by the veterinarian (see

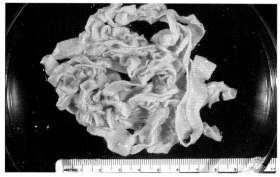

Figure 6-6   *Moniezia* species are large tapeworms. They can grow to 6 m long and up to 1.6 cm at the widest margins.

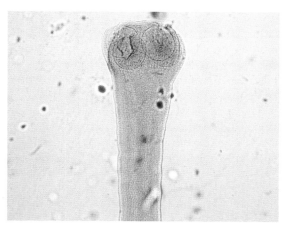

Figure 6-7   Scolex of *Moniezia* is unarmed; it lacks an armed rostellum.

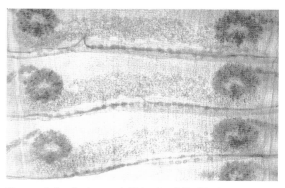

Figure 6-8   Each proglottid of adult *Moniezia* species contains two sets of laterally located genital organs and genital pores.

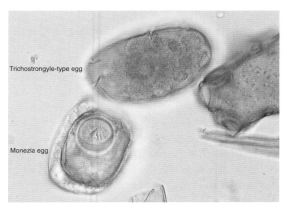
Trichostrongyle-type egg

Monezia egg

Figure 6-9 *Moniezia* species produce eggs with a characteristic square or triangular shape. Two species are common among ruminants, *M. benedini* in cattle and *M. expansa* in cattle, sheep, and goats. Eggs of both species can be easily differentiated using standard fecal flotation procedures. Eggs of *M. expansa* are triangular or pyramidal in shape and 56 to 67 µm in diameter. The eggs of *M. benedini* are square or cuboidal in shape and approximately 75 µm in diameter. Both eggs contain a pyriform apparatus.

Figure 6-5). For every cysticercoid that is ingested by the ruminant, one adult tapeworm will develop in the small intestine of that ruminant (Figure 6-10). It is important that the veterinarian recognize the oribatid mite as the source of this tapeworm and understand the importance of effective tapeworm therapeusis (morantel, niclosamide, albendazole, fenbendazole, or oxfendazole) in cattle. Pasture rotation in addition to therapeusis is essential in greatly reducing the transmission of this parasite.

THYSANOSOMA ACTINOIDES. Thysanosoma actinoides is the fringed tapeworm found in the bile ducts, pancreatic ducts, and small intestine of ruminants (Figure 6-11). The adult tapeworm measures 8 mm by 15 to 30 cm. As with *Moniezia* species, the proglottids are very short; however, these proglottids possess a unique feature: a very prominent fringe located on the posterior aspect of each proglottid. (See Figure 6-12 for the fringed adult *T. actinoides*.)

Eggs of this tapeworm occur in packets of 6 to 12 eggs, with individual eggs measuring 19 by 27 µm. These eggs do not possess a pyriform apparatus.

The metacestode (larval) stage of *T. actinoides* is the cysticercoid stage, which may be found within the proposed intermediate hosts, psocids. *Psocids* are primitive insects often associated with vegetation. These insects become infected by ingesting the hexacanth embryo, which develops into the cysticercoid stage within the body of psocid. Ruminants may become infected by accidentally ingesting cysticercoid-infected psocids that infest vegetation. The cysticercoid is a microscopic stage and probably will not be observed by the veterinarian. For every cysticercoid that is ingested by the ruminant, one adult tapeworm will develop in the small intestine of that ruminant. It is important that the veterinarian recognize psocids as the source of this tapeworm and understand the importance of effective tapeworm therapeusis (niclosamide or praziquantel, as well as pasture rotation) in cattle.

METACESTODE (LARVAL) STAGES FOUND IN MUSCULATURE OF FOOD ANIMALS

Cattle may serve as intermediate hosts for a tapeworm of humans, *Taenia saginata (Taeniarhynchus saginata)*. The larval stage for this tapeworm is a cysticercus, or bladder worm, called *Cysticercus bovis.* This condition in cattle is often referred to as "beef measles" or "measly beef." These infective metacestodes are found in the musculature (skeletal and cardiac muscles) of cattle. Humans become infected with this zoonotic tapeworm by ingesting poorly cooked beef. (See Figure 6-13 for the cysticercus of *C. bovis* within beef muscle.)

Pigs may serve as the intermediate host for a similar tapeworm of humans, *Taenia solium.* The larval stage for this tapeworm is a cysticercus, or bladder worm, known as *Cysticercus cellulosae.* This metacestode stage in pigs is often referred to as "pork measles" or "measly pork." These metacestodes are found in the musculature (skeletal and cardiac muscles) of pigs. Humans become infected with this zoonotic tapeworm by ingesting poorly cooked pork. It is also

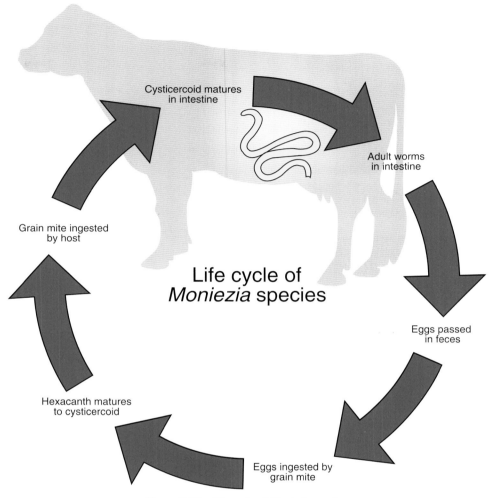

Cysticercoid matures
in intestine

Adult worms
in intestine

Grain mite ingested
by host

Life cycle of
Moniezia species

Eggs passed
in feces

Hexacanth matures
to cysticercoid

Eggs ingested by
grain mite

Figure 6-10   Life cycle of *Moniezia* species.

important to note that if humans ingest the eggs of *T. solium*, the cysticercus can develop within their muscles (Figure 6-14) and within nervous tissue such as the brain, eye, and spinal cord.

The adult stages of the metacestode stages (*C. bovis* and *C. cellulosae*) are found in the small intestine of humans. Because humans may become infected by ingesting poorly cooked beef or pork, these are important zoonotic tapeworms.

METACESTODE (LARVAL) STAGES FOUND IN ABDOMINAL CAVITY OF FOOD ANIMALS

For *Taenia hydatigena,* an adult tapeworm found in the small intestine of dogs, the larval stage is a ping-pong-ball–sized, fluid-filled bladder called *Cysticercus tenuicolis,* which is usually attached to the greater omentum or other abdominal organs of the ruminant intermediate host (Figure 6-15). To acquire this tapeworm,

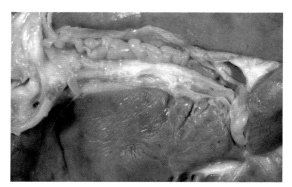

Figure 6-11 *Thysanosoma actinoides,* the fringed tapeworm, is unusual in that it is not found in the intestine (as are most adult tapeworms). Instead, it resides in the bile duct of sheep.

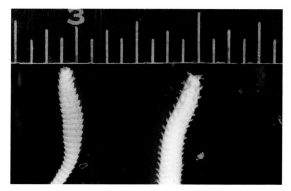

Figure 6-12 Adult *Thysanosoma actinoides* measures 8 mm by 15 to 30 cm. Note that proglottids are very short. They demonstrate a unique morphologic feature, a conspicuous fringe located on posterior aspect of each proglottid, thus the common name, "fringed tapeworm."

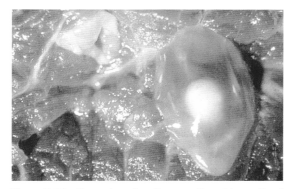

Figure 6-13 Gross view of cysticercus of larval form of beef tapeworm, *Taenia saginata (Cysticercus bovis)* within muscle of a beef cow.

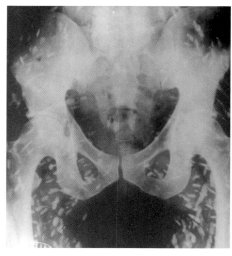

Figure 6-14 Radiographic view of cysticerci of larval form of pork tapeworm, *Taenia solium (Cysticercus cellulosae)* within human muscle.

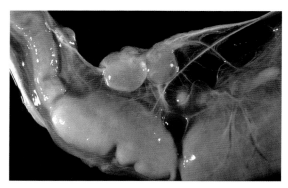

Figure 6-15 Larval stage for *Taenia hydatigena* is a ping-pong-ball–sized, fluid-filled bladder *(Cysticercus tenuicolis)* that is usually attached to greater omentum or other abdominal organs of ruminant intermediate host.

dogs become infected by ingesting the abdominal viscera of cysticercus-infected ruminants. For every cysticercus that is ingested by the dog, one adult tapeworm will develop in the small intestine of that dog. It is important that the veterinarian recognize the ruminant as the source of this tapeworm and understand the importance of preventing predation or ingestion of ruminant offal by the dog.

HORSES

Intestinal Tract

Anoplocephala perfoliata, Anoplocephala magna, and *Paranoplocephala mamillana* are the equine tapeworms. *A. perfoliata* is found in the small and large intestine and cecum; *A. magna* and *P. mamillana* are found in the small intestine and occasionally the stomach. *A. perfoliata* can measure from 5 to 8 cm in length and up to 1.2 cm in width. The scolex is oblong, 2 to 3 mm in diameter, with very prominent *lappets* behind each of the four suckers. The proglottids are wider than long, and each proglottid has only one set of male and female reproductive organs (Figure 6-16). *A. magna* can measure up to 80 cm in length and 2.5 cm in width. The scolex is large and oblong, 4 to 6 mm in diameter, but lacking the lappets of *A. perfoliata* (Figure 6-17). *P. mamillana,* also known as the dwarf tapeworm, is only 6 to

50 mm in length and 4 to 6 mm in width (Figure 6-18). The scolex is quite narrow.

The eggs of *A. perfoliata* are thick walled, with one or more flattened sides measuring 65 to 80 μm in diameter; those of *A. magna* are similar but slightly smaller, measuring 50 to 60 μm. The eggs of *P. mamillana* are oval and thin walled, measuring 51 by 37 μm. Eggs of all three species have a three-layered eggshell; the innermost lining is a pyriform apparatus. The hexacanth embryo can be visualized just inside the pyriform apparatus (Figure 6-19). Eggs of all equine tapeworms can be recovered using standard fecal flotation. The prepatent period for all three species ranges from 28 to 42 days.

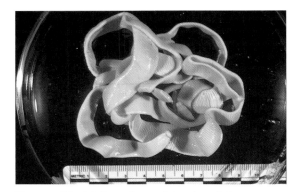

Figure 6-17 Adult specimen of *Anoplocephala magna,* an equine tapeworm. Scolex is quite large, 4 to 6 mm in diameter, and lacks prominent lappets.

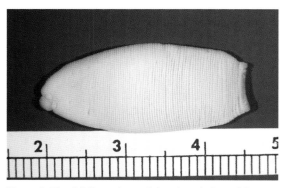

Figure 6-16 Adult specimen of *Anoplocephala perfoliata,* an equine tapeworm. Scolex is oblong, 2 to 3 mm in diameter, and has very prominent lappets behind each of four suckers. Proglottids are wider than long, and each has only one set of male and female reproductive organs.

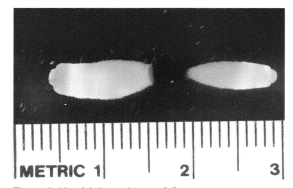

Figure 6-18 Adult specimens of *Paranoplocephala mamillana,* the dwarf equine tapeworm. Scolex is quite narrow and lacks prominent lappets.

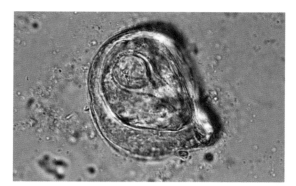

Figure 6-19 Fecal flotation revealing egg of *Anoplocephala perfoliata*. Egg is thick walled, with one or more flattened sides measuring 65 to 80 μm in diameter; those of *A. magna* are similar but slightly smaller, measuring 50 to 60 μm. Eggs have an innermost lining called the pyriform (pear-shaped) apparatus.

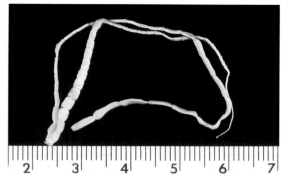

Figure 6-20 Adult specimen of *Dipylidium caninum*, the "double-pored" or "cucumber seed" tapeworm of dogs and cats. Adult tapeworm can grow to 50 cm long. This tapeworm usually demonstrates its presence by release of and appearance of motile, terminal, gravid proglottids, which are usually found on feces, hair coat, or bedding. In fresh state, proglottids resemble cucumber seeds, thus the common name, "cucumber seed" tapeworm.

As in *Moniezia* species in ruminants, the metacestode (larval) stage of equine tapeworms is the cysticercoid stage, which may be found within the intermediate hosts, oribatid grain mites. Intact proglottids and eggs are found in the feces of the equine definitive host. Mites become infected by ingesting the hexacanth embryo, which develops into the cysticercoid stage within the body of the grain mites. Horses become infected by ingesting cysticercoid-infected mites infesting the grain. The cysticercoid is a microscopic stage and probably will not be observed by the veterinarian. For every cysticercoid that is ingested by the ruminant, one adult tapeworm will develop in the small intestine of that ruminant (see Figure 6-10). It is important that the veterinarian recognize the oribatid mite as the source of this tapeworm and understand the importance of pasture rotation and effective tapeworm therapeusis (pyrantel pamoate and pyrantel tartrate; praziquantel has been used with success but is not FDA approved) in horses.

TRUE TAPEWORMS OF DOGS AND CATS

Tapeworms that infect dogs and cats are *Dipylidium caninum, Taenia pisiformis, T. hydatigena, T. ovis, T. taeniaeformis, Multiceps multiceps,*

M. serialis, Echinococcus granulosus, E. multilocularis, and *Mesocestoides* species.

Dipylidium caninum

Dipylidium caninum is often called the "double-pored" or "cucumber seed" tapeworm. This tapeworm is the most common tapeworm found in the small intestine of the dog and cat, because the dog or cat becomes infected by ingesting the flea intermediate host. Fleas often contain this parasite's infective cysticercoid stage. The adult tapeworm can grow to a length of 50 cm (Figure 6-20). The scolex of this tapeworm is armed and consists of a prominent proboscis covered with rearward-facing rose-thorn–like hooks (Figure 6-21). This tapeworm usually demonstrates its presence by the release of and the appearance of its motile, terminal, gravid proglottids, which are usually found on the feces (Figure 6-22). They may also be found on the pet's hair coat or in the bedding of the host. In the fresh state, these proglottids resemble cucumber seeds ("cucumber seed" tapeworm). These proglottids have a lateral pore located along the midpoint of each of their long edges ("double-pored" tapeworm)

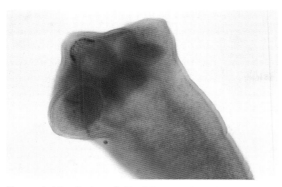

Figure 6-21   Scolex of *Dipylidium caninum* is armed and consists of prominent proboscis covered with rearward-facing rose-thorn–like hooks.

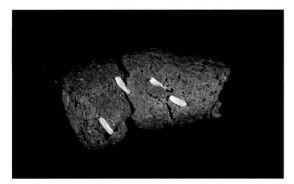

Figure 6-22   *Dipylidium caninum* usually demonstrates its presence by release of and appearance of motile, terminal, gravid proglottids, which are usually found on feces.

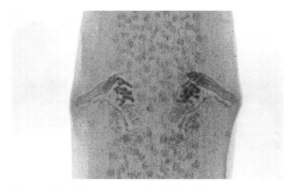

Figure 6-23   These proglottids of *Dipylidium caninum* have a lateral pore along midpoint of each long edge, thus the second common name, "double-pored" tapeworm.

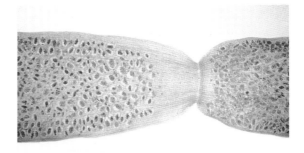

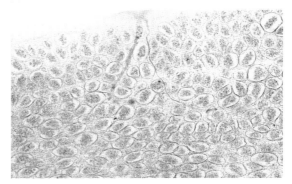

Figure 6-24   Gravid proglottids of *Dipylidium caninum* are filled with thousands of egg packets.

(Figure 6-23). Gravid proglottids contain thousands of unique egg packets, each containing 20 to 30 hexacanth embryos (Figure 6-24). (See Figure 6-25 for individual egg packet of *D. caninum* containing hexacanth embryos.) The proglottids of *D. caninum* often dry out in the external environment. As they lose moisture, they shrivel up, resembling uncooked grains of rice (Figure 6-26). If reconstituted with water, the dried proglottids usually assume their former cucumber seed appearance. The prepatent period for *D. caninum* is 14 to 21 days.

The metacestode (larval) stage of this tapeworm is the cysticercoid stage, which may be found within the flea intermediate host. Larval fleas become infected by ingesting the hexacanth embryo, which develops into the cysticercoid stage within the body of the adult flea. Dogs and cats become infected by ingesting cysticercoid-

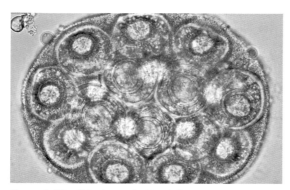

Figure 6-25 If fresh proglottids of *Dipylidium caninum* are teased or broken open, they may reveal thousands of egg packets, each containing 20 to 30 hexacanth embryos.

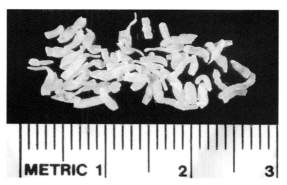

Figure 6-26 Dried proglottids of *Dipylidium caninum* resemble uncooked grains of rice. When water is added, they assume their natural state.

infected adult fleas (Figure 6-27). The cysticercoid is a microscopic stage and probably will not be observed by the veterinarian. For every cysticercoid that is ingested by the dog or cat, one adult tapeworm will develop in the small intestine of that dog or cat. If a human (e.g., child) ingests a flea containing the cysticercoid stage, this tapeworm will develop to the adult stage within the small intestine. It is a zoonotic parasite.

This tapeworm is typically diagnosed in one of two ways. The egg packets can be found on fecal flotation (see Figure 6-24) if the gravid proglottids dry up and release the egg packets. The gravid proglottids may also be seen by the client in the feces, on bedding, or in the hair coat. It is important that the veterinarian recognize the flea as the source of this tapeworm and understand the importance of flea control in effective tapeworm therapeusis. *Dipylidium caninum* is typically treated with a single dose of praziquantel or epsiprantel.

Taenia pisiformis, T. hydatigena, and T. ovis

Taenia pisiformis, T. hydatigena, and *T. ovis* are the canine taeniids. The canine taeniids measure from 1 to 2 cm *(T. ovis),* to 200 cm *(T. pisiformis),* and up to 75 to 500 cm *(T. hydatigena)* in length. These adult taeniids are found within the small intestine of the canine definitive host (Figure 6-28). The scolex of all these tapeworms is armed, consisting of two rows of rostellar hooks (Figure 6-29). As with *D. caninum,* the *Taenia* species manifest by the appearance of motile, terminal, gravid proglottids on the feces, on the pet's hair coat, or in the bedding of the host. In the fresh state, these proglottids have a single lateral pore located along the midpoint of either of their long edges (unlike the double-pored tapeworm) (Figure 6-30).

As with *D. caninum,* if the fresh proglottids are teased or broken open, they may reveal typical hexacanth embryos (Figure 6-31). These hexacanth embryos have a striated eggshell (called the *embryophore*) and contain six hooks (or teeth) within the interior of the egg. This egg is referred to as a *typical taeniid type of egg.* The proglottids of *Taenia* species also dry out in the external environment and resemble uncooked grains of rice. If reconstituted with water, they usually assume their former single-pored appearance. If gravid proglottids of *Taenia* species are recovered from a dog's or cat's feces, the proglottid should be torn open or macerated in a drop of saline solution on a glass slide to reveal the characteristic eggs under the compound microscope.

The eggs of the taeniid tapeworms are slightly oval and are 43 to 53 μm by 43 to 49 μm in diameter *(T. pisiformis),* 36 to 39 μm by 31 to 35 μm in diameter *(T. hydatigena),* and 19 to 31 μm by 24 to 26 μm *(T. ovis).* Eggs of *Taenia*

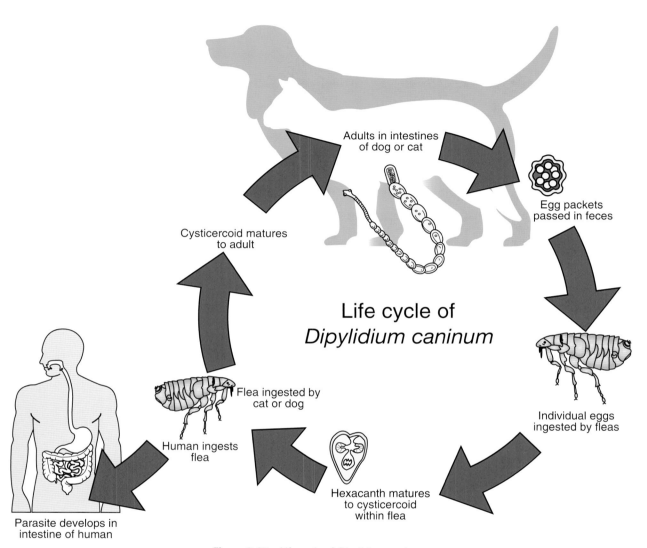

Figure 6-27 Life cycle of *Dipylidium caninum.*

species contain a single **oncosphere** with three pairs of hooks. The oncosphere is often called a "hexacanth embryo." The eggs of the taeniids are very similar to those of *Echinococcus* and *Multiceps* species.

The metacestode (larval) stage for *T. pisiformis, T. hydatigena,* and *T. ovis* is the cysticercus, or bladder worm, stage, which may be found within the respective rabbit, ruminant, or ovine intermediate hosts.

For *T. pisiformis* and *T. hydatigena,* the rabbit and the ruminant become infected by ingesting the taeniid eggs or hexacanth embryos, often found close to canine feces. These embryos hatch and develop into the cysticercus stage within the peritoneal cavity of the intermediate hosts. For *T. pisiformis,* the larval stage is a pea-sized, fluid-filled bladder (called *Cysticercus pisiformis*), usually attached to the greater omentum or other abdominal organs of the rabbit (Figure 6-32).

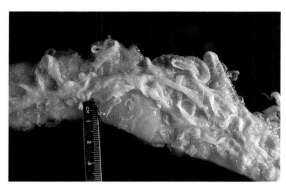

Figure 6-28 Adult canine taeniids are found in small intestine of canine definitive host.

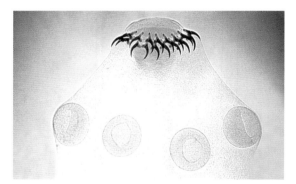

Figure 6-29 Details of scolex of canine taeniid. Note four suckers and armed rostellum.

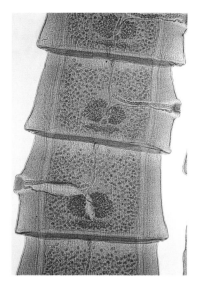

Figure 6-30 Mature proglottids of *Taenia* species demonstrating single lateral pore located along midpoint of long edges (as opposed to the double-pored tapeworm).

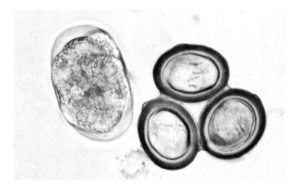

Figure 6-31 Typical taeniid egg with striated shell and six inner hooks. Because of the hooks, this egg is referred to as a **hexacanth** or **six-toothed** embryo. Egg is characteristic for tapeworms of genera *Taenia*, *Multiceps*, and *Echinococcus*.

Dogs become infected by killing and ingesting cysticercus-infected rabbits. For every cysticercus that is ingested by the dog, one adult tapeworm will develop in the small intestine of that dog (Figure 6-33). It is important that the veterinarian recognize the rabbit as the source of this tapeworm and understand the importance of preventing predation or the ingestion of rabbit carrion by the dog. *T. pisiformis* can be treated with praziquantel or epsiprantel.

For *T. hydatigena,* the larval stage is a ping-pong-ball–sized, fluid-filled bladder (called *Cysticercus tenicollis*), usually attached to the greater omentum or other abdominal organs of the ruminant intermediate host (Figure 6-34; see also Figure 6-15). To acquire this tapeworm, dogs become infected by ingesting the abdominal viscera of cysticercus-infected ruminants (see Figure 6-33). For every cysticercus that is ingested by the dog, one adult tapeworm will develop in the small intestine of that dog. It is important that the veterinarian recognize the ruminant as the source of this tapeworm and understand the importance of preventing preda-

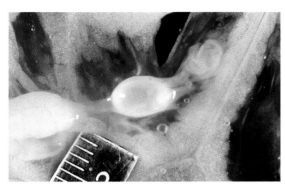

Figure 6-32   Larval stage for *Taenia pisiformis* is pea-sized, fluid-filled bladder *(Cysticercus pisiformis)*. Larval stage is usually attached to greater omentum or other abdominal organs of rabbit intermediate host.

tion or ingestion of ruminant offal by the dog.

For *T. ovis*, the larval stage is a fluid-filled bladder (called *Cysticercus ovis*) found within the musculature of the ovine intermediate host (very similar to the cysticerci of *Cysticercus bovis* and *C. cellulosae* described earlier) (see Figure 6-13). To acquire this tapeworm, dogs become infected by ingesting the musculature of cysticercus-infected sheep (see Figure 6-33). For every cysticercus that is ingested by the dog, one adult tapeworm will develop in the small intestine of that dog. It is important that the veterinarian recognize sheep muscle (uncooked mutton) as the source of this tapeworm and understand the importance of preventing predation and ingestion of sheep muscle by dogs.

Taenia taeniaeformis (Hydatigera taeniaeformis)

Taenia taeniaeformis, or *Hydatigera taeniaeformis*, is called the **feline tapeworm** or the **feline taeniid.** This tapeworm, which may be up to 60 cm in length, is observed infrequently in cats allowed to roam and prey on rabbits and rodents. The scolex is similar to that of the canine taeniids, as are the proglottids; however, in the fresh or intact state the terminal proglottids of *T. taeniaeformis* are said to be bell shaped. The egg of this tapeworm is 31 to 36 μm in diameter and contains a single oncosphere with three pairs of hooks. For this reason, the oncosphere is often called a "hexacanth" (or "six-toothed") embryo. As with the eggs of the canine taeniids, the egg is very similar to that of *Echinococcus* species. (See Figure 6-31 for unique features of this taeniid type of tapeworm egg.)

The metacestode (larval) stage for *T. taeniaeformis* is the **strobilocercus,** a morphologic variation of the cysticercus (bladder worm) stage. For *T. taeniaeformis* to develop, the rodent intermediate host becomes infected by ingesting the taeniid eggs, or hexacanth embryos, often found in proximity to feline feces. These embryos hatch and develop into the cysticercus stage within the liver of the intermediate host. For the first 42 days in this location, it develops as a cysticercus. On day 42, however, the cysticercus changes its form into that of a strobilocercus. For *T. taeniaeformis*, the strobilocercus is a scolex attached to a long neck, which connects to a bladder; this stage has a scientific name, *Cysticercus fasciolaris* (Figures 6-35, 6-36, and 6-37). The cat becomes infected by killing the rat and ingesting the strobilocercus. The neck and its connected bladder are digested, the scolex attaches, and the tapeworm begins to grow in the cat's intestine (see Figure 6-33). For every strobilocercus that is ingested by the cat, one adult tapeworm will develop in the small intestine of that cat. It is important that the veterinarian recognize the rat as the source of this tapeworm and understand the importance of preventing predation or the ingestion of rat or mouse carrion by the cat. The cat can be treated with praziquantel.

Multiceps multiceps and Multiceps serialis

Multiceps multiceps and *M. serialis* are also taeniid tapeworms of the small intestine of canids. The adults of *M. multiceps* are 40 to 100 cm in length; those of *M. serialis* can grow up to 72 cm. Both possess a scolex with a double row of rostellar hooks.

The eggs of *M. multiceps* are 29 to 37 μm in diameter, and those of *M. serialis* are elliptic and measure 31 to 34 by 29 to 30 μm. Both contain a

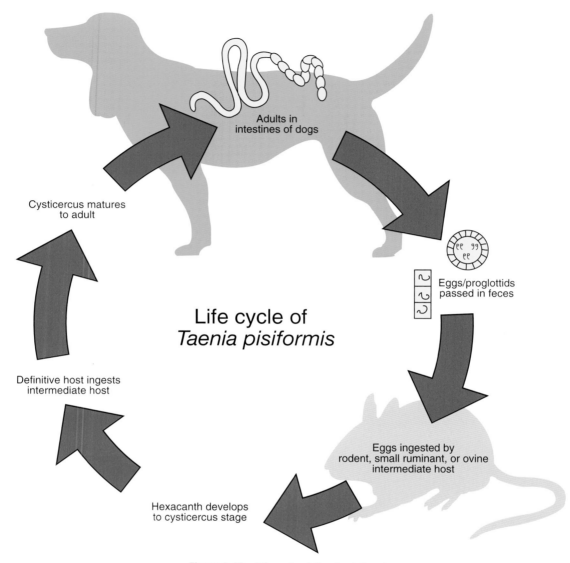

Figure 6-33 Life cycle of *Taenia pisiformis.*

single oncosphere with three pairs of hooks. As with the eggs of the canine and feline taeniids, the eggs of *Multiceps* species are very similar to those of *Taenia* and *Echinococcus* species. (See Figure 6-31 for unique features of this taeniid type of tapeworm.)

The metacestode (larval) stage for *M. multiceps* and *M. serialis* is the **coenurus** stage, which

may be found within the respective ovine or rabbit intermediate host. This coenurus also has a scientific name: *Coenurus cerebralis* for *M. multiceps* and *Coenurus serialis* for *M. serialis*. It is essentially a single, large bladder with several invaginated scolices attached to its inner wall. The coenurus is found within the tissues of the respective intermediate host. For each coenurus

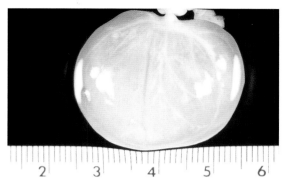

Figure 6-34   Larval stage for *Taenia hydatigena* is a ping-pong-ball–sized, fluid-filled bladder *(Cysticercus tenuicollis)*, usually attached to greater omentum or other abdominal organs of ruminant intermediate host.

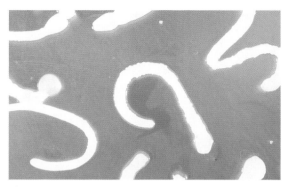

Figure 6-37   Detail of individual strobilocercus, *Cysticercus fasciolaris.*

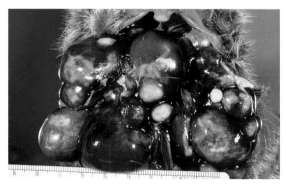

Figure 6-35   Larval stage for *Taenia taeniaeformis* is a strobilocercus *(Cysticercus fasciolaris)*. The strobilocercus is a scolex attached to a long neck, which connects to a bladder.

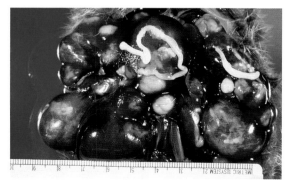

Figure 6-36   The strobilocercus is found in the liver of a rodent intermediate host.

that is ingested by the dog, several adult tapeworms will develop, one for each invaginated scolex ingested.

For *M. multiceps,* the sheep intermediate host becomes infected by ingesting taeniid eggs, or hexacanth embryos, which are often found close to canine feces. These embryos hatch and migrate to neurologic tissue (either brain or spinal cord tissue), where they develop into the coenurus stage within the tissue hosts. Naturally, the presence of these large, space-occupying lesions within the brain and spinal cord can produce neurologic signs in the infected sheep. The larval stage of *M. multiceps* may be up to 5 cm in diameter and is a fluid-filled bladder (called *C. cerebralis)* with many individual scolices lining the walls of the bladder. Dogs become infected either by killing the sheep and ingesting coenurus-infected neural tissue or by being fed such tissues by their sheepherder owners. For every coenurus that is ingested by the dog, many adult tapeworms will develop in the small intestine of that dog. It is important that the veterinarian recognize the sheep as the source of this tapeworm and understand the importance of preventing predation or the ingestion of sheep carrion or offal by the dog.

For *M. serialis,* the rabbit intermediate host becomes infected by ingesting the taeniid eggs or hexacanth embryos often found in proximity to

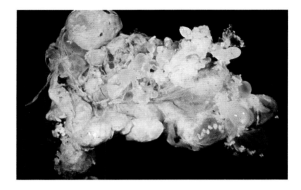

A

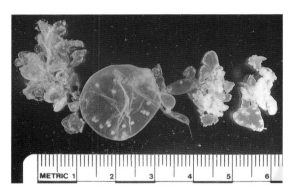

B

Figure 6-38 **A,** *Coenurus serialis* from subcutaneous connective tissues of a rabbit. **B,** Note individual invaginated scolices lining walls of bladder.

canine feces. These embryos hatch and migrate to the rabbit's subcutaneous tissues, where they develop into the coenurus stage. The presence of these large, bladderlike cysts within the subcutaneous tissues of the rabbit can interfere with movement and speed, making the rabbit easy prey. For *M. serialis,* the larval stage may be up to 4 cm in diameter and is a fluid-filled bladder (called *C. serialis*) (Figure 6-38) with many individual invaginated scolices lining the walls of the bladder. Dogs become infected either by killing the slow-moving rabbit and ingesting coenurus-infected subcutaneous tissues or by being fed such tissues by their rabbit-hunting owners. For every coenurus that is ingested by the dog, many

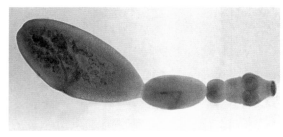

Figure 6-39 Adult *Echinococcus* species is a tiny tapeworm, only 1.2 to 7 mm in length. Entire tapeworm has only three proglottids: immature, mature, and gravid.

adult tapeworms will develop in the small intestine of that dog. It is important that the veterinarian recognize the rabbit as the source of this tapeworm and understand the importance of preventing predation or the ingestion of rabbit carrion or offal by the dog.

Echinococcus granulosus and *Echinococcus multilocularis*

Echinococcus granulosus and *E. multilocularis* are the hydatid disease tapeworms associated with unilocular and multilocular hydatid disease. *E. granulosus* is the hydatid cyst tapeworm of dogs, and *E. multilocularis* is the hydatid cyst tapeworm of cats. These are important parasites because of their extreme zoonotic potential.

The adult *Echinococcus* is a tiny tapeworm, only 1.2 to 7 mm in length. The entire tapeworm has only three proglottids: immature, mature, and gravid (Figure 6-39). When passed, the tiny gravid proglottids likely will be overlooked by the client, the veterinary technician, and the veterinarian. Definitive diagnosis of *Echinococcus* species infection is best achieved by identifying adult tapeworms taken from the host's intestinal tract. In the rare instances in which *Echinococcus* species infection is suspected, antemortem diagnosis is accomplished by purging the dog or cat using arecoline hydrobromide, 3.5 mg/kg body weight, and collecting its feces.*

---

*For source, contact the Centers for Disease Control and Prevention (CDC), Atlanta, GA.

This procedure is usually only performed when infection is strongly suspected. Entire worms or their proglottids may be collected from the final clear mucus. Because of serious zoonotic potential, all evacuated material should be handled with caution. After the feces have been examined, the evacuate should be incinerated. Rubber gloves should be worn when handling feces.

The egg of *E. granulosus* is ovoid, 32 to 36 μm by 25 to 30 μm, and contains a single oncosphere with three pairs of hooks. The egg of *E. multilocularis* is ovoid, 30 to 40 μm, and contains a single oncosphere with three pairs of hooks. Because of serious zoonotic potential (see Chapter 16), any "suspect" eggs of *Echinococcus* species should be handled with extreme caution. These eggs are very similar in appearance to those of *Taenia* and *Multiceps* species. (See Figure 6-31 for unique features of this taeniid type of tapeworm.)

The metacestode (larval) stage for *E. granulosus* and *E. multilocularis* is the **hydatid cyst** stage, which may be found within the respective ruminant or rodent intermediate host. The hydatid cyst for *E. granulosus* is a unilocular hydatid cyst found within the liver, lung, and other organs of the ruminant intermediate host. The hydatid cyst for *E. multilocularis* is a multilocular hydatid cyst found within the liver of the rodent intermediate host. Humans may also serve as an intermediate host for both these tapeworms. Humans become infected by ingesting eggs of these tapeworm species.

The unilocular (single-compartment) hydatid cyst of *E. granulosus* has a thick cyst wall, with a thin germinal membrane located just inside it. Brood capsules containing protoscolices "bud" from this germinal membrane. When a dog ingests the hydatid cyst containing the brood capsules and protoscolices, each protoscolex develops into an adult tapeworm (Figure 6-40).

The multilocular (multicompartment) hydatid cyst of *E. multilocularis* lacks the thick cyst wall of the unilocular hydatid cyst. It is often described as being "alveolar" or similar to a "bunch of grapes." Without the wall, the cyst is very invasive, often replacing normal tissue, similar to a malignant cancer. It also possesses a

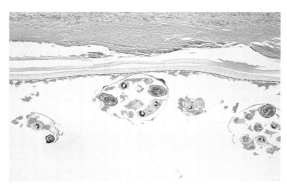

Figure 6-40 Photomicrograph of a unilocular hydatid cyst of *Echinococcus granulosus* has a thick, multilayered wall and a thin, granular germinal membrane. Spherical brood capsules containing protoscolices arise from the germinal membrane.

thin germinal membrane. Brood capsules containing protoscolices bud from the germinal membrane. When a cat ingests the hydatid cyst containing the brood capsules and protoscolices, each protoscolex develops into an adult tapeworm in the intestine of the cat.

Praziquantel can be used to treat adult *Echinococcus* worms but will not affect the hydatid cyst stage. The best treatment for the hydatid cyst stage of the parasites is preventing ingestion of the eggs.

Mesocestoides Species

Mesocestoides species may parasitize the small intestine of carnivores, including the dog and the cat. These are small- to medium-sized true tapeworms, ranging from 12 cm to more than 2 m in length (Figure 6-41). The scolex of this tapeworm is oblong, with four suckers, and is unarmed (Figure 6-42). Gravid proglottids of *Mesocestoides* have a unique appearance (Figure 6-43). The eggs of *Mesocestoides* species contain a single oncosphere (hexacanth embryo) with three pairs of hooks. (See Figure 6-44 for features of this egg.).

Mesocestoides is an unusual genus among the true tapeworms in that it is the only one that uses two intermediate hosts. (The pseudotapeworms described in the next section use two intermediate hosts.) The egg is a hexacanth embryo. If it is

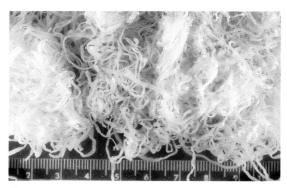

Figure 6-41 Adult *Mesocestoides* species are medium-sized tapeworms, ranging from 12 cm to over 2 m long.

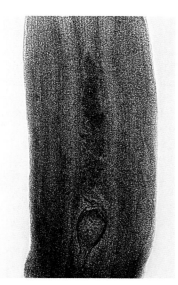

Figure 6-43 Gravid proglottids of *Mesocestoides* have a unique appearance.

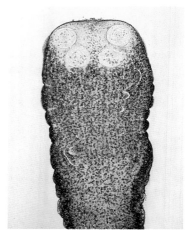

Figure 6-42 Scolex of *Mesocestoides* species is oblong, has four suckers, and is unarmed.

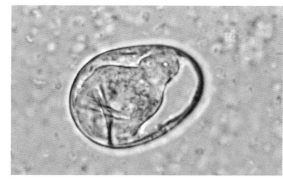

Figure 6-44 Eggs of *Mesocestoides* species contain a single oncosphere with three pairs of hooks. The oncosphere is often called a "hexacanth embryo."

ingested by an oribatid mite, it develops into a cysticercoid within that mite (much like the cysticercoid of *Dipylidium, Moniezia, Thysanosoma,* and *Anoplocephala* species). If this cysticercoid-containing mite is ingested by a mouse or reptile, the cysticercoid develops into a ***tetrathyridium,*** a solid-bodied metacestode stage with a deeply invaginated, acetabular scolex (Figure 6-45). This tetrathyridium is approximately 1 cm in diameter and is capable of multiplying exponentially; that is, one tetrathyridium becomes two, two become four, four become eight, and so on

(Figures 6-46 and 6-47). This type of asexual reproduction produces large numbers of tetrathyridia that are infective to the canine or feline definitive host. The tetrathyridia multiply in the body of the second intermediate host and are often confined to the serous cavities, particularly the peritoneal cavity (Figure 6-48), and other internal organs, such as the liver (Figures 6-49 and 6-50). Tetrathyridia often multiply so

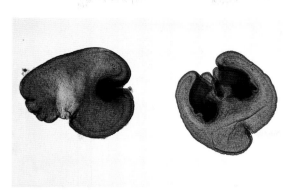

Figure 6-45   Metacestode stage for *Mesocestoides* species is a tetrathyridium, a solid-bodied metacestode stage with a deeply invaginated, acetabular scolex.

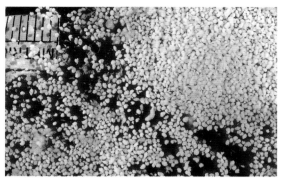

Figure 6-47   This type of asexual reproduction produces large numbers of tetrathyridia that are infective to canine or feline definitive host.

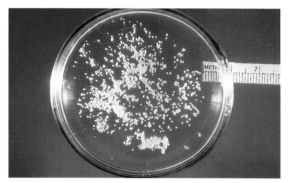

Figure 6-46   Tetrathyridium is about 1 cm in diameter and is capable of multiplying exponentially (i.e., one tetrathyridium becomes two, two become four, four become eight).

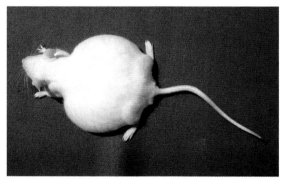

Figure 6-48   Tetrathyridia multiply in body of second intermediate host and are often confined to serous cavities, particularly peritoneal cavity.

much within the abdominal cavity that they greatly expand the girth of the intermediate host. When ingested by the definitive host, each tetrathyridium becomes an adult tapeworm within the intestine of that definitive host.

COTYLODA (PSEUDOTAPEWORMS)

Phylum: Platyhelminthes
  Class: Cestoda
    Subclass: Cotyloda
Members of the subclass Cotyloda, or pseudo-tapeworms, grossly resemble the members of the

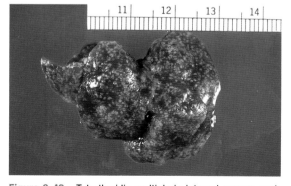

Figure 6-49   Tetrathyridia multiply in internal organs, such as the liver.

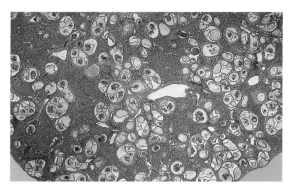

Figure 6-50   Histopathology of liver of rat infected with tetrathyridia.

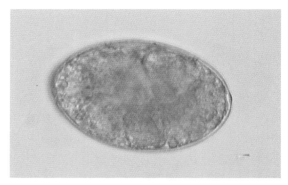

Figure 6-52   Operculated egg of pseudotapeworm is almost identical to egg of digenetic trematodes. Most pseudotapeworms release eggs directly from the uterus; eggs then pass out to external environment in feces of definitive host.

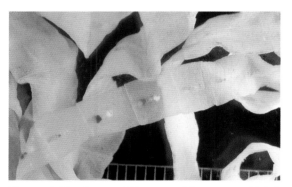

Figure 6-51   Representative pseudotapeworm *(Diphyllobothrium latum)*, with centrally located reproductive organs and genital pores.

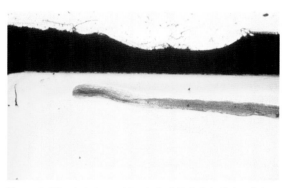

Figure 6-53   Anterior end (scolex) of *Diphyllobothrium latum.*

subclass Eucestoda. These flatworms are ribbonlike and divided into a long chain of proglottids. These are hermaphroditic tapeworms, but instead of possessing laterally located reproductive organs and genital pores, they have centrally located reproductive organs and genital pores (Figure 6-51). The egg for members of this subclass is operculated (Figure 6-52) and almost identical to the egg of the digenetic trematodes. Most pseudotapeworms release their operculated eggs directly from the uterus; the eggs then pass out to the external environment in the feces of the definitive host. The adult tapeworms occasionally release chains of gravid proglottids when these terminal proglottids have become

aged or spent. Instead of possessing four suckers and (possibly) a rostellum, the pseudotapeworm has two slitlike organs of attachment (known as **bothria**) on the lateral aspects of the scolex. Figure 6-53 shows the scolex of *Diphyllobothrium latum.*

During its life cycle, the pseudotapeworm uses two intermediate hosts. The pseudophyllidian-type operculated egg makes contact with water and releases a ciliated, hexacanth embryo. This stage is called a **coracidium.** The coracidium is ingested by a microscopic aquatic crustacean and, within that crustacean, develops into a stage called a *procercoid.* The crustacean, with the procercoid, is later ingested by a fish or an amphibian and, within the musculature of that host, develops into a solid-bodied metacestode stage called a *plerocercoid,* or *sparganum.* The definitive host becomes infected by ingesting the second intermediate host with this plerocercoid (sparganum) stage. The scolex attaches in the small intestine and begins to "grow" a new tapeworm.

The important pseudotapeworms of animals are *Spirometra* species and *Diphyllobothrium* species.

SPIROMETRA SPECIES

Spirometra species are often referred to as "zipper" or "sparganosis" tapeworms. These medium-sized tapeworms are often found in the small intestine of both the dog and the cat and are often found in pets residing in Florida and along the Gulf Coast of North America. This tapeworm is a clinical oddity because it produces an operculated egg. Each proglottid of *Spirometra* species possesses a centrally located, spiraled uterus and an associated uterine pore through which eggs are released. These tapeworms characteristically release eggs until they exhaust their uterine contents. Gravid segments are usually not discharged into the pet's feces. The tapeworm is unique because while it is attached to the host's jejunum, the mature proglottids often separate along the longitudinal axis for a short distance. The tapeworm appears to "unzip," thus its common name, the "zipper tapeworm." Spent "zipped" and "unzipped" proglottids often appear in the feces of the pet. (See Figure 6-54 for unique features of this pseudotapeworm.)

The egg of *Spirometra* species resembles that of a fluke (digenetic trematode). The egg has a distinct operculum at one end of the pole of the shell. The eggs are oval and yellowish brown. They average 60 by 36 µm, have an asymmetric appearance, and tend to be rather pointed at one end (Figure 6-55). When the eggs rupture, a distinct operculum is visible. The eggs are unembryonated when passed in the feces.

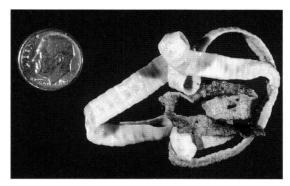

Figure 6-54 Adult *Spirometra* species with centrally located, spiraled uterus and uterine pore through which eggs are released. Gravid segments usually are not discharged into feces. This tapeworm is unique because while attached to host's jejunum, mature proglottids often separate along longitudinal axis for a short distance. Tapeworm appears to "unzip," thus its common name, "zipper tapeworm."

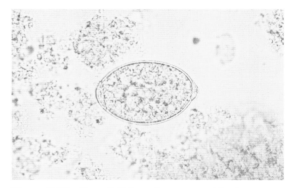

Figure 6-55 Egg of *Spirometra mansonoides* is operculated, resembling egg of a fluke (digenetic trematode).

The metacestode (larval) stage for *Spirometra* species is the sparganum, a solid-bodied stage with slitlike mouthparts. This stage is found in the musculature of its intermediate hosts, fish and amphibians such as frogs. Dogs and cats become infected by ingesting the fish and amphibian intermediate hosts. It is important that the veterinarian recognize the fish and the amphibian as the sources of this tapeworm and understand the importance of preventing

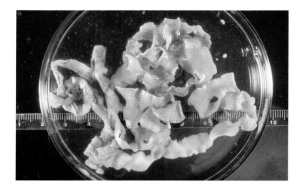

A

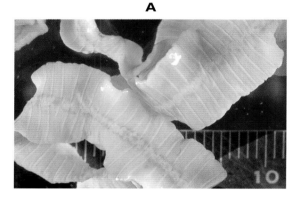

B

Figure 6-56 **A,** Adult *Diphyllobothrium* species can measure 2 to 12 m long, although this tapeworm probably does not attain maximum length in dogs and cats. **B,** Each proglottid has a centrally located, rosette-shaped uterus and an associated uterine pore through which eggs are released.

predation or the ingestion of carrion or offal by the dog and cat.

DIPHYLLOBOTHRIUM SPECIES

Diphyllobothrium species are often referred to as "broad fish tapeworms." This tapeworm can be 2 to 12 m in length; however, it probably does not attain this maximum length in dogs and cats. Each proglottid of this tapeworm has a centrally located, rosette-shaped uterus and an associated

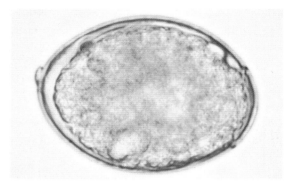

Figure 6-57 Egg of *Diphyllobothrium* species also resembles that of a fluke (digenetic trematode). Egg is oval, with distinct operculum at opposite end of pole of shell. Eggs are light brown and average 67 to 71 μm by 40 to 51 μm. Eggs tend to be rounded on one end, with operculum on opposite end. Eggs are unembryonated when passed in feces.

uterine pore through which the eggs are released (Figure 6-56). These tapeworms continually release eggs until they exhaust their uterine contents. The terminal proglottids become senile rather than gravid and detach in chains rather than individually. The egg of *Diphyllobothrium* species also resembles that of a fluke (digenetic trematode). The egg is oval and possesses a distinct operculum at one end of the pole of the shell. The eggs are light brown, averaging 67 to 71 μm by 40 to 51 μm, and tend to be rounded on one end (Figure 6-57). The operculum is present on the end opposite the rounded pole. The eggs are unembryonated when passed in the feces.

The metacestode (larval) stage for *Diphyllobothrium* species is the plerocercoid, a solid-bodied stage with slitlike mouthparts. This stage is found in the musculature of the fish intermediate host. Dogs and cats become infected by ingesting the fish intermediate host. It is important that the veterinarian recognize the fish as the source of this tapeworm and understand the importance of preventing predation or the ingestion of raw fish by the dog and cat.

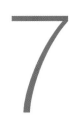

The Phylum Platyhelminthes, Class Trematoda

The phylum Platyhelminthes, the flatworms, includes two of the strangest classes in the animal kingdom, the *trematodes* (or flukes) and the *cestodes* (or tapeworms). The morphologic feature common to these two classes is that the worms are dorsoventrally flattened.

Members of the phylum Platyhelminthes, class Trematoda, are often referred to as trematodes or "flukes." Their bodies are often flattened, unsegmented, and leaflike. An example of a typical fluke is *Fasciola hepatica* (Figure 7-1). Within this class are two subclasses, the subclass Monogenea (the monogenetic trematodes) and the class Digenea (the digenetic trematodes). Monogenetic trematodes usually parasitize fish, amphibians, and reptiles, whereas digenetic trematodes are usually associated with wild and domestic animals and humans.

SUBCLASS MONOGENEA

Phylum: Platyhelminthes
    Class: Trematoda
        Subclass: Monogenea

Monogenetic trematodes are usually ectoparasites of fish, amphibians, and reptiles. They attach to the exterior surfaces, such as gills, skin, fins, and the mouth. These trematodes attach to the host with a posterior adhesive organ that may have suckers, hooks, or clamps (Figure 7-2). These parasites are usually diagnosed in veterinary practices that specialize in treating saltwater or freshwater aquarium fish or in aquacultural environments (e.g., fish farming). Because monogenetic trematodes are diagnosed so infrequently in veterinary practice, the emphasis in this chapter (and the text) is on the digenetic trematodes.

SUBCLASS DIGENEA

Phylum: Platyhelminthes
    Class: Trematoda
        Subclass: Digenea

Digenetic trematodes, or flukes, usually are endoparasites of both domestic and wild animals and occasionally humans. Digenetic flukes generally are broad, leaf-shaped,

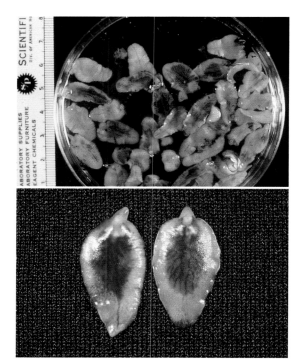

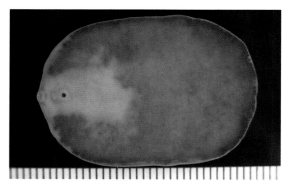

Figure 7-3 Digenetic flukes are usually broad, leaf shaped, and flattened (see Figure 7-1), although a few are thick and fleshy.

Figure 7-1 Representative flukes *(Fasciola hepatica)* with flattened, unsegmented, leaflike bodies.

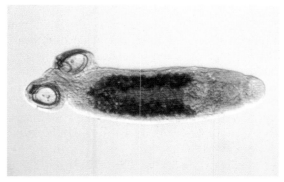

Figure 7-2 Representative monogenetic fluke with posterior adhesive organ that may have suckers, hooks, or clamps.

and flattened, although a few, such as *Fascioloides magna,* are thick and fleshy (Figure 7-3). One group of trematodes (the schistosomes) are long, thin, and wormlike, resembling the nematodes or roundworms.

KEY MORPHOLOGIC FEATURES

Figure 7-4 details the internal morphology of a representative digenetic fluke. On or near the anterior end is the fluke's mouth, which is surrounded by a muscular oral sucker. This mouth connects to a muscular pharynx, which in turn leads to an esophagus, which bifurcates into two blind ceca. Flukes do not possess an anus; to release digested food, they regurgitate their cecal contents back into the tissues or organs they infect. These contents are often observed in the tissues on histopathologic section and are colloquially referred to as "fluke puke." Flukes also possess a muscular organ of attachment called an *acetabulum,* or ventral sucker. This organ is used as a "holdfast organ" and is not associated with feeding.

With the exception of the schistosomes, or blood flukes, all flukes are hermaphroditic; that is, each fluke possesses complete sets of both male and female reproductive organs. The male reproductive organs consist of two testes, the vas efferens, the vas deferens, the seminal vesicle, and the cirrus (the fluke's version of a penis). The

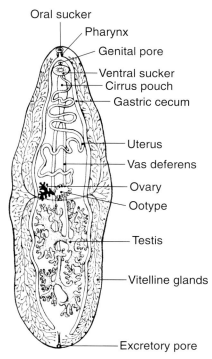

Figure 7-4   Internal morphology of representative digenetic fluke. Note that digenetic flukes are hermaphroditic; that is, they contain both male and female reproductive organs.

Oral sucker
Pharynx
Genital pore
Ventral sucker
Cirrus pouch
Gastric cecum
Uterus
Vas deferens
Ovary
Ootype
Testis
Vitelline glands
Excretory pore

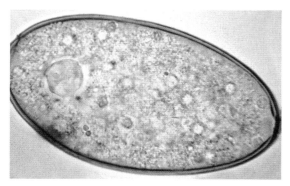

Figure 7-5   Fertilized operculated egg released by female portion of reproductive system of the hermaphroditic fluke. The operculum is a tiny "trapdoor" through which the miracidium emerges.

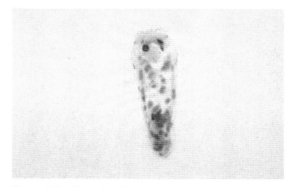

Figure 7-6   The miracidium is the motile, ciliated stage that emerges though the operculum and eventually penetrates the snail, the first intermediate host.

female reproductive organs consist of an ovary, an oviduct, a seminal receptacle, the yolk glands, the ootype, Mehlis' gland, vitelline glands, and the uterus. Self-fertilization usually takes place; however, cross-fertilization between two adult flukes also occurs.

LIFE CYCLE OF THE FLUKE

The female portion of the fluke's reproductive tract produces operculated eggs that have been stored in the uterus (Figure 7-5). Eggs pass out of the uterus through the genital pore and are usually passed out to the external environment within the host's feces. The operculated eggs embryonate in the external environment. If the egg makes contact with water, it will hatch and produce a motile stage called a *miracidium* (Figure 7-6). The miracidium is covered with tiny hairs called *cilia.* The movement of the cilia

allows the miracidium to swim in the water. The miracidium seeks out an aquatic snail (Figure 7-7), the first intermediate host, then penetrates the skin of the snail and develops to the next stage, the *sporocyst.* The sporocyst is merely a sack in which the next stage, the *redia,* develops. Many rediae develop within the sporocyst. Within each redia, many cercariae develop (Figure 7-8). The cercarial stage often has a tail and will emerge from the snail and swim in the water (Figure 7-9). Depending on the species of fluke, at this point the cercaria will take one of the following three paths:

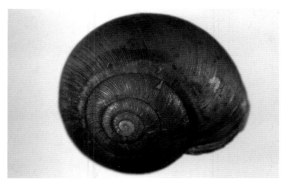

Figure 7-7 For most digenetic flukes, a snail is the first intermediate host.

1. The cercaria may directly penetrate the skin of the definitive host.
2. The cercaria may attach to vegetation, lose its tail, secrete a thick cyst wall around itself, and thus develop into a metacercaria (Figure 7-10). The vegetation with the attached, encysted metacercaria will be ingested by the definitive host.
3. The cercaria may lose its tail, penetrate the second intermediate host, secrete a thick cyst wall around itself, and develop into a metacercaria within the second intermediate host. The second intermediate host with the encysted metacercaria will be ingested by the intermediate host.

If the fluke takes the first option, the cercaria will migrate to its predilection site (the site of infection) and develop into the adult fluke. If the fluke takes the second option, the thick cyst wall will be digested by the host and the juvenile fluke released. The juvenile fluke then migrates to the predilection site and develops into an adult fluke. If the fluke takes the third option, the second intermediate host and the thick cyst wall are digested and the juvenile fluke released. The juvenile fluke then migrates to the predilection site and develops into an adult fluke. Most of the predilection sites of the flukes are associated with the digestive system. The exceptions are *Paragonimus kellicotti*, the lung fluke of dogs and

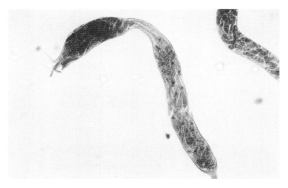

A

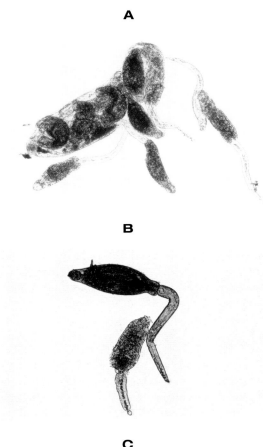

B

C

Figure 7-8 After penetration of the snail intermediate host, the next developmental stage, **A**, the sporocyst, is formed by the miracidium. **B**, The sporocyst stage forms many internal redial stages. **C**, Each redial stage forms many internal cercarial stages.

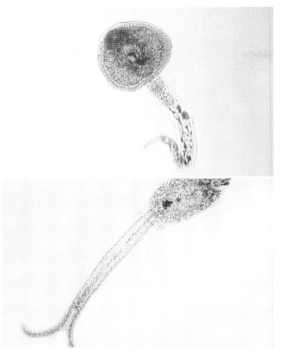

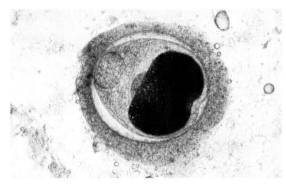

Figure 7-10   Metacercarial stage dissected from muscles of salmonid fish. Cercarial stage may swim to vegetation, drop its tail, secrete thick cyst wall, and develop into metacercarial stage; or cercarial stage may drop its tail, penetrate or be eaten by second intermediate host, secrete thick cyst wall around itself, and develop to metacercaria within the second intermediate host.

Figure 7-9   Cercarial stage is released from redial stage. This stage often has a tail and emerges from snail to swim in water. Rarely, cercarial stage penetrates skin of the definitive host.

cats, and the schistosomes, or blood flukes, which are flukes that reside in the blood vessels. Once the adult stage of the fluke is reached, self-fertilization and cross-fertilization occur, and the life cycle begins again, with operculated eggs being released to the outside environment.

Chapter 8 details some of the important flukes of domestic animals (and, in some cases, wild animals) in North America. As individual species, adult flukes can be quite distinctive in appearance. Flukes tend to be found in certain predilection tissue or organ sites within the host's body. Although some may "wander" off course in the developmental life cycle, adult flukes are usually associated with certain tissue or organ sites. It is important for the diagnostician to associate certain flukes with their predilection sites.

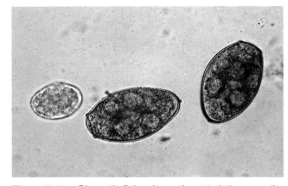

Figure 7-11   Digenetic flukes have characteristic ovum, the operculated egg, which is almost unique to this subclass. Most of these flukes possess this oval egg with a distinct operculum, or door, on one end of the egg. The egg of *Paragonimus kellicotti* has an operculum that is easily observed.

Finally, digenetic flukes have a characteristic ovum that is almost unique to this subclass, the operculated egg (Figure 7-11). Most of these flukes possess an oval egg with a distinct *operculum,* or door, on one pole (either end) of the egg. There are a few exceptions to this fact, and these are noted as these flukes are discussed.

8

Trematodes (Flukes) of Animals and Humans

The following organisms are flukes that may parasitize domesticated and wild animals. A few species are known to parasitize humans.

FLUKES OF RUMINANTS (CATTLE, SHEEP, AND GOATS)

Dicrocoelium dendriticum is commonly referred to as the "lancet fluke" of sheep, goats, and cattle. This tiny, flattened, leaflike fluke is only 6 to 10 mm long and 1.5 to 2.5 mm wide (Figure 8-1). These flukes are found in the fine branches of the bile duct and can produce hyperplasia of the bile duct's glandular epithelial lining. This fluke produces brown, embryonated eggs that are 36 to 46 μm by 10 to 20 μm. The egg possesses an *operculum* (similar to a hinged hatch) on one pole (end) of the egg. This operculum is said to be indistinct.

Rumen flukes comprise two genera of veterinary importance, *Paramphistomum* and *Cotylophoron* (Figure 8-2). Rumen flukes belong to a group of flukes called **amphistomes** (*amphi* means "on both sides" or "double," and *stome* means "mouth"); these flukes appear to possess a "mouth" at both ends of their bodies. Amphistomes have an oral sucker (the feeding organelle, or "true mouth") on the anterior end and a large ventral sucker (an organ of attachment) on the posterior end. In the fresh state, amphistomes are light colored to bright red and pear shaped, approximately 5 to 13 mm by 2 to 5 mm. They attach with the oral sucker to the lining of the rumen and reticulum of cattle, sheep, goats, and many other ruminants and expose the ventral suckers (Figure 8-3). The adult flukes are nonpathogenic; the pathogenicity of these flukes lies in the migration of the juvenile forms in the small intestine. These juvenile forms are known for the ability to ingest large plugs of intestinal lining. The eggs of *Paramphistomum* species measure 114 to 176 μm by 73 to 100 μm; the eggs of *Cotylophoron* species measure 125 to 135 μm by 61 to 68 μm. The prepatent period for *Paramphistomum* species is 80 to 95 days.

Fasciola hepatica is the liver fluke of cattle, sheep, and other ruminants. It is perhaps the most economically important fluke in veterinary medicine because it causes a "liver rot," or liver condemnation, at slaughter. This fluke is the best-known fluke among those parasitizing food animals; parasitologists have studied *F. hepatica* more

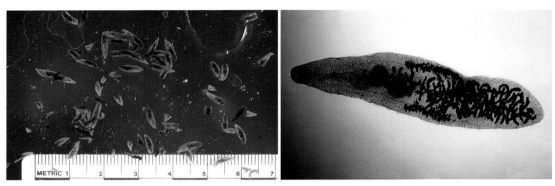

Figure 8-1 Adult *Dicrocoelium dendriticum,* commonly referred to as the "lancet fluke" of sheep, goats, and cattle. This tiny, flattened, leaflike fluke (6-10 mm long and 1.5-2.5 mm wide) is found in fine branches of bile duct.

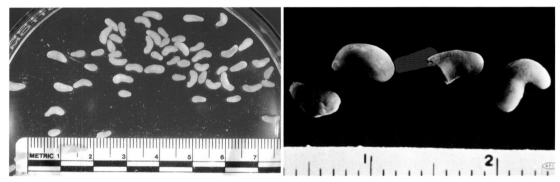

Figure 8-2 Rumen flukes, or amphistomes (*Paramphistomum* and *Cotylophoron* species), have an oral sucker (feeding organelle) on the anterior end and a large ventral sucker (organ of attachment) on the posterior end.

than any other fluke. Adult flukes are found in the bile ducts of the liver and possess a unique appearance. They are flattened and leaflike, measuring 30 by 13 mm (Figure 8-4). These liver flukes are broader in the anterior region than in the posterior region and possess an anterior cone-shaped projection that is followed by a pair of prominent, laterally directed shoulders. These flukes are tan to reddish brown in the fresh state; preserved specimen take on a grayish appearance. Their eggs are oval, yellow-brown, and measure 130 to 150 μm by 60 to 90 μm. Each egg will possess a distinct operculum (Figure 8-5).

Fascioloides magna is also a liver fluke; however, this fluke has the white-tailed deer as

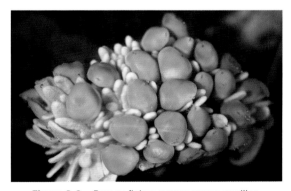

Figure 8-3 Rumen flukes among rumen papillae.

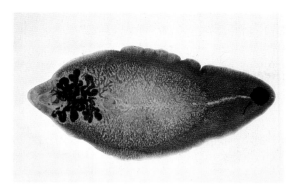

Figure 8-4   Adult liver flukes *(Fasciola hepatica)* are broader in the anterior region and have a prominent, anterior cone-shaped projection followed by prominent shoulders. In the fresh state, these flukes are grayish brown and measure 30 by 13 mm.

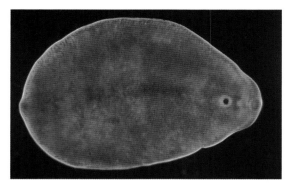

Figure 8-6   Adult *Fascioloides magna* are large, flattened, flesh-colored, oval flukes measuring up to 10 cm in length, 2.5 cm in width, and 4.5 mm in thickness. These flukes lack the anterior conelike projection of adult *Fasciola hepatica.*

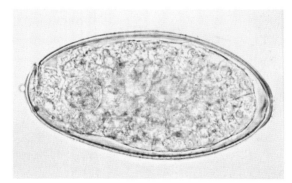

Figure 8-5   Egg of *Fasciola hepatica*. Eggs are oval, operculated, and yellow-brown and measure 130 to 150 μm by 60 to 90 μm.

its true definitive host. It may also use cattle, sheep, and pigs as incidental hosts. The adult flukes are found in the liver parenchyma and possess a unique appearance. They are large, flattened, flesh-colored, oval flukes, measuring up to 10 cm in length, 2.5 cm in width, and 4.5 mm in thickness (Figure 8-6). These flukes lack the anterior conelike projection of *F. hepatica*. The egg is operculated, up to 170 μm in length and 100 μm in width. *F. magna* flukes produce open cysts in the liver parenchyma of white-tailed deer. These cysts communicate with the bile

ducts, allowing eggs to be passed to the external environment. Thus, eggs are often found on fecal flotation solutions of these infected hosts. In incidental hosts such as cattle and sheep, however, these flukes produce closed cysts in the liver parenchyma. These cysts do not communicate with the bile ducts, so the egg of *F. magna* cannot pass to the external environment. Incidental hosts act as "dead end" hosts; that is, they are not capable of transmitting this parasite to other animals.

Eggs of the flukes just mentioned may be recovered from feces using either the fecal sedimentation procedure or a commercially available fluke egg recovery test.

FLUKES OF SMALL ANIMALS (DOGS AND CATS)

Platynosomum fastosum is the "lizard poisoning fluke" of cats. This fluke received this common name because cats became infected by ingesting the lizard second intermediate host that contains the infective metacercarial stages of the fluke. These adult flukes are found in the liver, gallbladder, bile ducts, and less often the small intestine of cats, producing signs such as diarrhea, vomiting, icterus, and even death. *P. fastosum* is a tiny, flattened, leaflike fluke, only 4 to 8 mm long and 1.5 to 2.5 mm wide, found in the fine branches of the bile duct of cats; it can produce desquamation (stripping) of the bile duct's glandular epithelial lining (Figure 8-7). The fluke's brownish, operculated eggs are oval, measuring 34 to 50 μm by 20 to 35 μm (Figure 8-8).

Nanophyetus salmincola is the "salmon poisoning fluke" of dogs in the Pacific Northwest region of North America. This fluke received its common name because dogs became infected by ingesting the salmon (fish) second intermediate host that contains the infective metacercarial stage of this fluke. The adult fluke inhabits the small intestine and serves as a vector for rick-

ettsial agents that produce "salmon poisoning" and "Elokomin fluke fever" in dogs. Whereas *F. magna* is the largest fluke of our domesticated animals, *N. salmincola* is the smallest, measuring only 0.5 to 1.1 mm in length (Figure 8-9). The color of adult flukes is white to cream. The eggs are yellowish brown, with an indistinct operculum and a small, blunt point at the end opposite to the operculum. Eggs are 52 to 82 μm by 32 to 56 μm (Figure 8-10).

Alaria species are intestinal flukes of dogs and cats and are found throughout the northern half of the North American continent. This fluke is 2 to 6 mm in length. It has a unique appearance

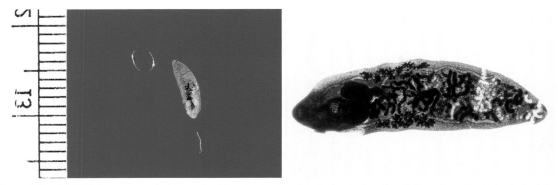

Figure 8-7 Adult *Platynosomum fastosum,* the "lizard poisoning fluke" of cats, is a tiny, flattened, leaflike fluke (only 4-8 mm long and 1.5-1.2 mm wide) found in fine branches of bile duct of cats.

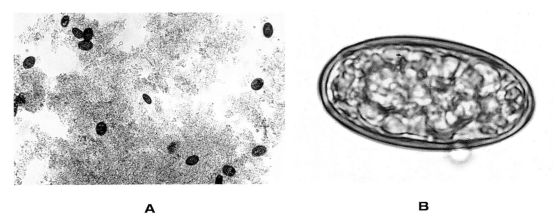

A   **B**

Figure 8-8 **A,** Eggs of *Platynosomum fastosum.* **B,** These oval, brown, operculated eggs measure 34 to 50 μm by 20 to 35 μm.

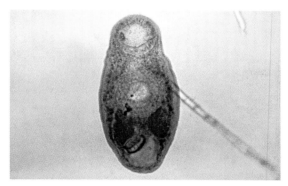

Figure 8-9 Adult *Nanophyetus salmincola,* the "salmon poisoning fluke" of the Pacific Northwest. This fluke measures only 0.5 to 1.1 mm in length. Color of adult flukes is white to cream.

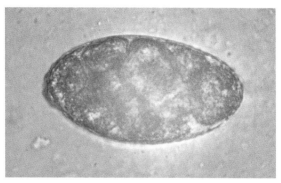

Figure 8-10 Egg of *Nanophyetus salmincola* is yellowish brown, with indistinct operculum and small, blunt point at end opposite operculum. Eggs are 52 to 82 μm by 32 to 56 μm.

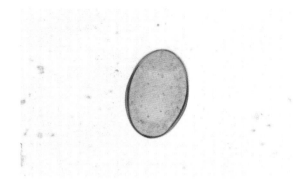

Figure 8-11 Egg of *Alaria* species is large, golden brown, and operculated, measuring 98 to 134 μm by 62 to 68 μm.

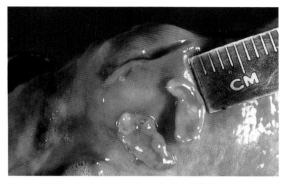

Figure 8-12 Adult *Paragonimus kellicotti* flukes are unusual in that they are found in the lung parenchyma, not the gastrointestinal tract.

among the flukes in that its anterior half is flattened and expanded and its posterior half is rounded and globose. The eggs are large, golden brown, and operculated. They measure 98 to 134 μm by 62 to 68 μm (Figure 8-11).

All the flukes covered in this chapter so far (in both ruminants and small animals) are parasites of portions of the digestive system, either the intestine or the ducts within the liver. The following flukes, however, are found in sites other than those associated with the digestive system. *Paragonimus kellicotti* is the lung fluke of dogs and cats found in cystic spaces in the lung

parenchyma. *Heterobilharzia americanum,* the canine schistosome, is a blood fluke that parasitizes the mesenteric veins of the small and large intestines and the portal veins of the dog.

Adult *Paragonimus kellicotti* flukes are found in cystic spaces within the lung parenchyma of both dogs and cats (Figure 8-12). These cystic spaces connect to the terminal bronchioles. The eggs are found in sputum or feces. Adults are thick, brownish-red flukes measuring up to 16 mm long by 8 mm wide (Figure 8-13). Eggs are yellowish brown, with a rather distinct operculum. The eggs are 75 to 118 μm by 42 to 67 μm; the shell at the pole opposite the operculum is somewhat thickened (Figure 8-14). These fluke

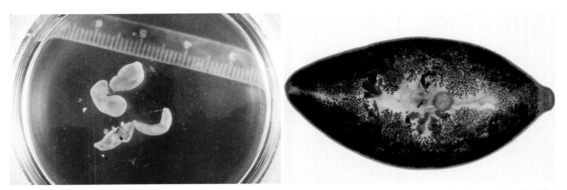

Figure 8-13 Adult *Paragonimus kellicotti* are thick, brownish red flukes measuring up to 16 mm long by 8 mm wide. Adult flukes are found within lung parenchyma.

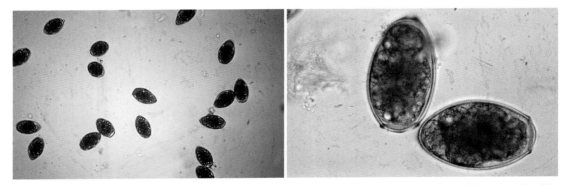

Figure 8-14 The distinctly operculated eggs of *Paragonimus kellicotti* are yellowish brown and 75 to 118 μm by 42 to 67 μm. The shell at the pole opposite the operculum is somewhat thickened.

eggs can be recovered using fecal sedimentation techniques; however, the eggs of *P. kellicotti* are usually recovered using standard fecal flotation solutions. These eggs can also be recovered in the sputum by tracheal washing. The adult flukes within the cystic spaces in the lung parenchyma can be observed with thoracic radiography.

Heterobilharzia americanum, the canine schistosome, is a blood fluke that parasitizes the mesenteric veins of the small and large intestines and the portal veins of the dog (Figures 8-15 and 8-16). The blood flukes, or **schistosomes,** are unique flukes in that they are not hermaphroditic. Separate sexes exist, so there are male schis-

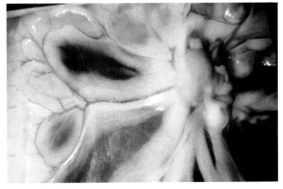

Figure 8-15 Gross necropsy revealing adult *Heterobilharzia americanum* in mesenteric veins of dog.

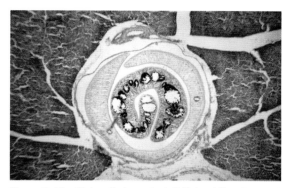

Figure 8-16   Histopathology of adult *Heterobilharzia americanum* in mesenteric veins of dog.

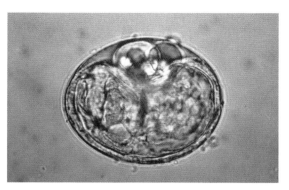

Figure 8-18   Thin-shelled egg of *Heterobilharzia americanum,* approximately 80 by 50 μm. Miracidium sometimes may be observed within egg.

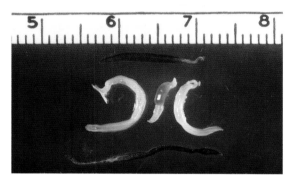

Figure 8-17   Adult male and female *Heterobilharzia americanum* recovered from mesenteric veins of dog.

tosomes and female schistosomes. Because these flukes reside in the fine branches of the mesenteric veins, they are long and slender. Females may be as long as 9 mm, and males are about 6.5 mm in length (Figure 8-17). This fluke is enzootic in the mudflats of the Mississippi delta and the coastal swampland of Louisiana. Although *H. americanum* inhabits the blood vasculature, it manifests its presence by a bloody diarrhea. Infected dogs also exhibit emaciation and anorexia. Diagnosis is by identification of the thin-shelled egg, about 80 by 50 μm, which contains a miracidium. (See Figure 8-18 for morphologic features of the egg of *H. americanum.*)

A few words about . . .

BOX 8-1   Flukes of Humans

Humans serve as definitive hosts for an important group of flukes called the **schistosomes** or the "blood flukes." These flukes are similar to *Heterobilharzia americanum* and inhabit the blood vasculature of the mesenteric veins and the blood vasculature associated with major organs (large and small intestine and urinary bladder) of the abdominal cavity of humans. These flukes are members of the genus *Schistosoma* (also known as *Bilharzia*) and are important parasites of humans in Africa, the Middle East, the Caribbean, and other areas of the world. These parasites are important in human medicine; however, other than this mention, they are beyond the scope of this textbook. The cercarial stage of this important fluke infects the definitive host by direct penetration of the skin of humans as they are wading or bathing in water. Some members of the genus *Schistosoma* infect the blood vasculature of the mesenteric and portal veins of cattle; however, these schistosomes occur in Africa, the Mediterranean, and the Middle East and are not usually associated with domesticated animals in North America. Schistosomes are species specific; that is, human schistosomes infect humans, and bovine schistosomes infect cattle. Schistosomes of domestic animals are not zoonotic. The veterinary technician who has interest in the schistosomes of humans should consult a textbook on the parasitology of humans.

A few words about...

BOX **8-2** Flukes of Wild Birds

Avian schistosomes occur in the blood vasculature of many wild birds (particularly aquatic birds) that migrate across the North American continent along seasonal "flyways." Migrating aquatic birds frequently rest in rivers and lakes of North America along their seasonal journeys. These birds are frequently infected with avian schistosomes in their blood vessels. The schistosomes produce eggs that pass to the external environment in the birds' feces. The eggs often make contact with water, hatch, and release the miracidia, the stage infective for the snail intermediate host. The miracidia penetrate aquatic snails and, within the snails, develop into the cercarial stage. The cercariae emerge from the snail, and to complete the life cycle, they usually penetrate the skin of the appropriate avian definitive host. However, if the cercariae penetrate the skin of a human (swimming or playing in the lake, river, or ocean), with repeated exposure, the cercariae can produce a severe papular or pustular dermatitis called **swimmer's itch** or **schistosome cercarial dermatitis** (Figure 8-19). This pruritic dermatitis is the only zoonotic parasite found among the digenetic trematodes. The dermatitis is quite pruritic and can ruin a vacation at the lake or the seashore.

A few words about...

BOX **8-3** Flukes of Game Fish

Birds near a lake or seashore may have flukes that reside in the gastrointestinal tract. As with the avian schistosomes described in Box 8-2, these flukes produce eggs that pass to the external environment and often make contact with water. The eggs hatch, releasing the miracidia. The miracidia penetrate aquatic snails and, within the snails, develop into the cercarial stage. The cercariae emerge from the snails and normally penetrate the skin of fish. When the cercariae penetrate the skin of fish, they produce a metacercarial stage. The metacercaria is actually a juvenile fluke. Fish often react to the presence of metacercaria by depositing melanin (black) pigment around the organism, producing a condition called **black spot** (Figure 8-20). Aquatic birds become infected with the fluke by ingesting the fish containing the metacercarial stage. Sometimes, fishermen catch these fish and during the cleaning process may notice these conspicuous black metacercarial stages in the skin or in the muscles of the fish. If the fish is properly cooked, it is safe for human consumption. Humans are not harmed when they ingest these stages; humans cannot become infected with this avian fluke. Therefore, this is not a zoonotic condition; however, it may not be aesthetically pleasing! The unsightly appearance of these metacercarial spots in the fish's tissues may prevail over the hungry fisherman's appetite.

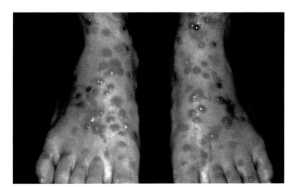

Figure 8-19 Severe papular or pustular dermatitis (swimmer's itch, or schistosome cercarial dermatitis) in human. This pruritic dermatitis is the only zoonotic digenetic trematode. (Courtesy Paul Honig, MD.)

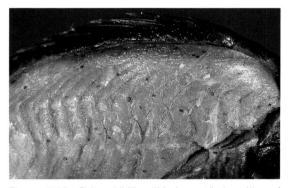

Figure 8-20 Fish exhibiting "black spot," deposition of melanin pigment in response to presence of metacercaria.

9

The Phylum Acanthocephala

The phylum Acanthocephala consists of the "thorny-headed worms," or "spiny-headed worms." With regard to number of acanthocephalan parasites that infect domesticated animals, the phylum Acanthocephala is very small.

COMMON ACANTHOCEPHALANS

Most acanthocephalans are parasites of marine and freshwater fish and aquatic birds; their predilection site is within the small intestine of the definitive host. Only two species, *Macracanthorhynchus hirudinaceus,* the thorny-headed worm of swine, and *Oncicola canis,* the canine acanthocephalan, are important to veterinary medicine.

KEY MORPHOLOGIC FEATURES

Members of the phylum Ancanthocephala are important parasites of domesticated and wild animals. Adult acanthocephalans are internal parasites, living in the small intestine of their vertebrate hosts. Acanthocephalans are typically elongate, cylindric worms, tapering on both ends. One acanthocephalan *(M. hirudinaceus)* can measure up to 70 cm in length. Acanthocephalans are dioecious; that is, they have separate sexes. Female acanthocephalans are typically larger than their male counterparts. The colloquial names "thorny-headed worm" and "spiny-headed worm" are derived from the fact that acanthocephalans possess a retractable proboscis, or "nose," on the anterior end (Figure 9-1). This proboscis is covered with tiny, backward-facing spines and serves as an organ of attachment (Figure 9-2). The proboscis embeds in the small intestinal mucosa and allows the acanthocephalan parasite to attach to the host, similar to the scolex of the true tapeworm. It is in this enteric site that acanthocephalans feed; however, these are unusual parasites in that they lack a mouth. Instead, these strange-looking helminths have a trait that is similar to the tapeworms: they do not possess an alimentary tract (a gut or intestinal tract). As a result, acanthocephalans must absorb nutrients through their body surface, or ***tegument.***

Another important organ system in the acanthocephalan is the reproductive tract. As with all helminths, acanthocephalans have a tremendous reproductive potential— one adult female worm can produce in excess of a quarter of a million eggs per day! These eggs pass out of the definitive host within its feces and embryonate in the external environment.

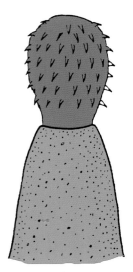

Figure 9-1 Anterior end of *Macracanthorhynchus hirudinaceus*, the thorny-headed worm of swine. This colloquial name is derived from acanthocephalans possessing a retractable proboscis, or "nose," on the anterior end.

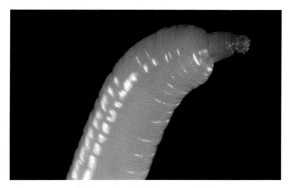
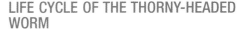

Figure 9-2 Proboscis of *Macracanthorhynchus hirudinaceus* is covered with tiny, backward-facing spines and serves as an organ of attachment.

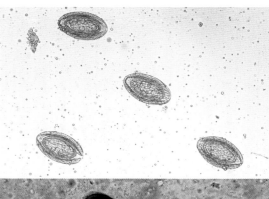
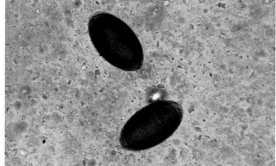
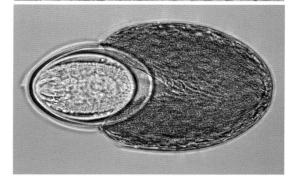

Figure 9-3 Egg of *Macracanthorhynchus hirudinaceus* is spindle shaped and has a shell of three layers. Egg contains the larval acanthocephalan, or acanthor.

LIFE CYCLE OF THE THORNY-HEADED WORM

The typical acanthocephalan has a unique life cycle. Because adult acanthocephalans are found attached to the small intestinal mucosa, the eggs are voided in the feces of the definitive host. The egg is spindle shaped and has a shell of three layers (Figure 9-3). This egg contains the larval acanthocephalan, or *acanthor.* The intermediate host, usually some type of arthropod (e.g., dung beetle), ingests the egg, and the acanthor larva hatches in that intermediate host. Within the intermediate host, the larva develops to the next stage, the *acanthella.* The acanthella develops into the *cystacanth* stage, which has an inverted proboscis. The definitive host ingests the arthropod intermediate host. Within the intestine of the definitive host, the acanthella everts its proboscis and attaches to the wall of the small intestine. This juvenile acanthocephalan grows to the adult stage, and the life cycle begins again (Figure 9-4).

ACANTHOCEPHALANS OF IMPORTANCE IN VETERINARY PARASITOLOGY

M. hirudinaceus and *O. canis* are the acanthocephalans of importance in veterinary medicine.

Macracanthorhynchus hirudinaceus

Macracanthorhynchus hirudinaceus, the thorny-headed worm of swine, is the acanthocephalan found attached to the lining of the small intestine of pigs (Figure 9-5). This parasite has the dubious distinction of having the longest scientific name among all the parasites of wild and domesticated animals. During postmortem examination, the prosector (pathologist) might, at first glance, make a diagnosis of the swine roundworm, *Ascaris suum* (see Chapter 4). On closer exami-

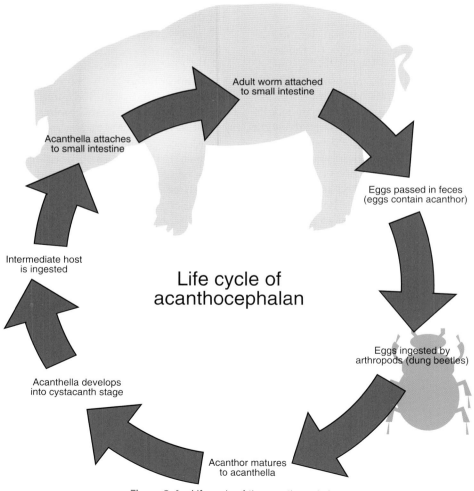

Life cycle of acanthocephalan

Adult worm attached to small intestine

Eggs passed in feces (eggs contain acanthor)

Eggs ingested by arthropods (dung beetles)

Acanthor matures to acanthella

Acanthella develops into cystacanth stage

Intermediate host is ingested

Acanthella attaches to small intestine

Figure 9-4   Life cycle of the acanthocephalan.

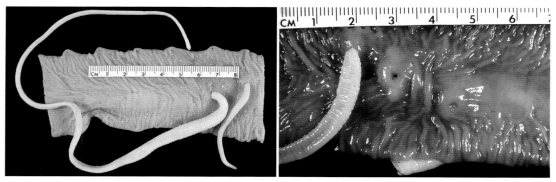

Figure 9-5   *Macracanthorhynchus hirudinaceus*, the thorny-headed worm of swine, is found attached to lining of small intestine of pigs.

nation, however, it is apparent that the parasite is firmly attached to the mucosa of the small intestine rather than free within the lumen. *A. suum* does not attach to the mucosa but remains within the lumen of the small intestine. *M. hirudinaceus* can grow up to 70 cm in length, although the males average up to 10 cm in length and the females up to 35 cm, and these worms are 4 to 10 mm thick. The proboscis is tiny and is covered with six rows of six hooks each. These backward-facing hooks are used to anchor the adult parasite to the mucosa. The eggs of *M. hirudinaceus* are 40 to 65 μm by 67 to 110 μm and have a three-layered shell; the second shell is brown and pitted (see Figure 9-3). Because humans seldom intentionally eat dung beetles (the intermediate host of *M. hirudinaceus*), this acanthocephalan is seldom identified as a zoonotic parasite.

Oncicola canis

Oncicola canis, the thorny-headed worm of dogs, is the acanthocephalan found attached to the lining of the small intestine of dogs. This is a tiny acanthocephalan, only 14 mm in length. The body is tapered posteriorly, and on the anterior end is the characteristic proboscis armed with hooks. As with *M. hirudinaceus,* these are backward-facing hooks used to anchor the adult parasite to the mucosa of the small intestine. The eggs of *O. canis* are brown and oval, approximately 65 by 45 μm.

Although with regard to domesticated animals the phylum Acanthocephala is extremely small, veterinarians should understand its importance, especially with regard to the swine industry.

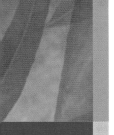

The Protozoans 10

Only two kingdoms of living creatures have members that are true parasites of domesticated animals. These parasites belong to the kingdom Animalia and the kingdom Protista. Most of the parasites of domesticated animals belong to the Animal kingdom (flukes, tapeworms, roundworms, thorny-headed worms, arthropods, and leeches). The rest of animal parasites belong to the kingdom Protista. This kingdom contains the unicellular, or one-cell, organisms (better known as the *protozoans*).

Most protozoans are free-living organisms; however, those protozoans that are parasitic may produce significant pathology in domesticated animals and humans. Within the kingdom Protista are several phyla, which contain (1) flagellated protozoans, (2) amoeboid protozoans, (3) apicomplexans, and (4) ciliated protozoans. These phyla contain the primary protozoans that may cause significant pathology in domesticated animals and humans.

CHARACTERISTICS OF THE PROTOZOANS

Protozoans are unicellular organisms; that is, they are one-cell organisms. Protozoans vary greatly in size, form, and structure; most are microscopic, and a very few are macroscopic, that is, visible to the naked eye. The kingdom Protista is divided into several phyla. These phyla differ in the manner in which the protozoans move within their tiny microenvironments. In veterinary parasitology, the most important phyla are Sarcomastigophora (containing the flagellates and amoebae), Ciliophora (containing the ciliates), and Apicomplexa (containing the coccidia, malarial organisms, and piroplasms).

MASTIGOPHORA (FLAGELLATES)

Kingdom: Protista
  Phylum: Sarcomastigophora
    Subphylum: Mastigophora (flagellates)
The flagellates are those protozoans that possess at least one *flagellum* (a long, whip-like or lashlike appendage) in their *trophozoite,* or moving, form. This flagellum allows the protozoan to move about in a fluid medium. As a result of this activity, parasitic flagellates live in the liquid world of the host's blood, lymphatic fluid, or cerebrospinal fluid. Flagellates are often pear shaped or bullet shaped and are able to swim in their host's body fluids, meeting very little resistance. These flagellates vary greatly in *pathogenicity* (disease-causing potential). Some flagellates are highly pathogenic, whereas others appear to cause little or no harm to the host. Some important genera

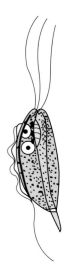

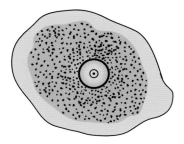

Figure 10-2 Diagram of motile trophozoite stage of a representative amoeba, *Entamoeba histolytica*, an amoeboid protozoan, with characteristic nucleus and "bull's-eye" nucleolus.

Figure 10-1 Diagram of representative flagellate, *Tritrichomonas foetus*, a flagellated protozoan of the reproductive tract of cattle. Note three anterior flagella, undulating membrane, and trailing posterior flagellum.

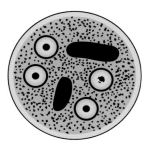

Figure 10-3 Diagram of resistant cyst stage of representative amoeba, *Entamoeba histolytica*, with thick cyst wall, four nuclei, and dark chromatoid bodies.

of parasitic flagellates of domestic animals are *Leishmania, Trypanosoma, Trichomonas, Histomonas,* and *Giardia* species. Figure 10-1 is a diagram of a representative flagellate, *Tritrichomonas foetus,* a flagellated protozoan of the reproductive tract of cattle.

SARCODINA (AMOEBAE)

Kingdom: Protista
　Phylum: Sarcomastigophora
　　Superclass: Sarcodina (amoebae)
The amoebae are protozoans that move via ***pseudopodia*** ("false feet"). Amoebae have two forms: the motile ***trophozoite*** form and the resistant ***cyst*** form. In their motile trophozoite form, amoebae glide or flow along a solid surface, usually the surface at the bottom of the liquid medium. Amoebae are amorphous (poorly defined, or bloblike, in shape). As with the flagellates, the amoebae vary greatly in their pathogenicity. Some amoebae are highly pathogenic, whereas others appear to cause little or no harm to the host. Amoebae demonstrate a resist-

ant cyst form that allows them to survive in adverse conditions in the external environment.

　The most important parasitic amoeba of humans is *Entamoeba histolytica. Entamoeba coli,* a nonpathogenic amoeba, may also be found in humans and pigs. Figure 10-2 is a diagram of the motile trophozoite stage of a representative amoeba, *E. histolytica,* an amoeboid protozoan. Figure 10-3 is a diagram of the resistant cyst stage of *E. histolytica.*

CILIOPHORA (CILIATES)

Kingdom: Protista
　Phylum: Ciliophora (ciliates)
Ciliates are protozoans that are covered with tiny, short hairs over most of their body surface. These tiny hairs are called ***cilia,*** thus the name ***ciliates.*** Ciliates move with these beating, undu-

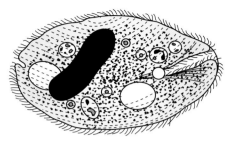

Figure 10-4 Diagram of motile trophozoite form of representative ciliate, *Balantidium coli,* a ciliated protozoan of the intestinal tract of pigs.

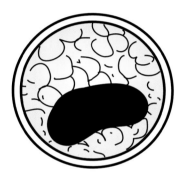

Figure 10-5 Diagram of resistant cyst stage of *Balantidium coli,* with thick cyst wall and large, dark nucleus.

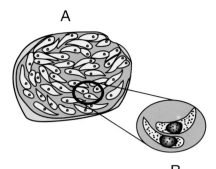

Figure 10-6 **A,** Diagram of cyst containing banana-, comma-, or boomerang-shaped sporozoites typical of apicomplexans of domestic animals, for example, *Eimeria, Isospora, Toxoplasma, Sarcocystis, Cryptosporidium, Plasmodium, Haemoproteus, Leukocytozoon, Babesia,* and *Theileria* species. **B,** Note enlarged banana-, comma-, or boomerang-shaped sporozoites.

lating hairs. As with amoebae, ciliates demonstrate two forms: the motile trophozoite form and the resistant cyst form. In their trophozoite, or moving, form, ciliates dart and twirl about speedily in liquid medium. Ciliates come in a variety of sizes and shapes, but all are covered with these tiny hairs. Figure 10-4 is a diagram of the motile trophozoite form of a representative ciliate, *Balantidium coli,* a ciliated protozoan of the intestinal tract of pigs. Some amoebae, such as *B. coli* and *Ichthyophthirius multifiliis,* are highly pathogenic to their hosts, whereas other ciliates, such as those in the rumen of the cow or sheep or the cecum of the horse, have beneficial roles. As with amoebae, ciliates demonstrate a resistant cyst form that allows them to survive in adverse conditions in the external environment. Figure 10-5 is a diagram of the resistant cyst stage of *B. coli.* The ciliates are unique among the protozoans in that they possess two types of nuclei: a macronucleus and a micronucleus.

APICOMPLEXA (APICOMPLEXANS)

Kingdom: Protista
 Phylum: Apicomplexa (apicomplexans)
Of the protozoans, the apicomplexans are the most diverse and the most complicated. The apicomplexans are parasites of almost every animal phylum. In domesticated animals, they are found primarily in the epithelium of the intestine, within blood cells, and within cells of the reticuloendothelial system. The life cycles of these protozoans vary among the genera that affect domesticated animals; however, they do have a common trait in that their life cycles are complex and intimately integrated into the physiology of the host's body. The locomotory organelles of the flagellates, amoebae, and ciliates (i.e., flagella, pseudopodia, and cilia) are discernible. In contrast, the locomotory organelles of the apicomplexans are not visible to the naked eye; their locomotory organelles are

internal. The apicomplexans are often banana, comma, or boomerang shaped (Figure 10-6) and move via undulations. Some of the most important genera of parasitic apicomplexans of domestic animals are *Eimeria, Isospora, Toxoplasma, Sarcocystis, Cryptosporidium, Plasmodium, Haemoproteus, Leukocytozoon, Babesia, Theileria, Cytauxzoon,* and *Hepatozoon.* These protozoans are perhaps the most diverse, complicated members of the Protista kingdom.

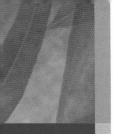

11

Common Protozoans That Infect Domestic Animals

This chapter is a continuation of Chapter 10 in that it details the common protozoans that infect domestic animals. The parasitic protozoans are discussed in the same sequential order as in Chapter 10: flagellates, amoebae, ciliates, and apicomplexans. These parasites are discussed in the same system-by-system manner, that is, those infecting the gastrointestinal tract, the circulatory system and peripheral blood, and the urogenital system. These parasites are discussed in the following species of domesticated animals: dogs and cats, ruminants (i.e., cattle and sheep), horses, pigs, pet and aviary birds, domestic fowl, rabbits, mice, rats, hamsters, guinea pigs, and fish.

DOGS AND CATS

GASTROINTESTINAL TRACT

Protozoans that infect the gastrointestinal tract of dogs and cats are flagellates, amoebae, ciliates, and apicomplexans.

Flagellates

Giardia species are flagellated protozoans often recovered from the feces of dogs and cats with diarrhea. They may also be recovered from animals with normal stools. These parasites occur in two morphologic forms: a rarely observed, motile feeding stage (the trophozoite) and a frequently observed, resistant cyst stage.

The motile trophozoite stage is pear shaped and dorsoventrally flattened and possesses four pairs of flagella. This stage is 9 to 21 µm by 5 to 15 µm. Two nuclei and a prominent adhesive disc are present on the anterior portion of the trophozoite, suggesting to the observer that a pair of eyes is "staring back." Figure 11-1 presents the motile trophozoite form of *Giardia* species.

The mature cysts of *Giardia* species are oval and are 8 to 10 µm by 7 to 10 µm. They have a refractile wall and four nuclei. Immature cysts, which represent recently encysted motile forms, contain only two nuclei. Figure 11-2 presents a cyst of *Giardia*

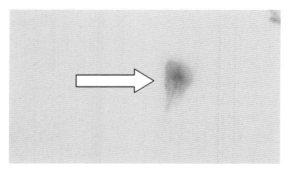

Figure 11-1 Motile trophozoite of *Giardia* species is pear shaped and dorsoventrally flattened and possesses four pairs of flagella. Two nuclei and prominent adhesive disc are present on anterior portion of the trophozoite, suggesting a pair of eyes staring back.

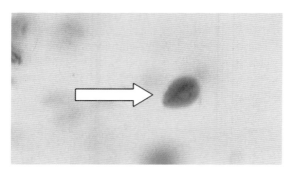

Figure 11-2 Mature cysts of *Giardia* species are oval and possess a refractile wall and four nuclei. Immature cysts, which represent recently encysted motile forms, contain only two nuclei.

species. In dogs, diarrhea may begin as early as 5 days after exposure to *Giardia,* with cysts first appearing in the feces at 1 week.

Diagnosis of *Giardia* species is by standard fecal flotation. Zinc sulfate (specific gravity, 1.18) is considered the best flotation medium for recovering cysts. Cysts are often distorted, with a semilunar appearance. The motile trophozoite occasionally can be found on direct smear of fresh feces using isotonic saline. Lugol's iodine stain may be used to visualize the internal struc-

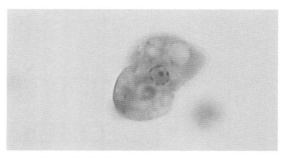

Figure 11-3 Motile feeding stage of *Entamoeba histolytica,* the trophozoite stage. Note single spherical nucleus with tiny pinpoint center, or endosome.

tures of both cysts and trophozoites. Fecal immunodiagnostic tests are also frequently used.

Amoebae

Entamoeba histolytica, the etiologic agent that produces amebic dysentery (an extremely severe dysentery) in humans may also produce sporadic infections in the dog. These cases usually have been acquired by association with infected humans. Although *E. histolytica* may produce acute or chronic diarrhea in the dog, it usually produces no pathology. Cats are rarely infected; most infections have been experimental.

E. histolytica occurs in two morphologic forms: a motile feeding stage (the trophozoite) and an environmentally resistant cyst stage. The motile trophozoite of *E. histolytica* ranges in size from 10 to 60 μm and has a single spherical nucleus that is 4 to 7 μm with a tiny pinpoint center, a structure called an ***endosome*** (Figure 11-3). The mature cysts are round and are 5 to 20 μm. They have a thin refractile wall and may demonstrate as many as four nuclei, each with its own endosome. Immature cysts, which represent recently encysted motile forms, contain only one nucleus (Figure 11-4).

Diagnosis of *E. histolytica* is by standard fecal flotation, which may be used to demonstrate both cyst and trophozoite forms. In a formed stool, usually the cyst form may be found; however, in diarrheic stool, both the cyst and the

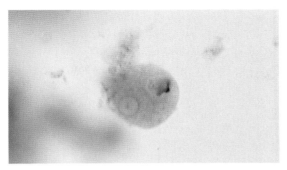

Figure 11-4   Cyst of *Entamoeba histolytica.* Cyst may demonstrate as many as four nuclei. Immature cysts, which represent recently encysted motile forms, contain only one nucleus.

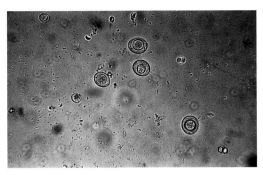

Figure 11-5   Unsporulated oocysts of *Isospora* species. *I. canis* (large oocysts) and *I. bigemina* (small oocysts) are present.

trophozoite forms may be observed. The direct smear technique may be used to observe motile forms in warm, freshly passed diarrheic stools. Lugol's iodine stain may be used to visualize the internal structures of both cysts and trophozoites. Zinc sulfate may be used to concentrate cysts. If infection with *E. histolytica* is suspected in a dog, a human pathology laboratory should be consulted for assistance with diagnosis. Because *E. histolytica* is primarily a human pathogen, great care should be taken with suspect feces.

E. histolytica also can be a significant problem in primates, such as monkeys and chimpanzees. Great care should be taken when handling suspect feces. Infection in monkeys has great public health significance.

Ciliates

Balantidium coli is the ciliated protozoan found occasionally in the cecum and colon of dogs. This parasite has been associated with diarrhea in dogs. *B. coli* is more intimately associated with pigs (see the section on swine protozoan parasites).

Apicomplexans

Isospora species (coccidians) are protozoan parasites of the small intestine of dogs and cats. They produce a clinical syndrome known as *coccidio-*

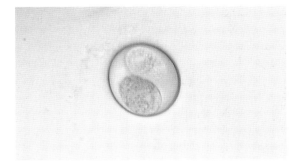

Figure 11-6   Sporulated oocyst of *Isospora rivolta* from older feces.

sis, one of the most commonly diagnosed protozoan diseases in puppies and kittens. Coccidiosis is rarely a problem in mature animals. The oocyst is the diagnostic stage observed in a fecal flotation of fresh feces; it is unsporulated in fresh feces and varies in size and shape among the common *Isospora* species. Figure 11-5 shows an unsporulated oocyst, and Figure 11-6 shows a sporulated oocyst. The canine coccidians and their measurements are *Isospora canis,* 34 to 40 μm by 28 to 32 μm; *I. ohioensis,* 20 to 27 μm by 15 to 24 μm; and *I. wallacei,* 10 to 14 μm by 7.5 to 9 μm. The feline coccidians and their measurements are *Isospora felis,* 38 to 51 μm by 27 to 29 μm, and *I. rivolta,* 21 to 28 μm by 18 to 23 μm. The prepatent period varies among species, but it is usually 7 to 14 days.

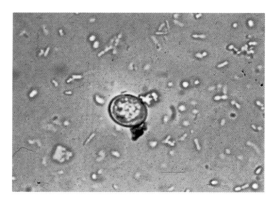

Figure 11-7 Unsporulated oocyst of *Toxoplasma gondii*, an intestinal coccidian of cats, from fresh feline feces. Its oocysts measure 10 by 12 μm.

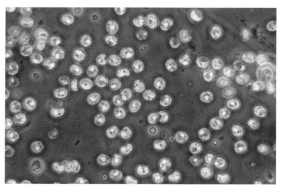

Figure 11-8 Numerous oocysts of *Cryptosporidium*, a coccidian parasite that parasitizes the small intestine of dogs and cats. Sporulated oocysts in feces are oval to spherical and measure 3 to 5 μm. Diagnosis is by standard fecal flotation. Oocysts are extremely small and may be observed just under coverslip, not in same plane of focus as other oocysts and parasite ova. Examination of fresh fecal smears using special stains (modified acid-fast stain) is also helpful.

Toxoplasma gondii is an intestinal coccidian of cats. Its oocysts are usually diagnosed using a standard fecal flotation solution. Oocysts of *T. gondii* are unsporulated in fresh feces and measure 10 by 12 μm (Figure 11-7). Several immunodiagnostic tests using whole blood or serum are available for diagnosis of *T. gondii*. The prepatent period is highly variable, ranging from 5 to 24 days, and depends on the infection route. Because this parasite can use humans (and many other warm-blooded vertebrates) as intermediate hosts, *T. gondii* is a very important zoonotic parasite.

T. gondii can be a significant pathogen in humans (particularly the pregnant woman and her developing fetus). It is important to discuss this parasite with clients. Great care should be taken when handling suspect feces. Infection in cats has great public health significance.

Cryptosporidium species is another coccidian parasite that parasitizes the small intestine of a variety of animals, including dogs and cats. The sporulated oocysts in the feces are oval to spherical and measure only 4 to 6 μm. Diagnosis is by standard fecal flotation. The oocysts are extremely small and may be observed just under the coverslip, not in the same plane of focus as other oocysts and parasite eggs (Figure 11-8). Examination of fresh fecal smears using special stains (modified acid-fast stain) is also helpful.

Because humans may become infected with *Cryptosporidium* species, feces suspected of harboring this protozoan should be handled with great care. *Cryptosporidium* is a zoonotic parasite.

Sarcocystis species are the final coccidian parasites cited here that are found in the small intestine. Several species infect dogs and cats, and identification of an individual species can be quite difficult. The oocysts of *Sarcocystis* species are sporulated when passed in the feces. Each oocyst contains two sporocysts, each with four sporozoites. These individual oocysts measure 12 to 15 μm by 8 to 12 μm and may be recovered in a standard fecal flotation of fresh feces.

CIRCULATORY SYSTEM AND BLOOD

Protozoans that infect the circulatory system and blood of dogs and cats are flagellates and apicomplexans.

Flagellates

Trypanosoma cruzi is a **hemoprotozoan** (a protozoan found circulating in the peripheral blood). It is primarily found in Central and South

America; however, it is occasionally reported in dogs in the southern half of the United States. This trypanosome is extracellular; it is not found within the red blood cell (RBC) itself. It "swims" within the blood. This swimming stage is called a *trypomastigote* and is 16 to 20 µm in length, approximately 3 to 10 times as long as an RBC is wide. It is banana shaped and possesses a lateral, undulating membrane and a thin, whiplike tail (the flagellum) that is used for swimming. These parasites are also transmitted by blood-feeding arthropods called *reduviid bugs,* or "kissing bugs" (see Chapter 13). *T. cruzi* also has a resting cyst stage (the *amastigote* stage) that may be found encysted within cardiac muscle and other tissues such as the esophagus. The encysted amastigote stage lacks the undulating flagellum of the swimming trypomastigote stage.

The trypomastigote stage of *T. cruzi* may be found swimming within the peripheral blood and may be demonstrated in direct blood smears. The amastigote stage must be confirmed using histopathologic sectioning. Suspect tissues should be submitted to a histopathology laboratory for diagnosis by a veterinary pathologist or parasitologist.

Leishmania species is another hemoprotozoan (blood protozoan). The parasite is primarily found in areas other than North America; however, it occasionally may be reported in dogs that have traveled or been born overseas. It can be rarely diagnosed in dogs that have never left the United States. This flagellate is intracellular and is found within reticuloendothelial cells of capillaries, the spleen, and other internal organs and in monocytes, polymorphonuclear leukocytes, and macrophages. Instead of having a flagellum and being called the trypomastigote stage, as with *T. cruzi,* this parasite lacks the flagellum and is called the amastigote stage. *Leishmania* is transmitted by blood-feeding arthropods called *phlebotomine sandflies* (see Chapter 13).

The amastigote stage of *Leishmania* must be confirmed using histopathologic sectioning of infected organs. Suspect tissues should be submitted to a histopathology laboratory for diagnosis by a veterinary pathologist or parasitologist.

Apicomplexans

Babesia canis is an intracellular parasite found within the RBCs of dogs. It has been referred to as the *canine piroplasm.* The parasite demonstrates pear-shaped organisms within canine RBCs. This protozoan parasite is spread by the bite of infected ticks. Diagnosis is by observing basophilic, pear-shaped organisms within RBCs in stained blood smears (Figure 11-9).

Cytauxzoon felis is another intracellular parasite that has been reported in the RBCs of cats in sporadic sites (Missouri, Arkansas, Georgia, and Texas) throughout the United States. It also produces piroplasms; however, these bodies have been described as being in the shape of a "bejeweled ring" and are referred to as the *ring form* in stained blood smears (Figure 11-10). This disease is spread by ticks, and its prognosis is poor. Diagnosis is made by observing the bejeweled-ring piroplasms within the RBCs in stained blood smears.

Hepatozoon canis and *Hepatozoon americanum* are intracellular, malaria-like parasites affecting dogs. The blood forms (the *gamonts*) of these protozoan parasites are found in the leukocytes. (Leukocytes containing gamonts of *H. canis* are common in peripheral blood smears, whereas those of *H. americanum* are rare.) Schizonts are

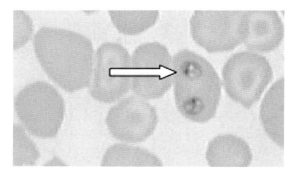

Figure 11-9   Trophozoites of *Babesia canis* within canine red blood cells.

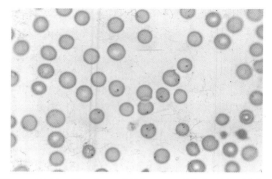

Figure 11-10 Ring form of *Cytauxzoon felis* in stained feline red blood cells.

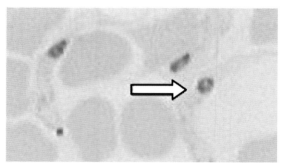

Figure 11-11 The "onion skin" tissue cysts of *Hepatozoon americanum* are found in skeletal muscle of dogs.

found in the endothelial cells of the spleen, bone marrow, and liver. The gamonts are surrounded by a delicate capsule and stain pale blue with a dark, reddish purple nucleus. Numerous pink granules are found in the cytoplasm of the leukocyte. The "onion skin" tissue cysts of *H. americanum* are found in skeletal muscle of dogs (Figure 11-11). This is an unusual parasite in that the dog becomes infected by ingestion of an infected tick, *Amblyoma americanum*. *H. canis* is well adapted to its canine host and varies from producing a subclinical to a mild disease. *H. americanum* produces a violent and frequently fatal course of disease; it is theorized to have crossed the species barrier from a wild animal host to the domestic dog.

RUMINANTS (CATTLE AND SHEEP)

GASTROINTESTINAL TRACT

Protozoans that infect the gastrointestinal tract of ruminants are ciliates and apicomplexans.

Ciliates

Nonpathogenic ciliates live in the rumen of all ruminants, including cattle and sheep. These are **commensals;** in this type of symbiotic relationship, both individuals benefit from the association. The cow provides a warm, moist, particulate medium in which the ciliates live; the ciliates, in exchange, aid in digestion by breaking down cellulose. Sometimes, ciliates may be observed in the diarrheic feces of cattle and sheep. These ciliates may be recovered on fecal flotation. Similar ciliates occur in the cecum of the horse and are often recovered from diarrheic feces.

Apicomplexans

Ruminants serve as host to many species of the coccidian parasite *Eimeria*. It is often difficult to identify the individual species of *Eimeria* because their oocysts are similar in size and shape. The two most common species of coccidia in cattle are *Eimeria bovis* and *Eimeria zuernii*; they can be differentiated on a standard fecal flotation. Oocysts of *E. bovis* are oval, have a micropyle, and measure 20 by 28 μm; the oocysts of *E. zuernii* are spherical, lack the micropyle, and measure 15 to 22 μm by 13 to 18 μm. When oocysts are recovered on fecal flotation, the observation is usually noted as **coccidia.** The coccidian oocysts of ruminants can be partially differentiated by size and appearance (Figure 11-12).

Cryptosporidium species is another coccidian that parasitizes the small intestine of a variety of animals, including cattle, sheep, and goats. The sporulated oocysts in the feces are colorless and transparent and measure only 3 to 5 μm. Diagnosis is by standard fecal flotation and stained fecal smears. Because humans may become infected with *Cryptosporidium* species, feces suspected of harboring this protozoan should be

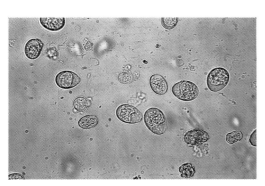

Figure 11-12   Unsporulated oocysts of *Eimeria* species recovered from fresh goat feces.

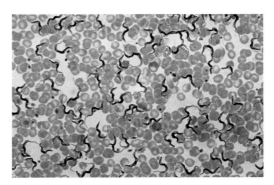

Figure 11-13   *Trypanosoma* species in bovine blood smear.

handled with great care. These oocysts are often recovered using Sheather's sugar solution. (See Figure 11-8 for features of the oocysts of *Cryptosporidium* species.)

CIRCULATORY SYSTEM AND BLOOD

Protozoans that infect the circulatory system and blood are flagellates and apicomplexans.

Flagellates

Trypanosoma species are hemoprotozoans found in the peripheral blood of many ruminants. This trypanosome has a long narrow body, a dark nucleus, anterior flagellum, and a sail-like undulating membrane (Figure 11-13). These protozoans may be observed among the RBCs in a thin blood smear. *Trypanosoma* species are not pathogenic and are very common but are seldom seen in a routine smear.

Apicomplexans

Babesia bigemina is an intracellular parasite found within the RBCs of cattle. This parasite is a large piroplasm, 4 to 5 µm in length by about 2 µm wide, and can be observed in a stained blood smear. These piroplasms are characteristically pear shaped and lie in pairs, forming an acute angle within the erythrocyte (Figure 11-14). The intermediate host for this protozoan parasite is the tick *Boophilus annulatus* (see Chapter 13). *If diagnosed, both the protozoan and its tick interme-*

diate host should be reported to state and federal authorities.

UROGENITAL SYSTEM

Tritrichomonas foetus is a protozoan parasite residing in the reproductive tract of cattle. These protozoans reside in the prepuce of infected bulls and in the vagina, cervix, and uterus of infected cows. *T. foetus* is pear shaped and approximately 10 to 25 µm long, with a sail-like undulating membrane and three rapidly moving, anterior whiplike flagella (Figure 11-15). In fresh specimens they move actively with a jerky movement. Diagnosis is by finding these protozoans in fluid freshly collected from the stomach of an aborted fetus, from uterine discharges, or from washings of the vagina and prepuce. Fluid material should be centrifuged at 2000 rpm for 5 minutes. The supernatant is then removed and a drop of sediment transferred to a glass slide for microscopic examination for the moving organisms. Several slides should be examined. For more accurate diagnosis, fluid material from the sources just mentioned can be cultured in special media. A specialized parasitology laboratory should be consulted for information on these techniques.

HORSES

GASTROINTESTINAL TRACT

Protozoan parasites that infect horses are flagellates, ciliates, and apicomplexans.

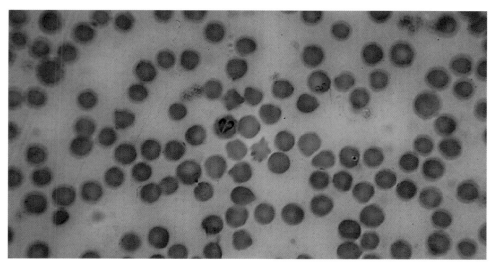

Figure 11-14 Trophozoites of *Babesia bigemina* within bovine red blood cells. Piroplasms are characteristically pear shaped and lie in pairs, forming an acute angle within the erythrocyte.

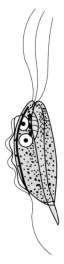

Figure 11-15 Diagram of *Tritrichomonas foetus.* This flagellated protozoan is pear shaped and approximately 10 to 25 μm long, with sail-like undulating membrane, trailing posterior flagellum, and three rapidly moving, anterior whiplike flagella.

Flagellates

Giardia equi is a flagellated protozoan of low incidence in horses. The trophozoites and cysts of this parasite are morphologically similar to those of the species found in dogs and cats (see Figure 11-1). *G. equi* invades the small intestine and causes chronic diarrhea. Normal flotation techniques rarely detect *G. equi,* but zinc sulfate will float the cysts.

Ciliates

As with the rumen ciliates of cattle and sheep, nonpathogenic ciliates live in the cecum of the horse. These commensals live in the warm, moist, particulate-rich medium of the cecum. Sometimes, ciliates may be observed in the diarrheic feces of horses and are often recovered on fecal flotation.

Apicomplexans

Eimeria leuckarti is the coccidian found in the small intestine of horses, particularly young ones, in the United States. Infections are usually asymptomatic and self-limiting. Horses rapidly become immune to further infection. This proto-

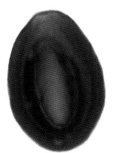

Figure 11-16   Unsporulated oocyst of *Eimeria leuckarti.* (350×.)

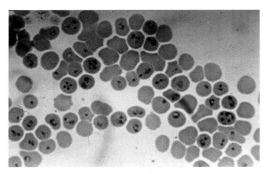

Figure 11-17   Basophilic, pear-shaped trophozoites of *Babesia equi* in red blood cells in stained equine blood smear. Trophozoites of *B. equi* may be round, ameboid, or pyriform (pear shaped). Four organisms may be joined, giving the effect of a Maltese cross. Individual organisms are 2 to 3 µm long.

zoan demonstrates unique oocysts that are quite large, 80 to 87 µm by 55 to 60 µm, and dark brown, with a thick wall and a distinct micropyle (opening) at the narrow end (Figure 11-16). These oocysts can be recovered on fecal flotation using saturated sodium nitrate (1:360) and saturated sugar solution (1:320); however, they also may be easily recovered using fecal sedimentation. The oocysts of *E. leuckarti* are the largest coccidian oocysts. They are frequently described in histopathologic examination.

CIRCULATORY SYSTEM AND BLOOD

Apicomplexans are the protozoans that infect the circulatory system and blood of horses.

Apicomplexans

Babesia equi and *Babesia caballi* are intracellular parasites found within the erythrocytes of horses. They are also referred to as the "equine piroplasms." These parasites are spread by the bite of infected ticks. Diagnosis is by observing basophilic, pear-shaped trophozoites in RBCs in stained blood smears. Trophozoites of *B. equi* may be round, ameboid, or pyriform (pear shaped). Four organisms may be joined, giving the effect of a Maltese cross (Figure 11-17). Individual organisms are 2 to 3 µm long. Trophozoites of *B. caballi* are pyriform, round, or oval and 2 to 4 µm long. They occur characteristically in pairs at acute angles to each other (Figure 11-18).

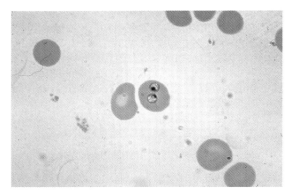

Figure 11-18   Trophozoites of *Babesia caballi* in red blood cells in stained equine blood smear. These piroplasms are pyriform, round, or oval and 2 to 4 µm long. They occur characteristically in pairs at acute angles to each other.

UROGENITAL SYSTEM

The protozoans that infect the urogenital system of horses are apicomplexans.

Apicomplexans

Klossiella equi is a nonpathogenic coccidian infecting the kidney of horses. Oocysts can occasionally be found during histopathologic examination of the kidney and in urine sediment.

There is no marked inflammatory response to infection with *Klossiella* in the horse.

NERVOUS SYSTEM

Apicomplexans are the protozoans that infect the nervous system of horses.

Apicomplexans

Sarcocystis neurona is sporadically found in the asexual, or schizogonous, stage of development in the nervous system, particularly the spinal cord, of horses. This stage can invade the central nervous system, producing a condition called *equine protozoal myeloencephalitis* (EPM). This disease most often affects Standardbreds and Thoroughbreds. Clinical signs are ataxia, weakness, stumbling, muscle wasting, and disorientation. EPM can resemble many other equine neurologic diseases, including wobbler syndrome, the neurologic form of herpesvirus infection, rabies, West Nile virus infection, and other equine viral encephalitis diseases (e.g., Eastern and Western equine encephalitis). These developmental stages cannot be seen antemortem. Diagnosis of this parasite is by histopathologic examination. Tissues suspected of harboring developmental stages of *S. neurona* should be submitted to a histopathology laboratory for diagnosis by a veterinary pathologist or parasitologist.

Sarcocystis neurona causes encephalomyelitis in many species of mammals and is the most important cause of neurologic disease in horses. Its complete life cycle is unknown, particularly its development and localization in the raccoon intermediate host.

SWINE

GASTROINTESTINAL TRACT

Protozoans that infect the gastrointestinal tract of swine are ciliates and apicomplexans.

Ciliates

Balantidium coli is the ciliated protozoan found in the large intestine of swine. Although it is often

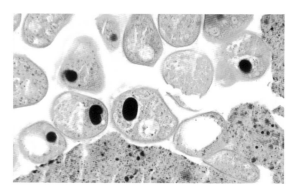

Figure 11-19 Motile trophozoite stage of *Balantidium coli*, ciliated protozoan found in the large intestine of swine, is often observed during microscopic examination of fresh diarrheic feces. It is covered with numerous rows of cilia and moves about the field of view with lively motility.

observed during microscopic examination of fresh diarrheic feces, it is generally considered to be nonpathogenic. Two morphologic stages can be found in feces: the cyst stage and the trophozoite stage. Both stages may vary in size. This is a very large protozoan parasite. The trophozoites may be 150 by 120 μm, with a sausage-to-kidney–shaped macronucleus. *B. coli* is covered with numerous rows of cilia and moves about the field with lively motility. The cyst is spherical to ovoid, 40 to 60 μm in diameter, and has a slight greenish yellow color. Both these stages may be easily recognized by microscopic examination of the intestinal contents of fresh, diarrheic feces. Figure 11-19 demonstrates the trophozoite stage of *B. coli* recovered on fecal flotation, and Figures 11-20 and 11-21 demonstrate *B. coli* in histopathologic section.

Apicomplexans

Isospora suis is the coccidian that parasitizes the small intestine of swine, especially young piglets. Oocysts are usually found on flotation of fresh feces. They are subspherical, lack the micropyle, and measure 18 to 21 μm. Postmortem diagnosis in piglets exhibiting clinical signs but not shedding oocysts can be achieved by direct smear of the jejunum stained with Diff-

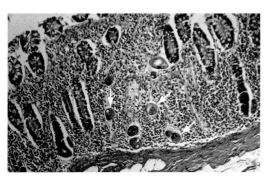

Figure 11-20 *Balantidium coli* of swine in histopathologic section. This photomicrograph was taken at low magnification. Note that *B. coli* is quite large and easily visible *(arrows)*.

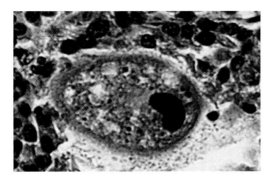

Figure 11-21 *Balantidium coli* of swine in histopathologic section. This photomicrograph was taken at higher magnification than Figure 11-20.

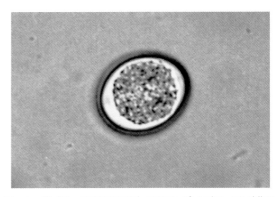

Figure 11-22 Unsporulated oocyst of swine coccidian, *Isospora suis,* recovered from swine feces. (560×.)

Quik. Diagnosis is by observation of the banana-shaped merozoites. The prepatent period is 4 to 8 days. (See Figure 11-22 for features of the oocyst of *I. suis.*)

Cryptosporidium species is another coccidian that parasitizes the small intestine of a variety of animals, including swine. The sporulated oocysts in the feces are colorless and transparent and measure only 3 to 5 μm. Diagnosis is by standard fecal flotation and stained fecal smears. Because humans may become infected with *Cryptosporidium* species, feces suspected of harboring this protozoan should be handled with great care. (See Figure 11-8 for features of the oocysts of *Cryptosporidium* species.)

PET AND AVIARY BIRDS AND OTHER DOMESTIC FOWL

GASTROINTESTINAL TRACT

Protozoans that infect the gastrointestinal tract of birds are flagellates and apicomplexans.

Flagellates

Giardia species is the most common protozoan seen in pet bird practices. This flagellated parasite is most often found in cockatiels, budgerigars, and lovebirds. The feces of affected birds often becomes voluminous and chunky, with a pea-soup consistency. Fresh saline mounts can demonstrate the motile trophozoites, with the characteristic "falling leaf" motility. Allergic skin conditions may be associated with giardiasis in cockatiels. It may be difficult to demonstrate *Giardia* in some of these cases.

The fecal trichrome stain can enhance visualization of *Giardia* species (Figure 11-23). Other stains used to enhance visualization of this flagellate include Lugol's iodine, Gram's iodine, and Wright's stain. Other stains, such as acid-fast stain or Gram's stain, may incidentally demonstrate trophozoites (Figure 11-24).

Histomonas meleagridis infects turkeys and peafowl, causing a fatal liver disease called *infectious enterohepatitis,* or "blackhead." Diagnosis is usually by histopathologic examination of the

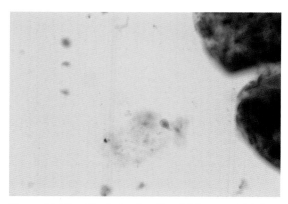

Figure 11-23 *Giardia* trophozoites (trichrome stain) from feces of cockatiel.

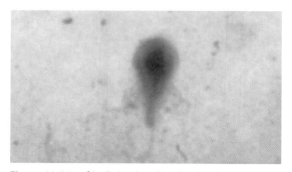

Figure 11-24 *Giardia* trophozoite, showing flagellar detail, in Gram-stained fecal smear. This was an incidental finding, because Gram's stain is not the stain of choice for flagellates.

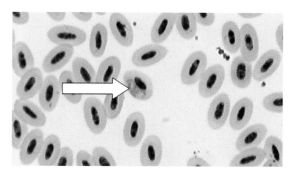

Figure 11-25 *Trichomonas gallinae* in crop wash from dove.

liver. Suspect tissues should be submitted to a histopathology laboratory for diagnosis by a veterinary pathologist or parasitologist. Suspicion of infection is increased by finding the eggs of the cecal worm, *Heterakis gallinarum,* which serves as the intermediate host for this parasite.

Trichomonas gallinae is frequently found in crop washes and crop swabs of pigeons, doves, and poultry. Occasionally, this parasite is associated with mortality in finches. In North America, trichomoniasis appears to be rare in psittacine birds but has been reported in budgerigars. The parasite is best demonstrated by a direct saline smear of crop contents and is characterized by four anterior flagella. An air-dried smear can be stained with Wright's stain. The parasite assumes an oval shape, staining blue with a red axostyle (Figure 11-25).

Apicomplexans

Coccidial infections are rare in pet birds, although *Isospora* and *Eimeria* have been reported. Coccidia are often observed in poultry and pigeons. A common error made by inexperienced veterinary technicians is to mistake normal urate crystals for coccidia. *Cryptosporidium* species has been reported in cockatiels. This tiny apicomplexan parasite is difficult to visualize in fecal samples and is usually diagnosed by histopathologic examination of the small intestine. Suspect tissues should be submitted to a histopathology laboratory for diagnosis by a veterinary pathologist or parasitologist.

CIRCULATORY SYSTEM AND BLOOD

Protozoans that infect the circulatory system and blood of birds are flagellates and apicomplexans.

Flagellates

Trypanosoma species is occasionally found in cockatoos and rarely produces clinical disease. As with the trypanosomes of mammals, this swimming, flagellated protozoan does not infect the RBCs. It has a very distinctive appearance, with posterior flagellum and an undulating membrane (Figure 11-26).

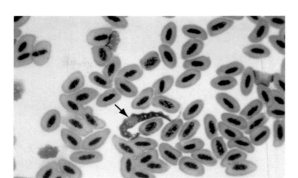

Figure 11-26 *Trypanosoma* species in blood of cockatoo.

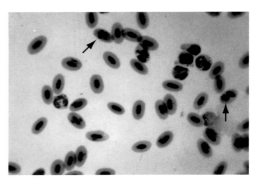

Figure 11-28 *Plasmodium* displacing nucleus of erythrocyte in blood of canary.

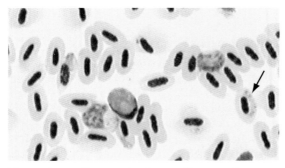

Figure 11-27 *Haemoproteus* is normally seen as "sausage-shaped body" within cytoplasm of avian red blood cell.

Apicomplexans

Haemoproteus species is often found within the RBCs of the white species of cockatoos, green-winged macaws, and some species of conures. This blood parasite is rarely associated with clinical disease, such as anemia. *Haemoproteus* is characterized by a bluish, sausage-shaped body in the cytoplasm of the RBC; sometimes the body is overlaid with blue dots (Figure 11-27). It infects a variety of wild waterfowl and can cause death in these birds.

Plasmodium species is the etiologic agent of avian malaria. It can cause mortality in canaries in some parts of the United States. This may be the result of the transmission of a local passerine strain by the mosquito intermediate host to susceptible canaries. The organism may not be observable in the peripheral blood cells; many of

the developmental stages of *Plasmodium* species occur in internal organs, such as the liver and spleen. A "signet ring" form, in which the body of the organism displaces the nucleus of the RBC, is the most frequently observed form (Figure 11-28). Diagnosis of infections with *Plasmodium* species is also by organ impression smears and histopathologic examination of the liver and the spleen. Tissues suspected of harboring developmental stages of *Plasmodium* should be submitted to a histopathology laboratory for confirmation by a veterinary pathologist or parasitologist.

Leucocytozoon species infects the white blood cells of raptors, birds of prey such as owls, hawks, and falcons. The presence of this large protozoan organism greatly distorts the shape and appearance of the white blood cell. A variety of forms can be present and can be associated with occasional leukocytosis and disease. The most common morphology of this protozoan is the fusiform, or spindle, shape (Figure 11-29).

Aegyptianella species is occasionally found in pet birds, such as the African gray parrot. This protozoan causes little clinical problem. The organism infects the RBCs, appearing as a marginated dot on the cells.

RESPIRATORY SYSTEM

The protozoans that infect the respiratory system of birds are apicomplexans.

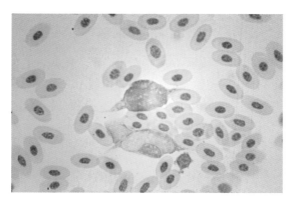

Figure 11-29 *Leucocytozoon* species in avian peripheral blood smear.

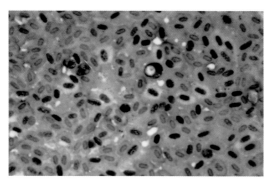

Figure 11-30 *Atoxoplasma serini* in mononuclear cell on lung impression smear from canary (Wright's stain).

Apicomplexans

Atoxoplasma serini is a protozoan parasite of canaries and finches (Figure 11-30). *Atoxoplasma* can affect several organs, causing respiratory signs. This parasite is best visualized on organ impression smears of the lung, liver, and spleen.

RABBITS

GASTROINTESTINAL TRACT

The protozoans that infect the gastrointestinal tract of rabbits are apicomplexans.

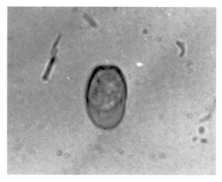

Figure 11-31 Unsporulated oocyst of rabbit intestinal coccidian, *Eimeria magna.*

Apicomplexans

Numerous species of *Eimeria* can infect rabbits. Most infect the intestine, causing intestinal coccidiosis, and one species, *Eimeria stiedai,* affects the bile ducts within the liver. The more pathogenic varieties of *Eimeria* species that affect the intestine are discussed in this section, and *E. stiedai* is considered separately. The intestinal coccidia of rabbits include *Eimeria irresidua, E. magna, E. media,* and *E. perforans.* All species of *Eimeria* infect the small intestine; *E. media* may also affect the large intestine.

The oocysts of *E. irresidua* are 38 by 26 μm and ovoid. The wall of the oocyst is smooth and light yellow. There is a wide micropyle, with no polar granules or residuum. Sporocysts within the oocyst are also ovoid, with both a body and residuum. Antemortem diagnosis depends on recognition of the mature oocyst, along with clinical signs, which may include severe hemorrhagic diarrhea, excessive thirst, and dehydration. Postmortem indications include inflammation of the intestines and sloughing of the lining of the intestine.

The mature oocyst of *E. magna* is 35 by 24 μm and ovoid, with a distinctive dark, yellow-brown wall (Figure 11-31). A wide micropyle appears built-up around the rim, with no micropyle cap. Oocysts and sporocysts contain a residuum (Figure 11-32). The sporocysts are ovoid and

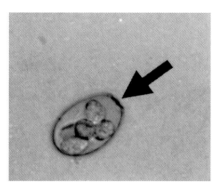

Figure 11-32   Oocyst of *Eimeria magna* after sporulation. Arrow indicates micropyle. Round darkened body in center of oocyst is residuum. Four oval lighter bodies are sporocysts.

have a body. *E. magna,* like *E. irresidua,* is highly pathogenic. Clinical signs include weight loss, anorexia, and mucoid diarrhea. Necropsy signs include inflammation and sloughing of the lining of the intestine.

E. media oocysts are ovoid and 31 by 18 µm, with a smooth wall and a light-pink color. There is a micropyle and a residuum. Sporocysts within the mature oocyst are ovoid, with a body and a residuum. *E. media* is moderately pathogenic and may cause enteritis and diarrhea. At necropsy, the intestinal wall may be edematous and contain gray foci of necrosis.

E. stiedai is a highly pathogenic coccidian that affects the bile ducts of rabbits. It causes variable mortality, which is highest in young rabbits. Oocysts of *E. stiedai* are 35 by 20 µm and ovoid, with a flattened pole at the micropyle end. The wall is smooth and yellow. There is no polar granule or residuum. Sporocysts are ovoid, with a body and a residuum.

Light infections with *E. stiedai* usually produce no clinical signs. Heavier infections may cause blockage of the bile ducts and impaired liver function, resulting in icterus and a distended abdomen caused by liver enlargement. Diarrhea or constipation and anorexia may be noted. At necropsy, white, dilated nodules are likely to be seen in the liver. Hyperplastic bile ducts contain a yellow-green creamy material, in which oocysts may be seen in impression smears when examined microscopically. Transmission of *E. stiedai* is by ingestion of sporulated oocysts passed in the feces. The prepatent period is 15 to 18 days. As in all *Eimeria* species, there is no cross-species contamination or public health significance.

MICE

GASTROINTESTINAL TRACT

Protozoans that infect the gastrointestinal tract of mice are flagellates and apicomplexans.

Flagellates

A few flagellates may be found by direct smear or fecal flotation from the mouse. They include *Giardia muris, Spironucleus muris, Tetratrichomonas microti,* and *Tritrichomonas muris.*

T. microti and *T. muris* are generally considered nonpathogenic in the mouse. Tritrichomonads and tetratrichomonads have three and four anterior flagella, respectively. Both genera have a trailing caudal flagellum. These trichomonads are frequently found in the small intestine, cecum, and colon of the mouse. Mice with diarrhea, regardless of the etiology, often have numerous tritrichomonads and tetratrichomonads because the diarrheic fluid medium secondarily provides an optimal habitat for the multiplication of these intestinal protozoa. Transmission of these trichomonads is by ingestion of organisms passed in the feces. *T. microti* is approximately 22 by 10 µm, and *T. muris* is approximately 7 by 5 µm.

G. muris and *S. muris* are the most common mouse flagellates and demonstrate the greatest potential for pathogenicity. Both *S. muris* and *G. muris* occur in the proximal small intestine and can produce enteritis, particularly in young weanling mice. The location of these flagellates in the intestines is proportional to the severity of the enteritis produced; the more severe the enteritis, the farther back (more distally) in the intestinal tract they are found. *G. muris* appears similar to other *Giardia* species. The trophozoite is pyriform (pear shaped), with two nuclei at the anterior end. Eight flagella emerge in symmetric pairs from different locations cranial to caudal in the organism. *Giardia* species may be suspected when motile forms are observed on a direct smear at 100× (high dry) magnification. *Giardia* species are identified by staining the direct fecal smear with Lugol's iodine, which will enhance the detail of the cranial nuclei and flagella.

Transmission of *G. muris* is by ingestion of cysts that have been passed in the feces. *G. muris* has also been found in the rat and hamster; therefore the owner of multiple species should be made aware of the possibility of cross-contamination. Although other species of *Giardia* are pathogenic to humans, the *Giardia* species found in rodents and rabbits have no known zoonotic potential.

S. muris appears somewhat similar to *Giardia* species except that the trophozoite of *S. muris* is uniformly slender, unlike the widened anterior end of *Giardia* species. *S. muris* has two anterior nuclei. There are three pairs of anterior flagella and one pair of trailing caudal flagella.

Apicomplexans

Several species of *Eimeria* infect mice, including *E. falciformis*, *E. ferrisi,* and *E. hansonorum*. *E. falciformis* and *E. hansorium* infect the small intestine, whereas *E. ferrisi* is found in the cecum. Although mixed infections can occur, little is known concerning the pathogenicity of *E. ferrisi* and *E. hansorium.*

E. falciformis is common in wild mouse populations. Oocysts are 14 to 26 µm by 11 to 24 µm, round to oval, smooth, and colorless. There is no micropyle or residuum. Sporocysts are oval and have a residuum and a small body. There are two sporozoites per sporocyst and four sporocysts per sporulated oocyst. Oocysts of *E. ferrisi* and *E. hansonorum* appear similar to those of *E. falciformis,* except they are small, 16 to 18 µm, and more spherical. *E. ferrisi* has a small body on the sporocysts, whereas *E. hansonorum* has a broad body.

Oocysts of *Eimeria* species can be detected by fecal flotation. As in coccidial infections in other species, finding oocysts on fecal flotation does not necessarily mean that *Eimeria* species is a primary cause of the disease. Diagnosis is made by considering clinical signs, enteric lesions, and identification of the coccidia in histopathologic section. Again, tissues suspected of harboring developmental stages of murine coccidiosis should be submitted to a histopathology laboratory for confirmation by a veterinary pathologist or parasitologist.

Clinical signs, if seen, are usually in younger animals that have developed little to no immunity and may include diarrhea, catarrhal enteritis, anorexia, hemorrhage, and epithelial sloughing.

As with other species of *Eimeria,* transmission is by ingestion of sporulated oocysts that have been passed in the feces. Oocysts passed in the feces sporulate in about 3 days. *Eimeria* species are host specific and thus are not considered zoonotic parasites.

UROGENITAL SYSTEM

The protozoans that infect the urogenital system of mice are apicomplexans.

Apicomplexans

Klossiella muris is a relatively nonpathogenic coccidian that occurs mainly in the kidneys of both wild and laboratory mice. This parasite has also been found in different stages of its life cycle in the adrenal and thyroid glands and in the brain, lung, and spleen. The oocyst of *K. muris* matures in the endothelial cells that line the arterioles and capillaries associated with the glomeruli of the kidney. At maturity, the oocyst is 40 µm in diameter. The oocyst grows and divides to form sporoblasts, which eventually rupture the host endothelial cell and pass through the urine as sporocysts. Other mice are then infected by ingestion of sporulated oocysts.

K. muris cannot be detected antemortem. On postmortem examination, the kidneys may appear enlarged and have small, gray necrotic areas on the surface. Histopathologic examination reveals that most of the necrotic areas are at the corticomedullary junction. Infection with *K. muris* is usually diagnosed from gross and microscopic lesions, including finding the organism in renal tissue. Tissues suspected of harboring developmental stages of renal coccidiosis should be submitted to a histopathology laboratory for confirmation by a veterinary pathologist or parasitologist.

Transmission of *K. muris* is by ingestion of the sporulated sporocysts passed in the urine. Because wild mice can carry this parasite, strict sanitation and prevention of wild mouse access to the pet population are necessary to control this parasite. *K. muris* is species specific and is not a zoonotic parasite.

RATS

GASTROINTESTINAL TRACT

The protozoans that infect the gastrointestinal tract of rats are flagellates and apicomplexans.

Flagellates

Although somewhat less susceptible than mice, rats may be infected with the flagellates discussed previously in the mouse section: *Giardia muris, Spironucleus muris, Tetratrichomonas microti,* and *Tritrichomonas muris.* Identification, detection, clinical signs, and transmission in rats are similar to those discussed for the mouse.

Apicomplexans

Eimeria nieschultzi is an intestinal coccidian uncommon in laboratory rats but common in wild rats. The sporulated oocyst of *E. nieschultzi* is oval, 16 to 26 µm by 13 to 21 µm, with no residuum. It has a smooth or colorless wall, with no micropyle. The sporulated oocyst contains four oval sporocysts, each with a small Stieda body and a residuum.

Antemortem, *E. nieschultzi* may be detected by finding the oocysts in fecal flotations or direct fecal smears. However, diagnosis is usually based on identification of the organism histopathologically in sections of the intestinal epithelium. Clinical signs of *E. nieschultzi* infections are usually seen in young rats less than several months of age. Signs include diarrhea, weakness, emaciation, and possibly death. Rats become infected with *E. nieschultzi* by ingestion of sporulated oocysts in the feces. *E. nieschultzi* is species specific and therefore is not considered a potential cross-contaminant or zoonotic problem.

HAMSTERS

GASTROINTESTINAL TRACT

The protozoans that infect the gastrointestinal tract of hamsters are flagellates.

Flagellates

Hamsters typically carry numerous intestinal flagellates without showing clinical signs. These parasites can be observed in fecal flotations or direct smear preparations. These flagellates include *Giardia* species, *Spironucleus muris, Tetranucleus microti,* and *Tritrichomonas muris (criceti).* Infected hamsters may serve as a source of infection for more susceptible rodents, such as in the transmission of *S. muris* to mice.

Identification, detection, clinical signs, transmission, and public health significance of this parasite in hamsters are similar to those discussed for the mouse.

GUINEA PIGS

GASTROINTESTINAL TRACT

The protozoans that infect the gastrointestinal tract of guinea pigs are flagellates, amoebae, and apicomplexans.

Flagellates

Trophozoites of *Giardia caviae* are similar to those of *G. muris,* as previously described. The body is pyriform, or pear shaped. Two nuclei lie at the anterior end, and four pairs of flagella emerge at various points of the body. Trophozoites are 8 to 15 µm by 6.5 µm. Cysts are about the same size as the trophozoites and contain two to four nuclei.

Cysts or trophozoites of *G. caviae* may be detected in a direct fecal smear or possibly in a fecal flotation preparation. If fecal flotation is used, zinc sulfate solution is preferred because sugar and salt solutions may distort the cysts. Diarrheic animals should be examined by direct smear for the presence of motile trophozoites; cyst forms will not be present.

There are no specific clinical signs in infected guinea pigs; however, mucoid diarrhea has been reported in other infected rodents. *G. caviae* is not considered a public health problem.

Tritrichomonas caviae is of little or no pathologic significance in the guinea pig. As with *T. muris*, *T. caviae* has three anterior flagella and a trailing posterior flagellum. *T. caviae* measures 10 to 22 µm by 6 to 11 µm and is larger than *G. caviae*. It has an undulating membrane that extends the length of its body. These trichomonads are usually found in the cecum of the guinea pig. The veterinary technician should be aware that in cases of protracted diarrhea produced by another pathogen, *T. caviae* protozoans proliferate secondarily because of the fluid medium produced by the diarrhea. *T. caviae* therefore may be observed on direct fecal smear, particularly in animals exhibiting clinical signs of diarrhea.

T. caviae is transmitted between guinea pigs by ingestion of the trophozoites passed in the feces of carrier animals. *T. caviae* is not seen in other species of animals and is not considered a public health hazard.

Amoebae

Entamoeba caviae is a relatively common nonpathogenic cecal organism in guinea pigs; it is mentioned in this chapter to make the veterinary technician aware that it should be disregarded as a pathogenic organism. The most frequently observed form of this protozoan is the motile trophozoite. Cysts are infrequently observed on concentration with zinc sulfate flotation medium. Mature cysts are 11 to 27 µm and have eight nuclei. The trophozoites are most often found in a direct fecal smear and measure 10.5 to 20 µm in diameter. The appearance of these trophozoite stages can be enhanced by staining the direct fecal smear with Lugol's iodine.

E. caviae is transmitted by ingestion of infective cyst forms that have been passed in the feces of chronic carrier guinea pigs. *Entamoeba caviae* is species specific and is not considered to be of zoonotic significance.

Apicomplexans

Eimeria caviae is a typical coccidian, with an oval to slightly subspherical oocyst that is 13 to 26 µm by 12 to 23 µm. Oocyst walls are brown and have no micropyle or polar granule. However, oocysts contain a residuum, as do sporocysts. *E. caviae* is commonly found in the guinea pig's large intestine, particularly the ascending or proximal colon.

E. caviae can be detected by fecal flotation. Repeated flotation should be done 4 to 5 days apart for 2 to 3 weeks. Diagnosis is made more consistently postmortem, at which time intestinal scrapings placed into saline may be examined microscopically for both intracellular intestinal stages and oocysts of *E. caviae*.

E. caviae is generally nonpathogenic, but young animals stressed by poor nutrition and husbandry may show clinical signs. Clinical signs are limited to diarrhea seen 11 to 13 days after exposure. The diarrhea ceases after a few days if the animal is not reinfected. Diarrhea may continue if reinfection occurs. As with the other protozoans of guinea pigs, *Eimeria caviae* is species specific and is not considered to be of zoonotic significance.

Cryptosporidium wrairi of guinea pigs is similar to *C. parvum* and *C. muris* of mice. However, *C. wrairi* is considered a distinct species. *C. wrairi* is most often seen lining the tips of the intestinal villi in the ileum of young guinea pigs. Examination of fresh mucosal scrapings by phase-contrast microscopy may provide the best results in the detection and identification of *C. wrairi*. Examination of paraffin-embedded materials is least satisfactory, especially when formalin is used as a fixative. The organisms appear to be extracellular but actually are within the microvilli of the intestinal epithelial cells. The only clinical sign of *C. wrairi* infection is weight loss. Younger guinea pigs at 250 to 300 g are most likely to carry the parasite. Older animals seem to be resistant or to have developed immunity to *C. wrairi*. *C. wrairi* is not found in other species of animals and is not considered a public health problem.

FISH

SKIN

Protozoans that infect the skin of fish are ciliates.

Ciliates

Ichthyophthirius multifiliis is a ciliate that infects the skin, gills, fins, and eyes of many freshwater tropical and ornamental fish in home aquaria and in hatcheries. This ciliated protozoan causes a skin disease called ***ichthyophthiriosis,*** or, more commonly, "ich." Ich is characterized by the formation of tiny white spots (the thin-walled trophozoite stage just beneath the epidermis) over many of the exposed surfaces of the fish. These parasites may be from 100 to 1000 μm in diameter, so they are grossly visible to the observer. Diagnosis is by observation of typical lesions; however, it is possible to perform skin scrapings on infected fish to reveal characteristic ciliates. A similar parasite, *Cryptocaryon irritans,* affects warm water marine (saltwater) fish. Other ciliates infecting fish include *Chilodonella, Tetrahymena,* and *Piscinoodinium.* As with *I. multifiliis,* there are marine counterparts for these genera. For details of these and other protozoan parasites of both freshwater and marine fish, a fish disease textbook should be consulted.

Introduction to the Arthropods

12

ARTHROPODA

The phylum Arthropoda is one of the largest phyla. There are more than a million species of arthropods, including the extinct trilobites, spiders, mites, ticks, crabs, crayfish, lobsters, water fleas, copepods, millipedes, centipedes, and other insects. The insects include the cockroaches, beetles, bedbugs, fleas, bees, ants, wasps, mosquitoes, butterflies, moths, grasshoppers, lice, silverfish, and dragonflies. With more than 900,000 species, insects are by far the largest class within the phylum Arthropoda.

KEY MORPHOLOGIC FEATURES

The name *arthropod* means "jointed foot" (*arthro* means "joint," and *pod* means "foot"). All adult arthropods have jointed appendages. All arthropods also are covered with a chitinous exoskeleton that is composed of segments; every arthropod has a segmented body covered with chitin. *Chitin* is a hard (yet elastic) body covering that envelops the entire body of all arthropods. Whenever you step on a cockroach, the chitin makes the "crunch" sound. Arthropods have a *hemocoel,* a body cavity filled with hemolymph. *Hemolymph* is a bloodlike fluid that bathes the internal organs of an arthropod. When a flying insect hits the windshield of a speeding car and "splats," hemolymph is the fluid that creates the "splat." Arthropods have a very simple circulatory system composed of a heartlike dorsal tube. This dorsal tube is actually a primitive heart that pumps the hemolymph to the arthropod's head. The digestive system of arthropods begins with a *ventral mouth* and ends with a *terminal anus.* Arthropods possess a variety of respiratory systems; they may use gills, book lungs, or tracheal tubes as respiratory organs. Arthropods have complex nervous and excretory systems. However, the most important organ system of the arthropods is the reproductive system. Arthropods have separate sexes; they are *dioecious.* Reproduction is by means of eggs. Arthropods have a tremendous reproductive capacity.

DIVISIONS OF THE PHYLUM ARTHROPODA

The phylum Arthropoda is made up of the following subphyla: Trilobitomorpha (the extinct trilobites), Onychophora (onychophorans, or "living fossils"), Tardigrada (water bears), Pycnogonida (sea spiders), Chelicerata (mites, ticks, spiders, scorpions, and others), and Mandibulata (crustaceans, centipedes and millipedes, and insects). Most of the arthropods that are important in veterinary parasitology are members of the *Chelicerata* and the *Mandibulata.*

Members of the phylum Arthropoda are important because (1) they may serve as causal agents themselves, (2) they may produce venoms or toxic substances, (3) they may serve as intermediate hosts for protozoan and helminth parasites, and (4) they may serve as vectors for bacteria, viruses, spirochetes, rickettsiae, chlamydial agents, and other pathogens.

CRUSTACEA (AQUATIC ARTHROPODS)

Phylum: Arthropoda
  Subphylum: Mandibulata
    Class: Crustacea (aquatic arthropods)
Members of the class Crustacea are always aquatic. Crustaceans are important because they serve as intermediate hosts for many helminth parasites, including flukes (e.g., *Paragonimus kellicotti*), tapeworms (e.g., *Spirometra mansonoides*), and roundworms (e.g., *Dracunculus insignis*). Crustaceans also serve as causal agents because they are ectoparasites of many fish, amphibians, and exotic reptiles.

MYRIOPODA (CENTIPEDES AND MILLIPEDES)

Phylum: Arthropoda
  Subphylum: Mandibulata
    Class: Myriopoda (centipedes and millipedes)
Members of the class Myriopoda are represented by centipedes and millipedes. Myriopodans are important because they produce venoms and toxic substances. Centipedes and millipedes are usually slow-moving arthropods. As defense

mechanisms, they are capable of producing venoms and toxic substances that can sting, blind, paralyze, burn, or even kill.

INSECTA (INSECTS)

Phylum: Arthropoda
  Subphylum: Mandibulata
    Class: Insecta (insects)
As mentioned earlier, the class Insecta has the largest number of members (>900,000 species) in the phylum Arthropoda. This is also the most diverse group. Members of the class Insecta are important because (1) they may serve as causal agents themselves, (2) they may produce venoms or toxic substances, (3) they may serve as intermediate hosts for protozoan and helminth parasites, and (4) they may serve as vectors for bacteria, viruses, spirochetes, rickettsiae, chlamydial agents, and other pathogens. Examples of all of these important pathogenic mechanisms are covered in Chapter 13.

KEY MORPHOLOGIC FEATURES

As members of the phylum Arthropoda, insects share the following morphologic characteristics: a segmented body with three pairs of segmented legs, bilateral symmetry, a chitinous exoskeleton, a dorsal heart, a ventral nerve cord, a digestive system from mouth to anus, an excretory system, and a reproductive system. As with all other arthropods, insects are dioecious (they, too, have separate sexes) and demonstrate a tremendous reproductive capacity.

The body of all adult insects is divided into three basic body sections: the head, thorax, and abdomen. The *head* is on the anterior, or front end, of the insect; the head contains the insect's brain and also has the antennae, the ventrally directed mouthparts, and the eyes (if eyes are present; some insects are eyeless). The *thorax* is the middle body section. The thorax of the adult insect always has three pairs of legs and may have either one or two pairs of wings; however, many insects, such as lice and fleas, are wingless.

The *abdomen* is the posterior, or the hind section, of the insect. It often contains the reproductive organs but has no ventral, segmented appendages (e.g., mouthparts of the head, legs of the thorax).

To achieve the size and development of the adult insect, the young insect must undergo changes in size, form, and structure. This series of changes is called *metamorphosis.* For the purposes of this text, there are two types of metamorphosis: simple metamorphosis and complex metamorphosis. *Simple metamorphosis* consists of three developmental stages: the egg stage, the nymphal stage, and the adult stage. In this form of metamorphosis, the nymphal stage resembles the adult stage in form, except that it is smaller and is not sexually mature (and therefore cannot reproduce). In winged insects the wings may be absent in the nymphal stage. An example of an insect that undergoes simple metamorphosis is the cockroach.

Complex metamorphosis consists of four developmental stages: the egg stage, the larval stage, the pupal stage, and the adult stage. None of these developmental stages bears a resemblance to any of the others. The egg stage does not resemble the larval stage, which in turn does not resemble the pupal stage, which in turn does not resemble the adult stage. The larval stage is described as "wormlike." To reach the adult stage, the insect must develop through the pupal stage, which is a resting stage. The adult stage emerges from the pupal stage and eventually becomes sexually mature and reproduces, producing large numbers of offspring.

ORDERS OF INSECTA

With regard to veterinary parasitology, the class Insecta is further divided into nine orders. The orders of greatest significance in parasitology are Dictyoptera (cockroaches and grasshoppers), Coleoptera (beetles), Lepidoptera (moths and butterflies), Hemiptera (true bugs), Hymenoptera (ants, bees, wasps, yellow jackets, and other stinging insects), Anoplura (sucking lice), Mallophaga (chewing lice), Diptera (two-winged flies), and Siphonaptera (fleas). Each of the orders within the class Insecta and their relative importance in veterinary medicine are discussed in detail in Chapter 13.

ACARINA (MITES AND TICKS)

Phylum: Arthropoda
  Subphylum: Chelicerata
    Class: Acarina (mites and ticks)

The subphylum Mandibulata comprises crustaceans, centipedes and millipedes, and insects. The members of the subphylum Chelicerata include mites, ticks, spiders, and scorpions. Within this subphylum are members of the class Arachnida, order Acarina, the mites and the ticks. Mites and ticks are often referred to as *acarines,* and infestation with mites or ticks is referred to as *acariasis.*

Mites and ticks are *not* insects; they are acarines. They are morphologically different from insects. First, the body segmentation of mites and ticks is different from that of insects. Insects are divided into head, thorax, and abdomen; mites and ticks, however, have lost all the external signs of body segmentation and are divided into two body components, the *capitulum* (the "mouthparts," or a fusion of the head and thorax) and the *idiosoma* (the abdomen). Discussions in this text refer to the two basic body parts of mites and ticks as the "mouthparts" and the "abdomen." Whereas insects may have antennae, wings, and compound eyes, acarines lack these structures. The mouthparts of the mites and ticks have two basic functions: sucking blood or tissue fluids or attaching or holding onto the host. The following organ systems are represented in mites and ticks: digestive, excretory, respiratory, nervous, and reproductive systems. As with the insects, mites and ticks are dioecious (have separate sexes) and possess a tremendous reproductive capacity.

In contrast to insects, mites and ticks do not undergo metamorphosis. There are four developmental stages in the life cycle of acarines: the egg stage, the larval stage, the nymphal stage, and the adult stage. The major difference among these life stages is that the larval acarine has three pairs of legs (or six legs), whereas both nymphal and adult acarines have four pairs of legs (or eight legs). Only the adult stage is capable of sexual reproduction.

Mites and ticks are significant in veterinary medicine and are discussed in detail in Chapter 13.

13

Arthropods That Infect and Infest Domestic Animals

The study of arthropods is referred to as *arthropodology.* Arthropods, members of the phylum Arthropoda, are important in veterinary parasitology for several reasons. Arthropods (1) serve as causal agents themselves by producing pathology or disease in domesticated or wild animals (or in humans); (2) serve as intermediate hosts for *helminths* (flukes, tapeworms, and roundworms) and *protozoans* (single-cell organisms) that infect domesticated or wild animals (or humans); (3) serve as vectors for bacteria, viruses, spirochetes, chlamydial agents, and other pathogens that produce disease in domesticated or wild animals (or humans); and (4) produce venoms and other substances that may be toxic to domesticated or wild animals (or humans). From one to four of these important criteria are true for each group of arthropods.

The phylum Arthropoda is broken down into several subphyla, two of which are important in veterinary parasitology. These two subphyla are the *Mandibulata* (crustaceans, myriopodans, and insects) and the *Chelicerata* (mites, ticks, spiders, and scorpions).

CRUSTACEANS

Kingdom: Animalia
  Phylum: Arthropoda (arthropods)
    Subphylum: Mandibulata (possess mandibulate mouthparts)
      Class: Crustacea (aquatic crustaceans)

Crustaceans are important in veterinary medicine for several reasons. First, crustaceans may be causal agents themselves when they serve as ectoparasites of fishes and amphibians. Tiny, microscopic crustaceans, such as *Argulus* species (Figure 13-1), parasitize the skin and gills of aquatic animals and can produce significant pathology. Crustaceans such as crabs can also be important as causal agents when they are swallowed by dogs that frequent beaches; in this scenario, crustaceans act as foreign bodies within the stomach or other portions of the gastrointestinal tract. Crustaceans may also serve as intermediate hosts for certain helminth parasites of domesticated animals. For example, the crayfish serves as the intermediate host for *Paragonimus kellicotti,* the lung fluke of dogs and cats. Certain aquatic copepods serve as first intermediate hosts for *Diphyllobothrium latum* and *Spirometra mansonoides,*

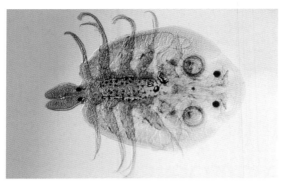

Figure 13-1. Tiny, microscopic *Argulus* species parasitizes skin and gills of fish.

pseudotapeworms of dogs and cats. Finally, certain freshwater crustaceans serve as the intermediate host for *Dracunculus insignis,* the guinea worm, a subcutaneous parasite of dogs.

MYRIOPODANS

Kingdom: Animalia
  Phylum: Arthropoda (arthropods)
    Subphylum: Mandibulata (possess
      mandibulate mouthparts)
      Class: Myriopoda (centipedes and
        millipedes)

The class Myriopoda comprises the centipedes and the millipedes. This strange class of arthropods is important because its members produce venoms or toxic substances.

Centipedes are usually small, terrestrial arthropods, predatory on creatures smaller than themselves. Centipedes have one pair of legs for every body segment. On the anterior end, they possess poison claws that connect to large poison glands. Centipedes often subdue their prey with these poison claws. It is important to note, however, that most of the truly poisonous centipedes are restricted to the jungles and areas of dense vegetation throughout the world and *not* to the continent of North America. Some pet stores sell exotic varieties of centipedes, and veterinarians are infrequently asked to "treat" these

exotic arthropods; however, a medical arthropodologist (or entomologist) might be consulted. Great care should be taken when handling all centipedes because they can bite. The bite of some of the larger centipede varieties has been likened to the sting of a hornet.

Millipedes are also small, terrestrial arthropods. Whereas centipedes are predatory on smaller creatures, millipedes are vegetarians. Millipedes have two pairs of legs for every body segment; remember that centipedes have only one pair. Beneath each pair of legs are repugnatorial glands that contain caustic substances capable of burning the skin. Millipedes are able to "squirt" these caustic, irritating substances onto the skin of any creature that might threaten them. As with the centipedes, most of the truly poisonous millipedes are restricted to the jungles and areas of dense vegetation throughout the world and *not* to the continent of North America. Some tribal people in these jungle areas grind up caustic millipedes and dip their arrow tips into the "juice" to make poisonous arrows. Although centipedes are sold as exotic pets in some pet stores, millipedes do not make good family pets.

INSECTS

Kingdom: Animalia
  Phylum: Arthropoda (arthropods)
    Subphylum: Mandibulata (possess
      mandibulate mouthparts)
      Class: Insecta (insects)

A major portion of this chapter discusses the orders of the class Insecta and their place in veterinary parasitology. The following orders are discussed:

Class: Insecta
  Order: Dictyoptera (cockroaches)
  Order: Coleoptera (beetles)
  Order: Lepidoptera (butterflies and moths)
  Order: Hymenoptera (ants, bees, and wasps)
  Order: Hemiptera (true bugs)
  Order: Mallophaga (chewing or biting lice)
  Order: Anoplura (sucking lice)

Order: Diptera (two-winged flies)
Order: Siphonaptera (fleas)

DICTYOPTERA (COCKROACHES)

Cockroaches are members of the order Dictyoptera. These disgusting creatures are perhaps the most commonly occurring insects that may actively "infest" a veterinary clinic. Because of their voracious feeding habits and their close association with stored food products (e.g., dried dog and cat food), cockroaches are often associated with the nocturnal environment of the veterinary clinic. Cockroaches habitually disgorge portions of their partly digested food and also defecate wherever they roam and feed. Under the proper circumstances, cockroaches may be incriminated in the natural transmission of pathogenic organisms, such as *Salmonella* species, to both humans and domesticated animals.

COLEOPTERA (BEETLES)

Members of the order Coleoptera, or beetles, are important because they may serve as intermediate hosts for certain parasites of domesticated animals. Dung beetles serve as intermediate host for *Spirocerca lupi,* the roundworm that produces esophageal nodules in dogs, and for *Gongylonema* species, a roundworm found in the tissues of the oral cavity and esophagus of goats and swine. Beetles can also serve as the intermediate host for the swine acanthocephalan, *Macracanthorhynchus hirudinaceus.*

Certain types of beetles, commonly called **blister beetles,** produce within their tissues a toxic substance called ***cantharidin*** (Figure 13-2). If these beetles are ingested by a mammalian host, they can produce a blistering of the skin, the oral mucosa, and the epithelium lining the alimentary tract. These beetles often infest the earth immediately below alfalfa hay, and when the hay is harvested, the beetles may be collected and subsequently fed to horses. When horses ingest these beetles, a fatal colic often results. Blister beetles have been referred to as "Spanish fly," a type of aphrodisiac or "love

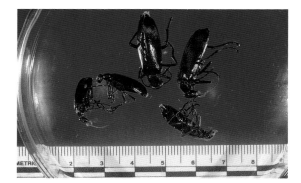

Figure 13-2   Blister beetles often infest alfalfa hay. They contain cantharidin, a toxic substance that produces colic in horses.

potion"; however, blister beetles are caustic and will burn living tissues and should not be used as an aphrodisiac.

LEPIDOPTERA (BUTTERFLIES AND MOTHS)

Members of the order Lepidoptera have two life cycle stages—the adult stage and the larval, or caterpillar, stage—that may be pathogenic to domestic animals. Some moths and butterflies in certain parts of Southeast Asia feed on the lachrymal (lacrimal) secretions (tears) of domestic and wild animals. These are exotic creatures, not native to North America. Some moths and butterflies from these exotic regions also have been known to suck blood.

Several species of larval moths and butterflies found in North America are covered with tiny, urticating, or stinging, hairs. Because caterpillars are often slow moving, these hairs serve as defense mechanisms against their predators. These stinging hairs cause significant stings in humans and domestic animals.

HYMENOPTERA (ANTS, BEES, AND WASPS)

The veterinarian should remember three basic facts about ants, bees, wasps, and hornets (members of the order Hymenoptera). First, "fire ants" are indigenous to the southeastern United States and can bite and sting almost any domesticated animal. "Downer cows" and newborn animals (weak, young lambs and calves and hatchling chicks) are particularly at risk to the perils of fire ants. Fire ants can attack any animal with which they come in contact. Second, bees, wasps, and hornets can sting domestic animals, particularly curious dogs and cats. These are minor envenomizations, seldom resulting in the death of an animal. Third, after being released in Brazil, Africanized honeybees, or "killer bees," have spread throughout South America and have crossed the border separating Texas and Mexico. Each year, these bees invade the United States to a greater extent. Almost any domestic animal (and humans) can be at risk of inadvertently disturbing a ground hive containing these bees and arousing its inhabitants. Death will often result from thousands of stings from these killer bees. Bees and wasps can cause anaphylactic reactions in allergic animals and humans. If not treated, these reactions can be severe enough to cause death.

If the veterinary diagnostician suspects that ants, bees, wasps, or hornets may be causing problems, the intact Hymenopteran should be collected in a sealed container containing 10% formalin or ethyl alcohol and submitted to an entomologist for identification.

HEMIPTERA (TRUE BUGS)

The veterinary diagnostician should remember the following basic facts about true bugs (members of the order Hemiptera). There are two groups of hemipterans that are of veterinary importance: reduviid bugs ("kissing bugs") and bedbugs. *Reduviid bugs* are *periodic* parasites; that is, they make frequent visits to the host to obtain a blood meal. Kissing bugs serve as intermediate hosts for *Trypanosoma cruzi,* a protozoan parasite that can produce a rare disease called *Chagas' disease* in humans and dogs. This disease is also called *South American trypanosomiasis* and is rarely diagnosed in the United States. *T. cruzi* infects a variety of internal organs; its infective stages swim in the blood of

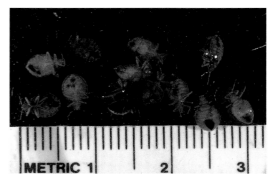

Figure 13-3 Bedbugs are periodic parasites of rabbit colonies, poultry houses, and pigeon colonies.

an infected host. Kissing bugs take blood meals from infected hosts and incubate the parasite in their intestinal tracts. The parasites are then transmitted to uninfected mammals as the bugs defecate. After taking a blood meal from a host, a kissing bug turns around and defecates on the feeding site. This inoculates the infective trypanosomes into the uninfected host. Kissing bugs play a key role in the transmission of Chagas' disease.

Bedbugs, Cimex lectularius, are the second type of hemipteran important in veterinary parasitology. Bedbugs are dorsoventrally flattened, wingless hemipterans that often infest human dwellings. They are periodic parasites, making frequent visits to the host to obtain a blood meal. Bedbugs are nocturnal feeders. Although bedbugs are most often incriminated as human parasites, they may also be found in rabbit colonies, poultry houses, and pigeon colonies, preying on domesticated animals (Figure 13-3). Unlike kissing bugs, bedbugs do not serve as intermediate hosts for pathogenic agents that infect humans or domestic animals.

If the veterinary diagnostician suspects that reduviid bugs or bedbugs may be causing problems, the intact hemipteran should be collected and stored in 10% formalin or ethyl alcohol and submitted to an entomologist for identification.

MALLOPHAGA (CHEWING OR BITING LICE) AND ANOPLURA (SUCKING LICE)

Lice are some of the most prolific ectoparasites of domesticated and wild animals. There are two orders of lice: **Mallophaga,** the chewing or biting lice, and **Anoplura,** the sucking lice. Lice are dorsoventrally flattened, wingless insects. As insects, lice have bodies divided into three divisions: (1) the head, with the mouthparts and antennae; (2) the thorax, with three pairs of legs and noticeable lack of wings; and (3) the abdomen, the portion that bears the reproductive organs. These body divisions and their relationship to each other are important in diagnostic veterinary parasitology.

Members of the order Mallophaga (chewing or biting lice) are usually smaller than members of the order Anoplura (sucking lice). Mallophagans are usually yellow and have a large, rounded head. The mouthparts are mandibulate and are adapted for chewing or biting. Characteristically, the head of every chewing louse is wider than the widest portion of the thorax. On the thorax are the three pairs of legs, which may be adapted for clasping or for moving rapidly among feathers or hairs. Chewing (biting) lice may parasitize birds, dogs, cats, cattle, sheep, goats, and horses. Chewing lice of cattle and fowl include *Damalinia bovis* (Figure 13-4), *Goniocotes*

gallinae (Figure 13-5), and *Menacanthus stramineus* (Figure 13-6).

Members of the order Anoplura (sucking lice) are larger than chewing lice. These lice range from red to gray; the color usually depends on the amount of blood that has been ingested from the host. In contrast to the large-headed mallophagans, anoplurans have a head that is narrower than the widest part of the thorax. Their mouthparts are of the piercing type and are adapted for sucking. Their pincerlike claws are adapted for clinging to the host's hairs. Interestingly, although they are found on many species of domestic animals, sucking lice do not parasitize birds or cats. Sucking lice of sheep, swine, monkeys, and dogs include, respectively, *Solenopotes capillatus* (Figure 13-7), *Haematopinus*

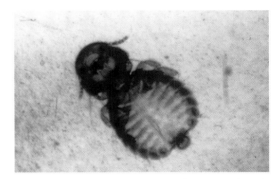

Figure 13-5 *Goniocotes gallinae*, the fluff louse of poultry.

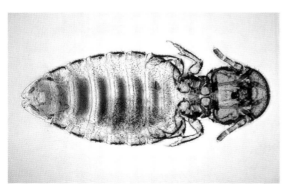

Figure 13-4 *Damalinia bovis*, the bovine biting, chewing louse.

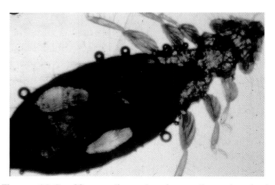

Figure 13-6 *Menacanthus stramineus*, the avian body louse.

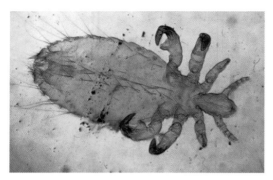

Figure 13-7 Sucking louse *Solenopotes capillatus* of sheep.

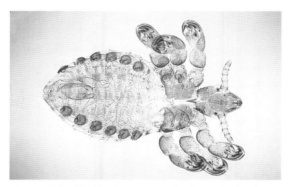

Figure 13-8 Sucking louse *Haematopinus suis* of swine.

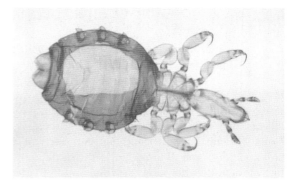

Figure 13-9 Sucking louse *Pedicinus obtusus* of monkeys.

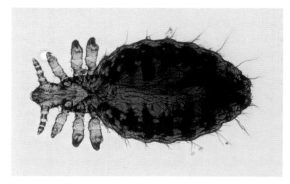

Figure 13-10 Sucking louse *Linognathus setosus* of dogs.

suis (Figure 13-8), *Pedicinus obtusus* (Figure 13-9), and *Linognathus setosus* (Figure 13-10).

Anoplurans and mallophagans have a life cycle consisting of three developmental stages. The *egg stage,* which is also called a *nit,* is tiny, approximately 0.5 to 1 mm in length. Nits are oval and white and are usually found cemented to the hair or feather shaft. Figure 13-11 shows *Linognathus setosus,* a gravid female sucking louse and an associated nit collected from a dog. Nits hatch about 5 to 14 days after being laid by the adult female louse. Thousands of nits can be "cemented" by female lice to the hair coat of domesticated animals (Figure 13-12). The *nymphal stage* is similar in appearance to the adult louse. However, the *nymph* is smaller and lacks functioning reproductive organs and genital openings. There are three nymphal

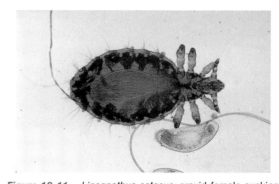

Figure 13-11 *Linognathus setosus;* gravid female sucking louse and associated nit on hair shaft collected from a dog. Nits are oval, white, and usually found cemented to hair or feather shaft of definitive host.

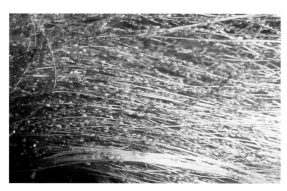

Figure 13-12 Thousands of nits can be cemented by female lice to hair coat of domesticated animals. This calf's tail contains thousands of nits.

stages, each progressively larger than its predecessor. The nymphal stage lasts from 2 to 3 weeks. The *adult stage* is similar in appearance to the nymphal stage, except that it is larger and has functional reproductive organs (Figure 13-13). The male and female lice copulate, the female louse lays eggs, and the life cycle begins again, taking 3 to 4 weeks to complete. Nymphal and adult stages may live no longer than 7 days if removed from the host. Eggs hatch within 2 to 3 weeks during warm weather, but seldom hatch off of the host.

Lice usually are transmitted by direct contact, but all life stages may be transmitted by *fomites,* inanimate objects such as blankets, brushes, and other grooming equipment. Lice are easily transmitted among young, old, and malnourished animals. Veterinarians often cannot determine why certain animals in a flock or herd are heavily infected, whereas others have only a few lice.

Infestation by lice (either mallophagan or anopluran) is referred to as *pediculosis* (Figure 13-14). Sucking lice can ingest blood to such a degree that they produce severe anemia in the parasitized host; fatalities can occur, especially in young animals. The packed cell volume can decrease as much as 10% to 20%. As many as a million lice may be found on a severely infested animal. Infested animals become more susceptible to other diseases and parasites and may succumb to stresses not ordinarily pathologic to uninfested animals. When animals are poorly fed and kept in overcrowded conditions, they often become severely infested with lice and quickly become anemic and unthrifty.

Careful examination of the hair coat or feathers of infested animals easily reveals the presence of adult lice and their accompanying nits. Hair clippings also serve as a good source for collecting lice. For those animals with a thick hair coat, pediculosis may be overlooked. A hand-held magnifying lens or a binocular headband magnifier (e.g., Optivisor) may assist in isolation of adult or nymphal lice crawling through or clinging to hair or feathers or tiny nits cemented to individual hairs.

When lice or nits are isolated, they may be collected with tiny thumb forceps and placed within a drop of mineral oil on a glass microscope slide. A coverslip should be placed over the specimen and the slide examined using the 4× or 10× objective of the microscope (Figure 13-15).

Identification of louse to genus and specific epithet is quite difficult. It is better to identify the specimen as being anopluran (sucking) versus mallophagan (chewing or biting). The veterinary diagnostician should remember that the head of every chewing louse is wider than the widest portion of its thorax. The typical sucking louse has a head that is narrower than the widest part of the thorax.

Lice of Mice, Rats, Gerbils, and Hamsters

Polyplax serrata is the house mouse louse. This louse is an anopluran (sucking louse), with mouthparts morphologically adapted for sucking blood from its host. Anoplurans are generally more debilitating than mallophagans (chewing lice). *P. serrata* is 0.6 to 1.5 mm long. It is a slender, yellow-brown to white louse with a head that is narrower than the widest part of the thorax. As with most lice, *P. serrata* is large enough to be detected by careful visual inspection of the hair coat or by microscopic examination of pulled hairs. The adult stage of *P. serrata*

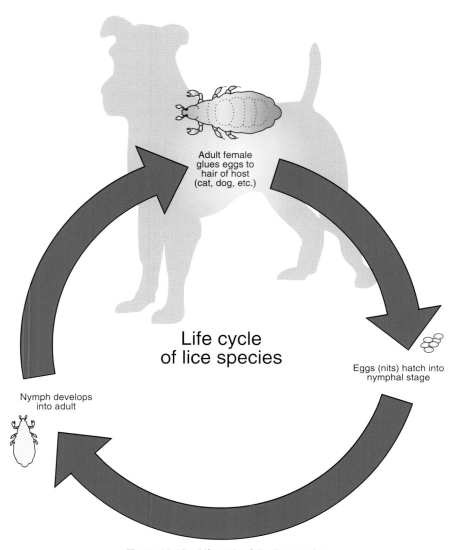

Figure 13-13 Life cycle of the lice species.

is most likely found on the forebody of the mouse. Oval nits may be seen attached near the base of the hair shafts.

Clinical signs associated with infestation by *P. serrata* include restlessness, pruritus, anemia, unthrifty appearance, and death. The diagnostician should not attribute dermal signs to pediculosis unless a louse or a nit is detected. The dermal signs may be the result of other causes, such as concurrent infestation with mites. Therefore it is wise to examine an animal or hair sample thoroughly, rather than ceasing when a single parasite has been identified.

P. serrata is transmitted by direct contact between mice. Because lice are species specific, cross-contamination of other species housed in

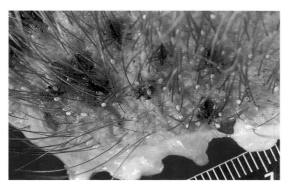

Figure 13-14 Pediculosis can be defined as infestation by either chewing or sucking lice, in this case, *Haematopinus suis* infestation in a pig.

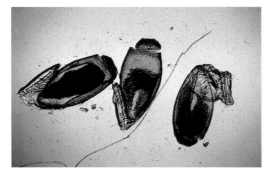

Figure 13-15 Appearance of operculated nits viewed with compound microscope.

the same area and transmission to humans are not considerations. However, *P. serrata* may serve as a vector for several rickettsial organisms and should therefore be handled with caution.

As with *P. serrata* in the mouse, the rat louse, *Polyplax spinulosa,* is an anopluran louse (sucking louse). *P. spinulosa* is similar to *P. serrata,* also having a narrow head compared with the thorax. Similarly, its mouthparts are adapted for sucking blood from the rat.

P. spinulosa may be detected by gross visual examination of the midbody and shoulders of the rat. Hair may be pulled from these areas and examined for nits, nymphs, and adults. Nits are often found attached to the base of the hair

shafts. Nymphs resemble small, pale adult lice. Clinical signs include restlessness, pruritus, anemia, and debilitation. Transmission of the rat louse is by direct contact. Ivermectin has been used successfully to treat lice in rodents. Because lice are species specific, transmission to other animals or humans is not a concern. *P. spinulosa* is a vector responsible for spread of *Haemobartonella muris* and *Rickettsia typhi* between rats. *R. typhi* also can be transmitted from infected rats to humans by rat fleas.

The louse found on the common pet store gerbil is *Hoplopleura meridionidis*. It is interesting that there are no records of lice reported from either the common pet store hamster, *Cricetus cricetus,* or the common laboratory hamster, *Mesocricetus auratus.*

Lice of Guinea Pigs

Gliricola porcelli and *Gyropus ovalis* are the lice of guinea pigs. Both species belong to the order Mallophaga (chewing lice). These lice differ from those of the order Anoplura (sucking lice) by their wide, triangular heads. Chewing lice have a strong pair of mandibles, which are used to abrade skin and obtain cutaneous fluids. *G. porcelli* and *G. ovalis* belong to the family Gyropidae, distinguished by having one or no claws on the second and third pairs of legs.

Gliricola porcelli, the slender guinea pig louse, is 1 to 1.5 mm by 0.3 to 0.44 mm (Figure 13-16). *Gyropus ovalis,* as its name implies, is more oval than *G. porcelli* and measures 1 to 1.2 mm by 0.5 mm (Figure 13-17). The head of *G. ovalis* is much broader than that of *G. porcelli*. Of these two lice, *G. porcelli* is the more common.

Guinea pig lice can be detected antemortem by careful inspection of the hair coat, either grossly or with a hand-held magnifying lens. Postmortem, a method similar to that used to detect lice in other species of animals may be useful. That is, a piece of the pelt from the dead animal may be placed in a covered Petri dish and placed under a mild heat source, such as a small reading lamp. In a short time, as the pelt cools, the lice migrate toward the warmth of the lamp,

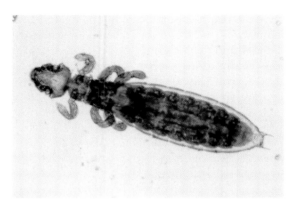

Figure 13-16 *Gliricola porcelli,* the slender, commonly found guinea pig louse.

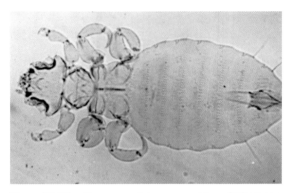

Figure 13-17 *Gyropus ovalis* is more oval than *Gliricola porcelli,* and its head is much broader.

to the tips of the hairs. The lice can be easily observed grossly or with a hand-held magnifying lens.

Light infestations of *G. porcelli* and *G. ovalis* usually cause no clinical signs. In heavy infestations, however, alopecia and scablike areas may develop, especially in the areas caudal to the ears of the guinea pig. Excessive scratching may be noticed. Ivermectin can be used to treat *G. porcelli* and *G. ovalis* in guinea pigs.

Transmission of *G. porcelli* and *G. ovalis* is by direct contact with another host guinea pig or bedding or other fomites from infested guinea pigs. As with other lice, lice of guinea pigs are

species specific and do not cross-infest other species, including humans.

Lice of Rabbits

Hemodipsus ventricosus is not typically found on domestic rabbits; however, when infestation does occur, it is especially debilitating. *H. ventricosus* is an anopluran louse, with a head narrower than the widest part of the thorax. Its mouthparts are specially designed for sucking blood from the host. It has a small thorax and a large, rounded abdomen covered with numerous long hairs. Adult *H. ventricosus* are 1.2 to 2.5 mm long and can be observed antemortem by careful visual examination of the hair coat, especially on the dorsal and lateral aspects of the rabbit. On postmortem examination, hairs may be pulled and placed in a Petri dish under a warm lamp and examined with a dissecting microscope or magnifying glass. Adult lice are drawn by the warmth of the lamp to the tips of the hairs. The oval nits of *H. ventricosus* are 0.5 to 0.7 mm in length and may be found attached to the base of the hair shafts by pulling the fur and examining it microscopically.

Clinical signs of *H. ventricosus* include alopecia and ruffled fur. Rabbit lice are avid bloodsuckers, so anemia may occur in severe infestations.

H. ventricosus is transmitted from rabbit to rabbit by prolonged direct contact. This mostly occurs between a doe and her litter. Although *H. ventricosus* is not considered zoonotic, it is a vector of *Francisella tularensis,* the etiologic agent that causes tularemia.

DIPTERA (TWO-WINGED FLIES)

The order Diptera is a very large, complex order of insects. As adults, all members have one pair of wings (two wings), thus the ordinal name **Diptera;** *di* means "two," and *ptera* means "wing." The members vary greatly in size, food source preference, and developmental stage or stages that parasitize animals or produce pathology. With regard to their roles as ectoparasites, dipterans produce two contrasting pathologic scenarios. As adults, they may feed intermittently on vertebrate blood, saliva, tears, and mucus; as larvae, they may develop in the subcutaneous tissues or internal organs of the host. When adult dipterans make frequent visits to the vertebrate host and intermittently feed on that vertebrate host's blood, they are referred to as *periodic parasites.* When dipteran larvae develop in the tissue or organs of vertebrate hosts, they produce a condition known as *myiasis.*

As periodic parasites, blood-feeding dipterans can be classified in several ways based on the way in which the adult male and female dipterans feed on vertebrate blood and on their food preference. There are certain dipteran groups in which only the females feed on vertebrate blood; these female flies require vertebrate blood for laying their eggs. Included in this group are biting gnats (*Simulium, Lutzomyia,* and *Culicoides* spp.), the mosquitoes (*Anopheles, Aedes,* and *Culex* spp.), the horseflies (*Tabanus* spp.) and the deerflies (*Chrysops* spp.).

In the second group of blood-feeding dipterans, both male and female adult flies require a vertebrate blood meal. These species include *Stomoxys calcitrans,* the stable fly; *Haematobia irritans,* the horn fly; and *Melophagus ovinus,* the sheep ked.

Another dipteran fly, *Musca autumnalis,* feeds on mucus, tears, and saliva of large animals, particularly cattle.

Periodic Parasites of Which Only Adult Females Feed on Vertebrate Blood

In the first dipteran group of periodic parasites, only the female dipterans feed on vertebrate blood. The tiniest members of this group are the biting gnats of *Simulium, Lutzomyia,* and *Culicoides* species.

SIMULIUM *SPECIES (BLACK FLIES).* Members of the genus *Simulium* are commonly called **black flies,** although they may vary from gray to yellow, or **buffalo gnats,** because their thorax humps over their head, giving the appearance of a buffalo's hump (Figure 13-18). These are tiny

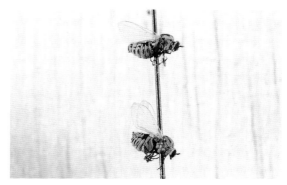

Figure 13-18   Members of the genus *Simulium* are commonly called black flies (but may be gray to yellow) or buffalo gnats (thorax humped over head gives appearance of buffalo's hump). Note small size compared with straight pin that is sticking them.

flies, ranging from 1 to 6 mm in length. They have broad, unspotted wings that have prominent veins along the anterior margins. They have serrated, scissorlike mouthparts, and thus their bites are very painful. Because the females lay eggs in well-aerated water, these flies are often found in the vicinity of swiftly flowing streams. They move in great swarms, inflicting painful bites and sucking the host's blood. These flies may keep cattle from grazing or cause them to stampede. The ears, neck, head, and abdomen are favorite feeding sites. Black flies also feed on poultry and can serve as an intermediate host for a protozoan parasite known as *Leucocytozoon* species.

Black flies prefer the daylight hours and tend to be active in open air. Repellents may offer some relief from these flies. The best method of preventing infestation with black flies is by keeping the equine or bovine hosts in the barn during daylight hours.

Black flies are most often collected in the field (usually in the vicinity of their breeding sites, swiftly flowing streams) and not found on animals presenting to a veterinary clinic. They are diagnosed by their small size, humped back, and strong venation in the anterior region of the wings. Identification of black flies to the level of genus is probably best left to an entomologist.

LUTZOMYIA *SPECIES (NEW WORLD SAND FLIES)*. Members of the genus *Lutzomyia* are commonly referred to as **New World sand flies.** They are tiny, mothlike flies, rarely more than 5 mm in length. A key feature for identification is that the body is covered with fine hairs. *Lutzomyia* species tend to be active only at night and are weak fliers. These tiny flies transmit a protozoan parasite known as *Leishmania* species.

As with black flies, sand flies most often can be collected in the field and are not found on animals presenting to a veterinary clinic. The adult flies are weak fliers and are often collected in rodent burrows, where they breed in moist organic debris. Phebotomine sand flies can be diagnosed by their small size and hairy wings and bodies. Identification of sand flies is probably best left to an entomologist.

CULICOIDES *SPECIES (NO-SEE-UMS)*. *Culicoides* gnats are also commonly known as **no-see-ums, punkies,** or **sand flies.** They are tiny gnats (1-3 mm in length) and similar to black flies in that they inflict painful bites and suck the blood of their hosts. They are active at dusk and at dawn, especially during the winter months. These gnats tend to feed on the dorsal or ventral areas of the host during dusk and evening hours; the feeding site preference depends on the species of biting gnat. Horses often become allergic to the bites of *Culicoides* species, scratching and rubbing these areas, causing alopecia, excoriations, and thickening of the skin. This condition has several names, including **Queensland itch, sweat itch,** and **sweet itch.** Because this condition is often seen during the warmer months of the year, it is also referred to as **summer dermatitis.** The best prevention for these flies is stabling animals during the hours between dusk and dawn. Repellents may offer some protection against *Culicoides* species. These flies also serve as the intermediate host for *Onchocerca cervicalis,* a nematode whose microfilariae are found in the skin of horses. These flies also transmit the blue-tongue virus of sheep.

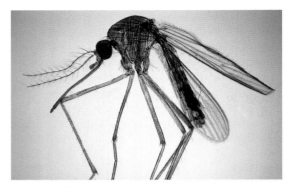

Figure 13-19 Female *Culex* species, one genus among several pathogenic genera of mosquitoes. Although mosquitoes are tiny, fragile dipterans, they are some of the most voracious blood-feeders known.

In contrast to the clear, heavily veined wings of black flies, the wings of *Culicoides* species are mottled. Identification of *Culicoides* species is probably best left to an entomologist.

ANOPHELES, AEDES, *AND* CULEX *SPECIES (MOSQUITOES)*. Although they are tiny, fragile dipterans, mosquitoes are some of the most voracious blood-feeders (Figure 13-19). Mosquitoes plague livestock, and as with black flies, swarms of mosquitoes have been known to keep cattle from grazing or cause them to stampede. The feeding of large swarms of mosquitoes can cause significant anemias in domestic animals. Because of their aquatic breeding environments, large numbers of mosquitoes can be produced from eggs laid in relatively small bodies of water. Although they are known for spreading malaria (*Plasmodium* spp.), yellow fever, and elephantiasis in humans, mosquitoes are probably best known in veterinary medicine as intermediate hosts for the canine heartworm, *Dirofilaria immitis.*

Many of the repellents on the market are effective against mosquitoes. The repellents must be applied to the entire body at labeled frequencies to provide protection to the animal. In addition, preventing the buildup of small bodies of water on the premises (e.g., water in old tires, small puddles after rains, cleaning water troughs frequently) will help reduce the breeding grounds available to mosquitoes.

Adult mosquitoes have wings and body parts covered by tiny, leaf-shaped scales. Identification of both adult and larval *Anopheles, Aedes,* and *Culex* species is probably best left to an entomologist.

CHRYSOPS *SPECIES (DEERFLIES) AND* TABANUS *SPECIES (HORSEFLIES). Chrysops* species (deerflies) and *Tabanus* species (horseflies) are large (up to 3.5 cm in length), heavy-bodied, robust, swift dipterans with powerful wings. These flies also have very large eyes. Horseflies and deerflies are the largest flies in this dipteran group in which only the females feed on vertebrate blood (Figure 13-20). Horseflies are much larger than deerflies. Deerflies have a dark band passing from the anterior to the posterior margin of the wings.

Adult flies lay eggs in the vicinity of open water. Larval stages of horseflies and deerflies are found in aquatic to semiaquatic environments, often buried deep in mud at the bottom of lakes and ponds. Adults are seen in summer and prefer sunlight. The female flies feed in the vicinity of open water and have reciprocating, scissorlike mouthparts, which they use to lacerate the tissues of vertebrates and lap up the oozing blood. These flies feed primarily on large

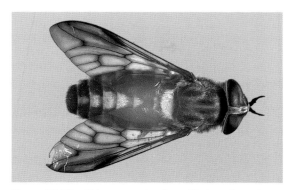

Figure 13-20   *Tabanus* species (horseflies) are large (up to 3.5 cm in length), heavy-bodied, robust dipterans with powerful wings. Horseflies are swift, speedy dipterans. These flies have very large eyes. Horseflies are much larger than deerflies.

animals, such as cattle and horses. Site preferences include the underside of the abdomen around the navel, the legs, and the neck and withers. Horseflies and deerflies feed several times in multiple sites before becoming filled with blood. When disturbed by the animal's swatting tail or by the panniculus reflex, the flies leave the host, although blood often continues to ooze from the open wound. The bites of these flies are very painful. Cattle and horses become restless in their presence. Stabling cattle and horses during the day will help reduce the annoyance of these parasites. The newer varieties of insect repellents offer a degree of relief to those animals turned out during the day. These flies may act as mechanical transmitters of anthrax, anaplasmosis, and the virus of equine infectious anemia.

The veterinary diagnostician can probably best identify these flies by their large, scissorlike mouthparts. Species identification of intact adult horseflies and deerflies is probably best left to an entomologist.

Periodic Parasites of Which Both Adult Males and Females Feed on Vertebrate Blood

In the second group of bloodfeeding dipterans, both male and female adult flies require a vertebrate blood meal. These species include *Stomoxys calcitrans,* the stable fly; *Haematobia irritans,* the horn fly; and *Melophagus ovinus,* the wingless sheep ked.

STOMOXYS CALCITRANS *(STABLE FLY).* The stable fly, *Stomoxys calcitrans,* is often called the **biting housefly.** It is approximately the size of the housefly, *Musca domestica,* but instead of having a sponging type of mouthpart, the stable fly has a bayonet-like proboscis that protrudes forward from its head (Figure 13-21). These flies are found worldwide. In the United States, they are found in the central and southeastern states, areas known for raising cattle. As mentioned previously, both male and female flies are avid bloodfeeders, preying on most domestic animals. They usually attack the legs and ventral abdomen but also may bite the ears. These flies tend to feed

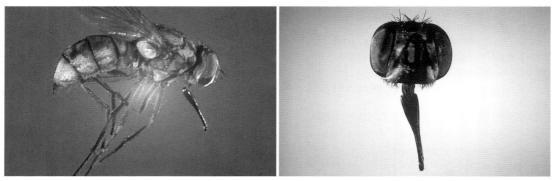

Figure 13-21 *Stomoxys calcitrans*, the stable fly or biting housefly, is approximately the size of the housefly, *Musca domestica*. It has a bayonet-like proboscis that protrudes forward from its head.

on the tips of the ears of dogs with pointed or raised ears (commonly called "fly strike"), such as German shepherds. This problem can be resolved by applying topical repellents to the ear tips.

S. calcitrans also feeds on horses and cattle, with horses being the preferred host. The fly usually lands on the host with its head pointed upward. It is a sedentary fly, not moving on the host. The flies inflict painful bites that puncture the skin and bleed freely. Stable flies stay on the host for short periods, during which they obtain their blood meals. This is an outdoor fly; however, in late fall and during rainy weather, it may enter barns or other enclosed areas. Topical insect repellents made for large animals work well against *S. calicitrans*. The repellents should be applied as recommended on the label for adequate protection.

Stable flies are mechanical vectors of anthrax in cattle and equine infectious anemia. This fly is the intermediate host for *Habronema muscae*, a nematode found in the stomach of horses. When large numbers of stable flies attack dairy cattle, a decrease in milk production can result. Beef cattle may refuse to graze in the daytime when attacked by large numbers of flies; as a result, these cattle do not gain the usual amount of weight.

Stable flies use decaying organic material for laying eggs. Removing piles of leaves, grass

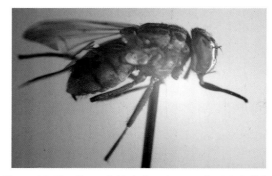

Figure 13-22 *Haematobia irritans* is approximately half the size of the stable fly, *Stomoxys calcitrans*. It also possesses a bayonet-like proboscis that protrudes forward from its head.

clippings, soiled bedding, and other decaying matter from the premises will reduce the stable fly breeding areas and reduce the *S. calcitrans* population.

The veterinary diagnostician can easily identify the stable fly by its size (approximately the same size as a housefly) and the bayonet-like proboscis that protrudes forward from the head.

HAEMATOBIA IRRITANS *(HORN FLY)*. *Haematobia irritans* is often called the **horn fly.** It is a dark-colored fly, approximately 3 to 6 mm in length, half the size of *Stomoxys calcitrans*, the biting housefly. As with the stable fly, the horn fly has a bayonet-like proboscis that protrudes forward from the head (Figure 13-22). These flies are found almost exclusively on cattle throughout North America.

When the air temperature is below 70° F, horn flies cluster around the base of the horns, thus the common name "horn fly." In warmer climates, horn flies often cluster in large numbers on the host's shoulders, back, and sides; these are the areas least disturbed by tail swishing. On hot sunny days, horn flies often accumulate on the host's ventral abdomen. Use of insecticides effective against *H. irritans* will help reduce the horn fly population on the individual cow. This may be accomplished with a fly spray or pour-on solution. A walk-through fly-removing apparatus will help reduce the individual population by half through mechanically removing the flies on the animal.

Adult horn flies spend most of their life on cattle; females leave the host to deposit their eggs in fresh cow manure. Using their tiny, bayonet-like mouthparts, they feed frequently, sucking blood and other fluids, and cause considerable irritation. Females flies are more aggressive than males. The energy lost in disturbing the feeding flies coupled with the loss of blood often results in reduced weight gain and milk production. Horn flies probably cause greater losses in cattle in the United States than any other blood-feeding fly. Adult horn flies also cause focal midline dermatitis on the ventral abdomen of horses. These flies serve as the intermediate hosts for *Stephanofilaria stilesi,* a filarial parasite that produces ventral plaquelike lesions on the underside of the abdomen of cattle.

The veterinary diagnostician can easily identify *H. irritans* by its dark color and size (approximately half the size of a stable fly). As with the stable fly, the horn fly's bayonet-like proboscis protrudes forward from the head.

MELOPHAGUS OVINUS *(SHEEP KED).* *Melophagus ovinus* is often referred to as the **sheep ked.** As mentioned earlier, members of the order Diptera usually possess one pair of wings; sheep keds are exceptions to that rule: they are wingless dipterans. Sheep keds have an unusual appearance; they are hairy and appear leathery and measure

approximately 4 to 7 mm in length (Figure 13-23). The head of this dipteran is short and broad. The thorax is brown, and the abdomen broad and grayish brown. The legs are strong and armed with stout claws (Figure 13-24). Keds are often described as having a "louselike" appearance, but they definitely are not lice.

Keds are permanent ectoparasites of sheep and goats. Their pupal stages are often found attached to the wool or fleece of the host. Keds are avid blood-feeders. Heavy infestation can reduce the condition of the host considerably and even cause significant anemia. The bites of *M. ovinus* cause pruritus over much of the host's

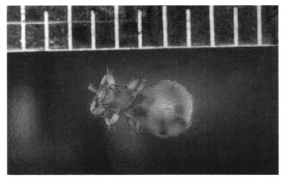

Figure 13-23 *Melophagus ovinus,* the sheep ked, is a wingless dipteran that is hairy, leathery, and approximately 4 to 7 mm in length.

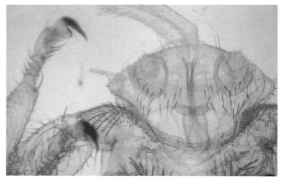

Figure 13-24 The head of *Melophagus ovinus* is short and broad. The legs are strong and armed with stout claws. Some say keds have a louselike appearance.

body; the infested sheep will often bite, scratch, and rub itself, thus damaging the wool. Ked feces is dark brown, stains the wool, and does not wash out readily. Keds are most numerous in the cold temperatures during the fall and winter months. Their numbers decline as the temperatures rise in the spring and summer months. Close inspection of the wool and underlying skin reveals infestation by these wingless dipterans. Infested wool often has a dark-brown appearance because of discoloration by ked feces. Control of *M. ovinus* may be accomplished by applying an effective insecticide to the sheep after shearing.

Sheep keds are closely related to the **hippoboscid flies,** winged dipterans that parasitize wild birds. These flattened, swiftly flying, blood-feeding dipterans are often found among the feathers of wild birds. Two important hippoboscid flies are *Lynchia* and *Pseudolynchia* species (Figure 13-25). They can serve as intermediate hosts for *Haemoproteus* species, a malaria-like parasite of wild birds.

Periodic Parasites That Feed on Mucus, Tears, and Saliva

The final periodic parasite among the dipteran flies discussed here is one that is not a blood-feeder but instead feeds on the mucus, tears, and saliva of large animals, particularly cattle. This fly is known as *Musca autumnalis,* or the **face fly.**

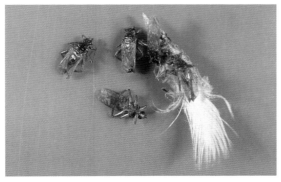

Figure 13-25 Louse flies, *Lynchia* or *Pseudolynchia* species, often parasitize wild birds.

MUSCA AUTUMNALIS *(FACE FLY).* Face flies, *Musca autumnalis,* are so named because they gather around the eyes and muzzle of livestock, particularly cattle. They may also be found on the withers, neck, brisket, and sides. Face flies feed mostly on saliva, tears, and mucus. They usually are not considered blood-feeders because their mouthparts are not piercing or bayonet-like. Instead, their mouthparts are adapted for sponging up saliva, tears, and mucus (Figure 13-26). These flies often follow flies that feed on blood, disturb them during their feeding process, and

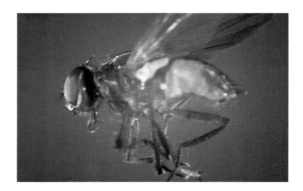

A

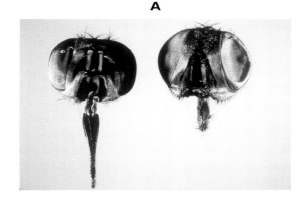

B

Figure 13-26   **A,** *Musca autumnalis,* the face fly. These flies gather around the eyes and muzzle of livestock, particularly cattle. Their mouthparts are adapted for sponging up saliva, tears, and mucus. **B,** Left, *Stomoxys calictrans;* right, *Musca atumnalis.*

then lap up the blood and body fluids that ooze and accumulate on the host's skin. Face flies are found on animals that are outdoors; they usually will not follow animals into barns or other enclosures.

Face flies produce considerable pathology because of their annoyance of the host. The irritation around the host's eyes stimulates the flow of tears, which attracts more flies. The flies' activity produces annoyance, which ultimately interferes with the host's productivity. Face flies may be vectors in the transmission of *Moraxella bovis,* a bacterium that causes infectious keratoconjunctivitis, or pinkeye, in cattle. Face flies may be controlled with the application of an insecticide to the animal's body to offer a degree of relief. Spraying potential breeding sites with insecticide will help reduce fly populations.

Grossly, the face fly is morphologically similar to the housefly, *Musca domestica.* These two species in the genus *Musca* can be differentiated only through minor differences in eye position and color of the abdomen. The veterinary diagnostician should probably not attempt to speciate this fly; speciation requires the skills of a trained entomologist. Rather, the veterinary diagnostician should remember this rule of thumb: if a fly with sponging mouthparts is found around the face of a cow or horse, it is most probably a face fly.

Myiasis-Producing Flies

With regard to their roles as ectoparasites, larval dipterans may develop in the subcutaneous tissues of the skin of many domestic animals. When dipteran larvae develop in the tissues or organs of vertebrate hosts, these larvae produce a condition known as *myiasis.* Based on degree of host dependence, there are two types of myiases: (1) facultative myiasis, in which the fly larvae are usually *free-living,* and (2) obligatory myiasis. In *facultative myiasis* the normally free-living larvae adapt themselves to a parasitic dependence on a host. In *obligatory myiasis* the fly larvae are completely parasitic; that is, they are dependent on the host during development

through the life cycle. In other words, without the host, the obligatory parasites will die.

DIPTERAN FLY LARVAE THAT INFEST THE SKIN

Facultative Myiasis-Producing Flies. The dipteran larvae capable of producing facultative myiasis in the skin are *Musca domestica,* the housefly; *Calliphora, Phaenicia, Lucilia,* and *Phormia* species, the blow flies, or bottle flies; and *Sarcophaga* species, the flesh flies. Larval stages of these flies are usually associated with skin wounds contaminated with bacteria or with a matted hair coat contaminated with feces.

Under normal conditions, adult flies of these genera lay their eggs in decaying animal carcasses or in feces. In facultative myiasis the adult flies are attracted to an animal's moist wound, skin lesion, or soiled hair coat. These sites provide the adult fly with moist media on which to feed. As adult female flies feed in these sites, they lay eggs. The eggs hatch, producing larvae (maggots), which move independently about the wound surface, ingesting dead cells, exudate, secretions, and debris, but not live tissue. This condition is known as *fly strike,* or *strike.* These larvae irritate, injure, and kill successive layers of skin and produce exudates. Maggots can tunnel through the thinned epidermis into the subcutis. This process produces tissue cavities in the skin that measure up to several centimeters in diameter (Figure 13-27). Unless the process is halted by appropriate therapy, the infested animal may die from shock, intoxication, histolysis, or infection. A peculiar, distinct, pungent odor permeates the infested tissue and the affected animal. Advanced lesions may contain thousands of maggots. It is important to remember that as adults, these flies can be pestiferous in a veterinary clinical setting. These flies are "vomit drop" feeders and fly from feces to food, spreading bacteria on their feet and within their disgorged stomach contents.

A tentative diagnosis of maggot infestation in any domestic animal can easily be made by a veterinary diagnostician, because maggots can be observed in an existing wound or among the soiled, matted hair coat. A specific diagnosis can

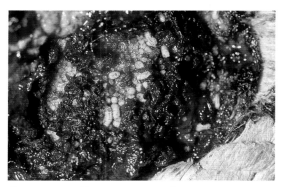

Figure 13-27 Fly strike in a Hereford cow. The fly larvae (maggots) move independently about the wound surface, ingesting dead cells, exudate, secretions, and debris, but not live tissue. This condition is known as fly strike, or strike.

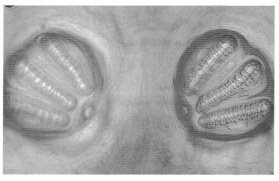

Figure 13-28 Diagnostic spiracular plates on the posterior end of fly maggot. This plate can be used for positive identification of the fly maggot.

be made by examining the *spiracular plate* on the posterior end of the fly maggot. Each species of fly maggot has its own distinctive spiracular plate, much like a fingerprint (Figure 13-28). As soon as a diagnosis of facultative myiasis has been made, the veterinary diagnostician must rule out the possibility of obligatory myiasis caused by *Cochliomyia hominivorax.*

Obligatory Myiasis-Producing Flies. The dipteran larvae capable of producing obligatory myiasis in the skin are *Cochliomyia hominivorax*, *Cuterebra* species, and *Hypoderma* species. In obligatory myiasis the dipteran larvae lead a parasitic existence.

Cochliomyia hominivorax. Only one fly in North America, *Cochliomyia hominivorax*, is a primary invader of fresh, uncontaminated skin wounds of domestic animals. These larvae must not be confused with the larvae of the facultative myiasis-producing flies just described. *C. hominivorax* is often referred to as the **screw-worm fly.** In economic terms, it is the most important of the flies that attack livestock in the southwestern and southern United States. Adult female flies are attracted to fresh skin wounds on warm-blooded animals, where they lay batches of 15 to 500 eggs in a shinglelike pattern at the edge of wounds. The female fly lays several thousand eggs during her lifetime. The cream-colored, elongated eggs hatch within 24 hours. Larvae enter the wound, where they feed for 4 to 7 days before they become third-stage (fully grown) larvae. These larvae can be as long as 1.5 cm; at this stage they resemble a wood screw, thus the name "screw-worm." When fully grown, the larvae drop to the ground, after which the adult flies emerge. The adult male and female fly breed only once during their lifetime, a key fact that is used to control these flies biologically.

Adult screw-worm flies are shiny, greenish blue with a reddish orange head and eyes, and 8 to 15 mm long. Larvae are often identified by their wood-screw shape and by the two deeply pigmented tracheal tubes on the dorsal aspect of the caudal ends of third-stage larvae (Figure 13-29).

Because of the obligatory nature of the screw-worm with regard to breeding in the fresh wounds of warm-blooded animals, *the veterinary diagnostician must report the parasite to both state and federal authorities. C. hominivorax* has been eradicated from the United States but occasionally enters the country surreptitiously in imported animals.

Cuterebra species (Wolves, Warbles). Larvae of the genus *Cuterebra* (commonly called **wolves** or **warbles**) infest the skin of rabbits, squirrels,

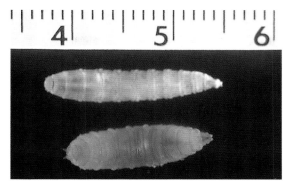

Figure 13-29 Larvae of *Cochliomyia hominivorax* can be identified by wood-screw shape and two deeply pigmented tracheal tubes on dorsal aspect of caudal ends of third larval stage.

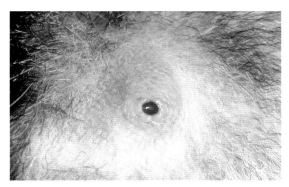

Figure 13-30 Larval *Cuterebra* species are usually found in swollen, cystlike subcutaneous sites, with a fistula (pore, or hole) communicating to outside environment.

mice, rats, chipmunks, and occasionally dogs and cats. A large discrepancy exists concerning the morphologic descriptions of larval *Cuterebra.* Most of the specimens recovered in a clinical setting are of the second-stage or third-stage larvae. Second-stage larvae are grublike, 5 to 10 mm long, and cream to grayish white; this stage is often sparsely covered with tiny, black, toothlike spines. Third-stage larvae are large, robust, and coal black, with a heavily spined appearance; they are up to 3 cm in length. Larval stages are usually found in swollen, cystlike subcutaneous sites, with a fistula (pore or hole) communicating to the outside environment (Figure 13-30). It is through this pore that the larval *Cuterebra* breathes.

Adult flies lay eggs near the entrance to rodent burrows. Pets usually contract this parasite while investigating or seeking out rodent prey. As a result, the most frequently affected cutaneous sites in dogs and cats are the subcutaneous tissues of the neck and head. Most cases occur during the late summer and early fall. Among the myiasis-producing flies, this dipteran larva is known for its aberrant or erratic migrations, having been found in a variety of extracutaneous sites, such as the cranial vault, the anterior chamber of the eye, and the pharyngeal regions. Clinical signs will vary with the site of infection or infestation. Larval *Cuterebra* species are often discovered in cutaneous sites during physical examination. They are usually removed surgically by enlarging the breathing pore and removing the larva with thumb forceps. Great care must be taken not to crush the larva during the extraction process because anaphylaxis might result.

Cuterebrosis is diagnosed by observing the characteristic swollen, cystlike subcutaneous lesion with its fistula or central pore that communicates to the outside environment. Second-stage or third-stage larvae are usually removed from these cutaneous lesions. These larvae are usually covered with tiny black spines (Figure 13-31).

Hypoderma species (Ox Warbles). Two larval species of *Hypoderma* flies (**ox warbles** or **cattle grubs**) infect cattle: *Hypoderma lineatum* and *H. bovis. H. lineatum* is found in the southern United States, and both species are found in the northern United States and Canada. The adult flies are heavy and resemble honeybees; they are often called **heel flies.**

The entire life cycle is almost a year in length. Adult flies are bothersome to cattle as they approach to lay eggs. Animals often become apprehensive and disturbed and attempt to escape this pesky fly by running away, an action called **gadding.** The eggs are about 1 mm long

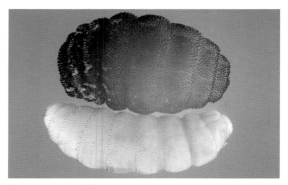

Figure 13-31 Different developmental stages of *Cuterebra* species. Larval *Cuterebra* are either sparsely or thickly covered with tiny black spines.

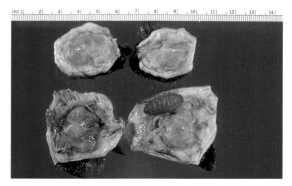

Figure 13-32 Mature larvae of *Hypoderma* species are 25 to 30 mm long, cream to dark brown, and covered with small spines. Lesions consist of large, cystlike swellings on back, with central breathing pore.

and are attached to hairs on the legs of cattle. *H. lineatum* deposits a row of six or more eggs on an individual hair shaft; *H. bovis* lays its eggs singly on the hair shaft. The larvae hatch in about 4 days and crawl down the hair shaft to the skin, which they penetrate. The larvae wander through the subcutaneous connective tissues in the leg, migrating through the esophagus *(H. lineatum)* or the region of the spinal canal and epidural fat *(H. bovis)*, until they reach the subcutaneous tissues of the back. Here the larvae create breathing holes in the skin of the dorsum; it is through these pores that they later exit and fall to the ground to pupate. The adult flies emerge from the pupae.

Adult *Hypoderma* species are beelike and are covered with yellow-to-orange hairs. Mature larvae are 25 to 30 mm long, cream to dark brown, and covered with small spines. Lesions consist of large, cystlike swellings on the back, with a central breathing pore (Figure 13-32). As with *Cuterebra* species, great care must be taken not to crush the *Hypoderma* larva during the extraction process because anaphylaxis might result.

DIPTERAN FLY LARVAE THAT INFECT THE GASTROINTESTINAL TRACT. *Gasterophilus* species (**horse bots** or **stomach bots**) have three developmental stages that may be associated with pathology in the horse. Just as adult *Hypoderma* species are

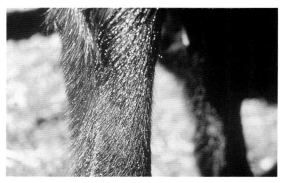

Figure 13-33 Numerous eggs cemented to forelimb of a horse.

annoying to the host, adult *Gasterophilus* species are similarly annoying. These adult flies resemble honeybees. During the late summer and early fall, the adult females fly in around the fetlocks of the forelegs and the chin and shoulders of the horse to oviposit eggs on the hairs in these regions (Figure 13-33). This fly's activity and the accompanying oviposition cause extreme annoyance to the host. Some horses will panic because of the egg-laying activity of these flies. Once the eggs have been laid on the hairs, the horses lick themselves. The abrasive tongue and accompanying saliva are a stimulus for the larvae to hatch from the eggs (Figure 13-34). The

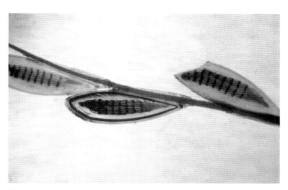

Figure 13-34 Individual egg of *Gasterophilus* species cemented by adult female fly to hairs on a horse's leg. Friction and moisture of horse's licking causes the egg to hatch. Note emergence of larval bot.

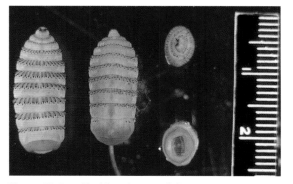

Figure 13-35 Final larval stage of *Gasterophilus* species is often found within feces of equine host. Note presence of anterior hooks, with larva attached to gastric mucosa.

larvae penetrate the mucosa of the lips, tongue, and buccal cavity and migrate through the oral mucosa. They eventually emerge and migrate to the cardiac portion of the stomach, where they remain attached for 10 to 12 months. The larvae measure up to 20 mm in length, are brown, and possess dense spines on the anterior border of each body segment. There is a pair of indistinct mouth hooks (organs of attachment) on the anterior end of the first body segment and a spiracular plate on the posterior end. These larvae usually pass out of the host in the spring (Figure 13-35) and pupate on the ground for 3 to 5 weeks.

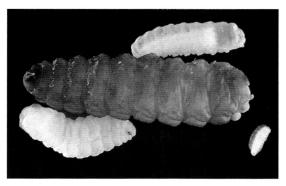

Figure 13-36 Several larval stages of *Oestrus ovis* extracted from nasal passages of sheep.

The adult flies emerge from the pupal case and live during the latter half of the summer. The larval stage of the *Gasterophilus* species can be treated with dichlorvos, trichlorfan, or ivermectin dewormers in the fall and spring seasons. A bot knife may be used on the legs of the animal to remove the eggs before they are able to infect the animal.

The veterinary diagnostician should be able to identify the annoying adult female flies seen around the horse in the fall. The telltale egg stages contain tiny larvae, and the dark-brown bots pass out with the feces. It is through the feces that the third larval stage exits the gastrointestinal tract; therefore this parasitic stage may be recovered in horse feces.

DIPTERAN FLY LARVAE THAT INFECT THE RESPIRATORY TRACT

***Oestrus ovis* (Nasal Bots).** *Oestrus ovis* (**nasal bots** or **nasal bot flies**) produce a respiratory myiasis in sheep. The adults are beelike flies and, like both *Hypoderma* and *Gasterophilus* species, are quite annoying to the sheep. The adult female fly flies into the area of the nostrils, where she deposits a tiny, first-stage larva. This tiny, white-to-yellow larva crawls upward into the nostrils and sinuses of the sheep, often producing a purulent rhinitis or sinusitis. The larvae grow rapidly into 3-cm, dark-brown larvae with large, black oral hooks (Figure 13-36). When fully developed, the larvae drop out of the nostrils and pupate in the ground; the adults then emerge from the pupa. Ivermectin has been shown to be very effective against *O. ovis.*

The veterinary diagnostician should be able to identify the large, dark-brown bots as they pass out of the nostrils.

SIPHONAPTERA (FLEAS)

Of all the orders of arthropods discussed thus far, members of the order Siphonaptera, or fleas, are perhaps the most important insect with respect to veterinary economics. Treating for fleas can be a veterinary practice builder. Because of the extreme popularity of dogs and cats and the prolific nature of the flea (and thus its ability to return after populations are exterminated on the animal and within the animal's environment), the veterinarian should pay special attention to diagnosing the various life cycle stages of fleas both on the pet and in the pet's environment (Figure 13-37).

Fleas, or *siphonapterans,* are small (4-9 mm in length), laterally compressed, wingless insects with powerful hind legs that are used for jumping onto hosts. Adult fleas have piercing-sucking (siphonlike) mouthparts that are used to suck the blood of their hosts (Figure 13-38). More than 2000 species of fleas have been identified throughout the world. Adult fleas are always parasitic, feeding on both mammals and birds (Figure 13-39). Dogs and cats are host to comparatively few species of fleas.

The flea life cycle consists of four stages: (1) adult stage, (2) egg stage, (3) larval stage, and (4) pupal stage. The female flea can lay up to several thousand eggs in her lifetime. The eggs may be laid on the infested animal or in the environment. Eggs laid on the animal will drop to the ground or bedding. The eggs will hatch into larvae within 2 weeks. The larvae eat organic debris (e.g., dead skin, dead hair, flea feces) from the environment. The larva will begin to form a

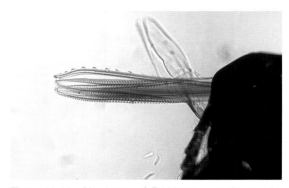

Figure 13-38   Mouthparts of *Echidnophaga gallinacea*, the stick-tight flea of poultry. Adult fleas are placed in the order Siphonaptera because they possess piercing-sucking (siphonlike) mouthparts used to suck host's blood.

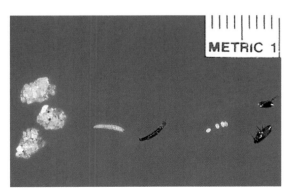

Figure 13-37   Life stages of *Ctenocephalides felis*, the cat flea: adult males and females, eggs, larvae, and pupae.

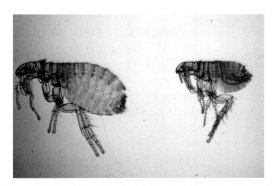

Figure 13-39   Morphologic details of adult male and female *Ctenocephalides felis*, cat fleas. Note penis rods of male and spermatheca of female.

cocoon as it passes into the pupal stage. The pupal stage is carried out entirely within the cocoon and can last for months. The cocoon keeps the pupa from desiccating over long periods (Figure 13-40). The flea will only emerge from the pupal stage if environmental signs (air pressure, vibrations, warmth) indicate a host is present. The adult flea can survive only up to 1 week without a blood meal. Once emerged, the adult flea will find a host, take a blood meal, and begin the life cycle again.

Ctenocephalides felis, the cat flea, is the most common flea found on dogs and cats. The dog flea, *Ctenocephalides canis,* is uncommon and occurs much less frequently on dogs than does the cat flea.

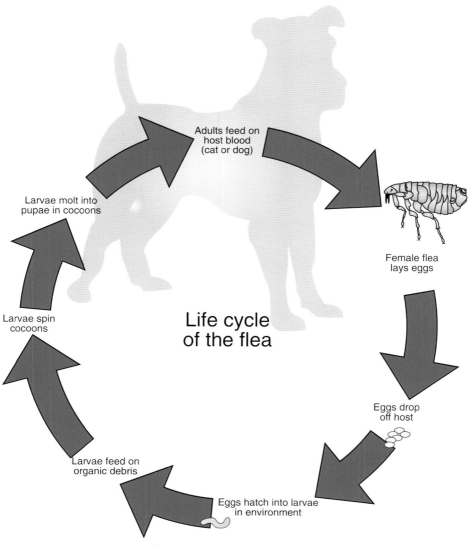

Figure 13-40   Life cycle of the flea.

When flea infestation is suspected in domestic rabbits, a complete physical examination of the rabbit hair coat should be performed, because different species of fleas prefer different areas of the body surface. *Cediopsylla simplex,* the **common eastern rabbit flea,** is often found around the face and neck of domestic rabbits. *Odontopsylla multispinosus,* the **giant eastern rabbit flea,** is often found over the "tail-head" region at the base of the tail of domestic rabbits (when they curl in sleep with head close to tail).

Echidnophaga gallinacea is also known as the **stick-tight flea of poultry** (Figure 13-41; see also Figure 13-38). A common flea of chickens and guinea fowl, *E. gallinacea* also feeds on dogs and cats. This flea has unique feeding habits. The female flea inserts her mouthparts into the skin of the host and remains attached at that site. On first observation, these specimens resemble attached ticks; however, they are indeed fleas.

Fleas are not typically found on either horses or ruminants. In barns where "barn cats" abound and excessive straw is present, large numbers of fleas have been found on calves. Under these conditions, fleas can produce significant anemias in young calves. *Pulex irritans,* the flea of humans, has been recovered from dogs and cats, especially in the southeastern United States.

Although the adult flea is the life cycle stage most often encountered, the veterinary diagnostician may also be presented with flea eggs or with larval fleas from the pet's environment. Flea eggs and larvae are frequently found in the owner's bedclothes, the pet's bedding, travel carriers, doghouses, and clinic cages. Flea eggs resemble tiny pearls; they are nonsticky, 0.5 mm long, white, oval, and rounded at both ends (Figure 13-42). Flea larvae resemble tiny fly maggots; they are 2 to 5 mm long, white (after feeding they become brown), and sparsely covered with hairs (Figures 13-43 and 13-44).

Adult fleas are usually encountered on the animal but may also be collected in the pet's

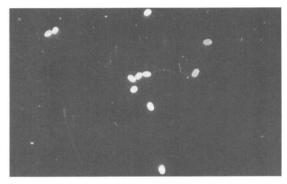

Figure 13-42 Eggs of *Ctenocephalides felis,* the cat flea. Flea eggs resemble tiny pearls; they are nonsticky, 0.5 mm long, white, oval, and rounded at both ends.

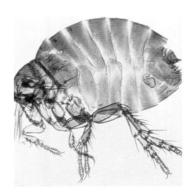

Figure 13-41 Adult *Echidnophaga gallinacea,* the stick-tight flea of poultry. Note angular profile. A common flea of chickens and guinea fowl, it also feeds on dogs and cats.

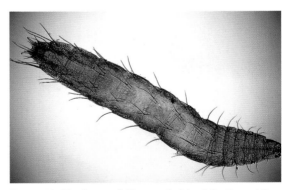

Figure 13-43 Larva of *Ctenocephalides felis,* the cat flea. Flea larvae resemble tiny fly maggots; they are 2 to 5 mm long, white (after feeding they become brown), and sparsely covered with hairs.

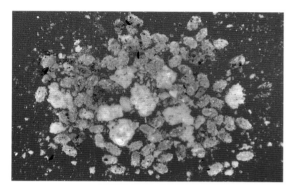

Figure 13-44 Sand-covered pupae of *Ctenocephalides felis*, the cat flea.

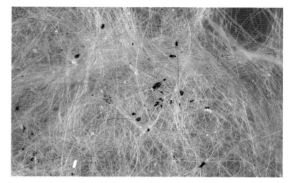

Figure 13-45 Flea dirt (flea feces or flea frass) of *Ctenocephalides felis*, the cat flea. Flea dirt can be used to diagnose current or recent infestations by fleas. If water is slowly dropped onto flea dirt on a gauze sponge, the flea dirt will reconstitute to host's blood.

environment. Observed on recovery from the pet, the larger fleas with an orange-to-light-brown abdomen are females; the smaller, darker specimens are males.

Because adult fleas spend most of their time on the host, diagnosis of flea infestation is usually obvious. However, in animals with flea-allergy dermatitis, fleas may be so few on the pet that the diagnosis of flea infestation is quite difficult.

Definitive diagnosis of flea infestation requires demonstration of the adult fleas and/or their droppings (flea dirt, flea feces, or flea frass) (Figure 13-45). Flea dirt can be used to diagnose current or recent infestations by fleas. Fleas can be easily collected by spraying the pet with an insecticide. After a few minutes, dead fleas drop off the animal. Alternatively, fleas may be collected using a fine-toothed flea comb, available from any veterinary supply company or pet store.

Adult fleas defecate large quantities of partially digested blood, commonly called *flea dirt.* These feces are reddish black and can appear as fine pepperlike specks, comma-shaped columns, or long coils. To collect a sample of flea dirt, the diagnostician must comb the pet with a flea comb and place the collected debris on a piece of white paper towel moistened with water. Rubbing the flea dirt with a fingertip causes the flea dirt to dissolve, producing a characteristic blood-red or rust-red color.

Flea control is important because fleas not only cause discomfort and irritation to the pet but also serve as intermediate hosts to certain helminth parasites. Fleas serve as intermediate host for *Dipylidium caninum,* the double-pored tapeworm of dogs and cats, and for *Dipetalonema reconditum,* the filarial parasite that resides in the subcutaneous tissues of dogs. Some types of fleas can also transmit diseases, such as bubonic plague and endemic typhus, to humans.

Flea control makes up a large part of pet care costs in the United States. There are many different types and styles of flea prevention products on the market. Flea prevention should encompass three different areas to ensure proper control: (1) the yard, (2) the house, and (3) the animal. The yard is the major source of initial flea infestation. A good-quality yard spray approved for fleas will reduce the flea population in the outside environment, thus reducing the chances of the pet bringing new adult fleas into the home. The house is a major source of animal reinfestation. Once the adult fleas breed and the female lays eggs, the eggs are present in the house. The pupae that result from the life cycle of the flea remain in the house and hatch as adults to reinfest the pet. Several types of products are available for use in the house, including foggers, sprays, and powders. Each of these products may incorporate an *adulticide* to kill the adult fleas and an *insect growth regulator* (IGR) to prevent the other life stages from developing to maturity. Although many products can be used to treat the yard and home, great improvements have been made in the products for animal application. There are daily or weekly sprays and powders available. However, the greatest advancements have been made to include once-a-month applications. Topical products such as Frontline TopSpot,* Advantage,[†] and Advantix[†] can be applied once a month, are resistant to water, and contain adulticide or adulticide and IGR. Other products, such as Program[‡] and Sentinel[‡] (also contains heartworm prevention), contain IGR and are given monthly in pill form for dogs. Program can also be given as a 6-month injection to cats. Capstar[‡] can be given to dogs and cats orally for the treatment of adult fleas over a 24-hour period; however, there is no residual activity after 36 hours. Regardless of the product used, all three forms of flea prevention (yard, house, animal) should be used for proper control of the flea population.

MITES AND TICKS

Kingdom: Animalia
   Phylum: Arthropoda (arthropods)
      Subphylum: Chelicerata (possess chelicerate mouthparts)
         Class: Acarina (mites and ticks)

Because mites and ticks belong to the class Acarina, any infestation of domestic animals by either mites or ticks is referred to as *acariasis.* The four developmental stages in the typical life cycle of the mite or tick are (1) the egg stage, (2) the six-legged larval stage, (3) the eight-legged nymphal stage, and (4) the eight-legged adult stage.

*Merial, 1-888-637-4251.
[†]Bayer Animal Health Corporation, Bedford, NH.
[‡]Novartis Animal Health, Greensboro, NC.

MITES OF VETERINARY IMPORTANCE

The first group of parasitic mites can be classified as *sarcoptiform mites.* As sarcoptiform mites, they have the following key features in common:
1. These mites can produce severe dermatologic problems in a variety of domestic animals. This dermatitis is usually accompanied by a severe pruritus, or itching.
2. Typically, sarcoptiform mites are tiny mites barely visible to the naked eye, approximately the size of a grain of salt.
3. In silhouette, the bodies of sarcoptiform mites have a round-to-oval shape.
4. Sarcoptiform mites have legs that have *pedicels,* or stalks, at the tips. The pedicels may be long or short. If the pedicel is long, it may be straight (unjointed) or jointed. At the tip of each pedicel, there may be a tiny sucker. Veterinary diagnosticians should use the description of the pedicel (long or short, jointed or unjointed) to identify sarcoptiform mites.

Sarcoptiform mites can be broken down into two basic families: the *Sarcoptidae* family, sarcoptiform mites that burrow or tunnel within the epidermis, and the *Psoroptidae* family, sarcoptiform mites that reside on the surface of the skin or within the external ear canal. Sarcoptidae includes *Sarcoptes, Notoedres, Cnemidocoptes,* and *Trixacarus* species. Psoroptidae includes *Psoroptes, Chorioptes,* and *Otodectes* species.

Family Sarcoptidae (Mites)

Members of the family Sarcoptidae burrow or tunnel within the epidermis of the infested definitive host. The entire four-stage life cycle is spent on the host. Male and female mites breed on the skin surface. The female mite penetrates the keratinized layers of the skin and burrows or tunnels through the epidermis. Over a 10- to 15-day period, she deposits 40 to 50 eggs within the tunnel. After egg deposition, the female dies. Six-legged larvae emerge from the eggs in 3 to 10 days and exit the tunnel to wander on the skin surface. These larvae molt to the eight-legged nymphal stage within tiny pockets in the epidermis. Nymphs become sexually active adults in 12 to 17 days, and the life cycle begins again.

SARCOPTES SCABEI *(SCABIES MITE).* The disease caused by *Sarcoptes scabei* is called **scabies,** or **sarcoptic acariasis.** Sarcoptic acariasis is extremely pruritic.

With regard to the host specificity of *Sarcoptes* species, varieties of these infest specific hosts. For example, *Sarcoptes scabei* variety *canis* affects only dogs, and *Sarcoptes scabei* variety *suis* affects only pigs. Almost every domestic animal has its own distinct variety of this mite, which does not infest other hosts.

Canine scabies is caused by *Sarcoptes scabei* variety *canis,* which produces lesions consisting of an erythematous, papular rash. Scaling, crusting, and excoriations are common. The ears, lateral elbows, and ventral abdomen are sites that are likely to harbor mites. The animal's entire body, however, may be infested. These mites are spread by direct contact and can affect all dogs in the household. *Sarcoptes scabei* variety *canis* is extremely contagious. The dog owner can become infested with this mite, but the disease is self-limiting. The mites burrow into the skin of humans, producing a papulelike lesion; however, the mites will not establish a full-blown infestation in humans. Therefore, *Sarcoptes scabei* variety *canis* is considered to be a zoonosis. Some dogs may be asymptomatic carriers of *Sarcoptes scabei* variety *canis.*

Cats also are parasitized by a variety of this mite, *Sarcoptes scabei* variety *felis.* Feline scabies caused by this variety is an extremely rare condition.

Among large animals, pigs are most often affected by scabies. Lesions caused by *Sarcoptes scabei* variety *suis* include small red papules, alopecia, and crusts, most frequently on the trunk and ears. Scabies in cattle (*Sarcoptes scabei* variety *bovis*) is rare. The main areas of infestation are the head, neck, and shoulders. Scabies in horses (*Sarcoptes scabei* variety *equi*) is an even

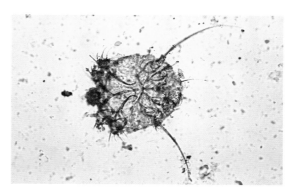

Figure 13-46 Adult *Sarcoptes scabei* mite. Anus is located on caudal end of body.

rarer entity. The main area of infestation is the neck. *Sarcoptes scabei* variety *ovis* affects the face of sheep and goats, rather than the fleece.

Areas with an erythematous, papular rash and crust should be scraped, especially the areas most associated with sarcoptic infestation in dogs, that is, the ears, lateral elbows, and ventral abdomen. Adult sarcoptic mites are oval and approximately 200 to 400 μm in diameter, with eight legs. The key morphologic feature used to identify this species is the long, unjointed pedicel with a sucker on the end of some of the legs. The anus is located on the caudal end of the body (Figure 13-46). The eggs of *Sarcoptes* mites are oval (Figure 13-47).

Sarcoptes scabei can be treated with ivermectin, lime-sulfur dips, or amitraz (not used for horses).

NOTOEDRES CATI *(FELINE SCABIES MITE) AND* NOTOEDRES MURIS. Although cats may be parasitized by *Sarcoptes scabei* variety *felis,* the mite most often associated with feline scabies is *Notoedres cati.* This mite infests mainly cats but occasionally also parasitizes rabbits. This sarcoptiform mite is found chiefly on the ears, back of the neck, face, and feet; in extreme cases, however, the entire body may be affected. The life cycle is similar to that of *Sarcoptes scabei,* with the mite burrowing or tunneling in the superficial layers of the epidermis. The characteristic lesion of notoedric acariasis is a yellowing crust in the region of the ears, face, or neck.

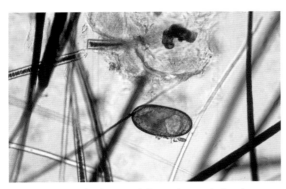

Figure 13-47 Oval eggs of *Sarcoptes scabei;* note emergence of six-legged larval mite.

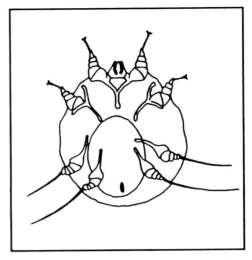

Figure 13-48 Drawing of female *Notoedres muris,* showing dorsal subterminal anal opening.

Notoedric mites are easier to demonstrate in cats than are sarcoptic mites in dogs. Again, likely infestation sites should be scraped. As with *Sarcoptes* species, *Notoedres* mites have a long, unjointed pedicel with a sucker on the end of some of the legs. Adult notoedric mites are similar to sarcoptic mites but are smaller, with a dorsal subterminal anus. The eggs of notoedric mites are oval.

Notoedres cati mites are treated with ivermectin. The best prevention is avoiding contact between infected cats and uninfected cats.

A related species, *Notoedres muris,* produces otic acariasis in rats (Figure 13-48). This mite resembles *Sarcoptes scabei,* with a rounded body and suckers on the first two pairs of legs of female mites and on the first, second, and fourth pairs of legs of male mites. Female *N. muris* can be distinguished from female *S. scabei* by the dorsal subterminal anal opening of *N. muris.* The anal opening of *S. scabei* is terminal (Figure 13-49).

The burrowing mite, *N. muris,* usually can be detected and diagnosed before and after death by collecting deep skin scrapings from the edges of suspected lesions. Lesions are usually on the unfurred parts of the body, such as the ear pinnae, tail, nose, and extremities. Lesions appear as crusted areas with reddened vesicles. *N. muris* is quite common in wild rodents. Transmission is by direct contact, so owners should be

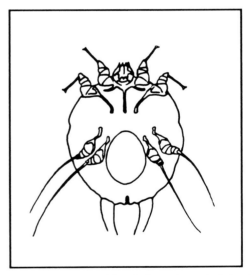

Figure 13-49 Drawing of female *Sarcoptes scabei,* showing terminal anal opening.

cautioned to keep pet rats safely away from wild rodent contact. This mite is also known to infest guinea pigs, but it does not infest humans.

Rabbits can be infested by notoedric and sarcoptic acarines. These mites cause similar lesions, usually on the head, neck, and legs. Lesions may also appear on the pinnae, making it necessary to distinguish *Notoedres cati* and *Sarcoptes scabei* (see Figure 13-49) from the guinea pig mite *Trixacarus caviae* (Figure 13-50) and the rabbit ear mite *Psoroptes cuniculi* (Figure 13-51).

In general, notoedric mites are smaller than sarcoptic mites, and *P. cuniculi* is larger than both. Except for size, the major distinguishing characteristic of *N. cati* and *S. scabei* is the location of the mite's anus. The anus is dorsal and subterminal in *N. cati* and terminal in *S. scabei*. In both *N. cati* and *S. scabei*, suckers are found at the end of long, unjointed stalks on the first two pairs of legs in adult females and on the first, second, and fourth pairs of legs in adult males. Psoroptic mites are distinguished by suckers at the end of long, jointed stalks on the first, second, and fourth pairs of legs in adult females and on the first, second, and third pairs of legs in adult males.

Diagnosis of infestation by *N. cati* and *S. scabei* is by identification of larval, nymphal, or adult mites or the eggs from deep skin scrapings. Deep skin scrapings from the edges of lesions are necessary to detect the burrowing mites. Lesions normally begin near the nose or lips, spread over the face, and may eventually involve the external or lateral pinna, extremities, and genital region. Both *N. cati* and *S. scabei* cause intense pruritus that may result in self-mutilation. A crust or scale may develop over infested areas, and the skin may become thick and wrinkled. Secondary bacterial infection may occur.

Transmission of notoedric and sarcoptic mites is by direct contact. *Sarcoptes scabei* is extremely contagious from rabbit to rabbit and from rabbit to human. The pet owner can become infested with this mite, but the disease is self-limiting. The mites burrow into the skin of humans, producing a papulelike lesion; however, the mites will not establish a full-blown infestation. Both *Notoedres cati* and *Sarcoptes scabei* are considered to be zoonotic.

CNEMIDOCOPTES PILAE *(SCALY LEG MITE OF BUDGERIGARS).* *Cnemidocoptes pilae* is the sarcoptiform mite that causes scaly leg or scaly face in budgerigars or parakeets. This mite tunnels in the superficial layers of the epidermis, affecting the pads and shanks of the feet; in severe cases, it may also affect the beak and the cere, the junction of the feathers and the beak. The mite characteristically produces a yellow–to–gray-white mass resembling a honeycomb. This condition can be quite disfiguring to the parakeet. The parasites pierce the skin underneath the scales, causing an inflammation with exudate that hardens on the surface and displaces the scales upward. This process causes the thickened

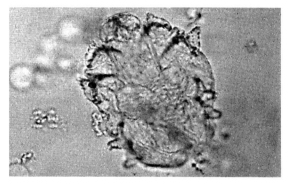

Figure 13-50   *Trixacarus caviae,* typical sarcoptiform mite of guinea pigs.

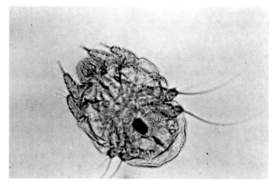

Figure 13-51   Adults of *Psoroptes cuniculi,* occurring most often in external ear canal of rabbits but also collected from horses, goats, and sheep. Mites exhibit characteristic long, jointed pedicels with suckers on ends of some legs.

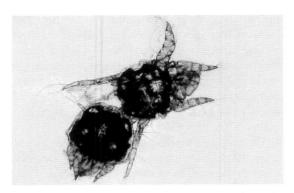

Figure 13-52 Adult *Cnemidocoptes pilae*, sarcoptiform mite that causes scaly leg or scaly face in budgerigars or parakeets. Adults are eight-legged, round to oval in silhouette, and about 500 μm in diameter. Adult females have very short legs and lack suckers. Adult male has longer legs and long, unjointed pedicel with sucker on the end of some legs.

scaly nature of the skin. In canaries, *Cnemidocoptes* species produces a syndrome called **tasselfoot,** a proliferation of the toes and feet. A related species, *C. mutans,* produces a condition called **scaly leg** in chickens, turkeys, and wild birds.

Infestation sites should be scraped. Great care should be taken in handling the infested birds because parakeets and canaries are fragile creatures. The adult mites are eight-legged, round to oval in silhouette, and about 500 μm in diameter (Figure 13-52). The adult female mites have very short legs and lack suckers. The adult male has longer legs and possesses the long, unjointed pedicel with sucker on the end of some of the legs.

Treatment for *Cnemidocoptes pilae* is accomplished with ivermectin.

TRIXACARUS CAVIAE. A burrowing or tunneling mite that infest guinea pigs is *Trixacarus caviae* (see Figure 13-50). *T. caviae* is a typical sarcoptiform mite with a rounded body and suckers on long, unjointed stalks on the first two pairs of legs of females and on the first, second, and fourth pairs of legs of males.

Deep skin scrapings from the edge of suspected lesions around the back, neck, and shoulders is necessary to detect this mite both antemortem and postmortem. Lesions include dry, scaly skin, with pruritus, alopecia, and dermatitis.

Other burrowing mites that may infest guinea pigs are *Sarcoptes scabei* (see Figure 13-49) and *Notoedres muris* (see Figure 13-48). *S. scabei* can be transmitted from rabbits to guinea pigs, in which they produce scabby lesions on the nose and lips. Young guinea pigs are particularly susceptible and may become anorectic to the point of death if not treated. (See previous discussion on identification, detection, and transmission of *S. scabei* in rabbits.) *N. muris* is generally associated with rats but has also been reported in guinea pigs. This mite produces red, crusty lesions on the face of guinea pigs. (See previous discussion on identification, detection, and transmission of *N. muris* in rats.)

Psoroptidae

Members of the family Psoroptidae reside on the surface of the skin or within the external ear canal. The entire five-stage life cycle (egg, larva, protonymph, deutonymph or pubescent female, and adult ovigerous female) is spent on the host. Adult male and female mites breed on the skin surface. The female produces 14 to 24 elliptic, opaque, shiny white eggs that hatch within 1 to 3 days. The six-legged mites are small, oval, soft, and grayish brown. Eight-legged nymphs are slightly larger than larvae. Larval and nymphal stages may last 7 to 10 days. The life cycle is completed in about 10 to 18 days. Under favorable conditions, mites can live off the host for 2 to 3 weeks or longer. Under optimum conditions, mite eggs may remain viable for 2 to 4 weeks.

PSOROPTES CUNICULI *(EAR CANKER MITE OF RABBITS).* *Psoroptes cuniculi* occurs most often in the external ear canal of rabbits but has also been collected from horses, goats, and sheep. These nonburrowing mites reside on the surface of the skin and feed on the rabbit host by puncturing the epidermis to obtain tissue fluids. Within the external ear canal of the infested host are the characteristic dried crusts of coagulated serum.

(In chronic cases, the rabbit's ears appear to be packed with dried corn flakes cereal). Affected animals shake their head and scratch their ears. Although usually associated with otitis media produced by secondary infection with *Pasteurella multocida*, the ear mites themselves are not responsible for this condition. Lesions sometimes occur on the head and legs. Severely infested animals may become debilitated. Loss of equilibrium may occur with torticollis.

The *Psoroptes cuniculi* mites within the corn flake–like crusty debris inside the ear can be easily isolated. The brownish-white female mite is large, 409 to 749 μm by 351 to 499 μm; males are 431 to 547 μm by 322 to 462 μm (see Figure 13-51). The mites exhibit characteristic long, jointed pedicels with suckers on the ends of some of the legs (Figure 13-53). The anus is in a terminal slit. In addition, mites can be observed with the unaided eye or with a hand-held magnifying glass.

Transmission of *P. cuniculi* is by direct contact. This parasite has no zoonotic potential. Treatment may be accomplished with the use of ivermectin otic (not approved for rabbits), milbemycin otic, or thiabendazole-dexamethasone–neomycin sulfate solution.

PSOROPTES OF LARGE ANIMALS. Psoroptes ovis, P. bovis, and *P. equi* are the scab mites of large animals, residing on sheep, cattle, and horses, respectively. These mites are host specific and reside within the thick-haired or long-wooled areas of the animal. They are surface dwellers and feed by puncturing the host's epidermis to feed on lymphatic fluid. Serum exudes through the puncture site; after the serum coagulates and forms a crust, wool is lost. The feeding site is extremely pruritic, and the animal excoriates itself, producing further wool loss. Mites migrate to undamaged skin. As *Psoroptes* mites proliferate, tags of wool are pulled out, and the fleece becomes matted. Finally, patches of skin are exposed, and the skin becomes parchment-like, thickened, and cracked and may bleed easily. Infested sheep constantly rub against fences, posts, farm equipment, and any object that might serve as a scratching post. The disease is spread by direct contact or infested premises.

Psoroptes bovis produces lesions on the withers, neck, and rump that consist of papules, crusts, and wrinkled, thickened skin. *Psoroptes equi* in horses is rare and affects the base of the mane and the tail.

Because of the intense pruritus and the highly contagious nature of this infestation, the occurrence of *Psoroptes* species in large animals should be reported to both state and federal authorities. This disease is reportable to the United States Department of Agriculture.

Mites of *Psoroptes* species that infest large animals are host specific. Adults are up to 600 μm in length. The mites exhibit characteristic long, jointed pedicels with suckers on the ends of some of the legs.

Large-animal *Psoroptes* species can be treated with lime-sulfur dips or ivermectin.

CHORIOPTES *SPECIES (FOOT AND TAIL MITE, ITCHY LEG MITE). Chorioptes equi, C. bovis, C. caprae,* and *C. ovis* are the **foot and tail mites** of large animals, residing on horses, cattle, goats, and sheep, respectively. As with *Psoroptes,* these mites are found on the skin surface. Their predilection sites are on the lower part of the hind legs, but they may spread to flank and shoulder areas. On cattle, they are frequently found in the tail region, especially in the area of the escutcheon. These mites do not spread rapidly or extensively.

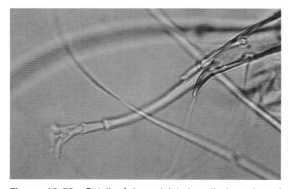

Figure 13-53 Detail of long, jointed pedicel on leg of *Psoroptes cuniculi.*

They puncture the skin, causing serum to exude. Thin crusts of coagulated serum form on the skin surface. The skin eventually wrinkles and thickens, although pruritus is not severe.

Infested horses stamp, bite, and kick, especially at night. Mites typically infest the pasterns, especially those of the hind legs.

Characteristic mites of the genus *Chorioptes* can be identified from skin scrapings of infested areas. The mites have characteristic short, unjointed pedicels with suckers on the ends of some of the legs. The female mites are about 400 μm long (Figure 13-54).

Ivermectin and lime-sulfur dips are used to treat *Chorioptes equi, C. bovis, C. caprae,* and *C. ovis.*

OTODECTES CYNOTIS *(EAR MITES).* Ear mites, *Otodectes cynotis,* are a common cause of otitis externa in both dogs and cats. Although they occur primarily in the external ear canal, ear mites may be found on any area of the body. A common infestation site is the tail-head region, because as dogs and cats curl up to sleep, their heads (and ears) are often close to the base of the tail. These mites are spread by direct contact and are highly transmissible both among and between dogs and cats.

Mites are found within the external ear canal, where they feed on epidermal debris and produce intense irritation. Infestation is usually in both ears. The host responds to the mite infestation by shaking its head and scratching its ears. In severe infestations, otitis media, with head tilt, circling, and convulsions, may occur. Auricular hematomas may develop.

Ear mites are usually identified with an otoscope, through which the mites appear as white, motile objects. Exudate collected by swabbing the ear may be placed in mineral oil on a glass slide and the mites observed under a compound microscope using the 10× objective. These mites are fairly large, approximately 400 μm (Figure 13-55); they can also be easily seen with the unaided eye. The mites exhibit characteristic short, unjointed pedicels with suckers on the ends of some of the legs (Figure 13-56). The anus of *O. cynotis* is terminal.

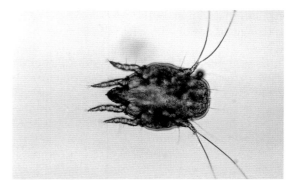

Figure 13-55 Adult male ear mite, *Otodectes cynotis.*

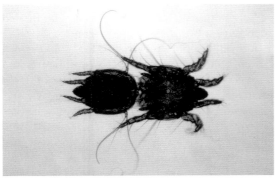

Figure 13-54 Female and male *Chorioptes* species. Note short, unjointed pedicels.

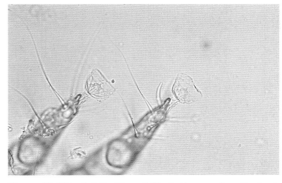

Figure 13-56 Detail of leg of *Otodectes cynotis* with short, unjointed pedicel.

Ivermectin otic, milbemycin otic, and thiabendazole-dexamethasone–neomycin sulfate solution are used to treat *Otodectes cynotis*. In addition to medication, the ears should be cleaned to remove the debris and mites from the ears.

Nonsarcoptiform Mites

The following group of parasitic mites are discussed together because they are not sarcoptiform mites. They can, however, produce severe dermatologic problems in a variety of domestic animals. These mites lack the pedicels or stalks on their legs that are so important in diagnosing the sarcoptiform mites.

DEMODEX *SPECIES.* Mites of the genus *Demodex* reside in the hair follicles and sebaceous glands of humans and of most domesticated animals. In many species, mites of the genus *Demodex* are considered normal, nonpathogenic fauna of the skin. These mites are host specific and are not transmissible from one species of host to another. The clinical disease caused by many of these mites is called *demodicosis.*

Demodex mites resemble eight-legged alligators; these mites typically are elongated mites with very short, stubby legs. Adult and nymphal stages have eight legs, and larvae have six. Adult *Demodex* mites are approximately 250 μm long (Figure 13-57). The eggs are spindle shaped or tapered at each end (Figure 13-58).

Of all the domestic animals infested with *Demodex* species, the dog is the most often and the most seriously infested. These mites are considered to be part of the normal skin flora of all dogs; in some dogs with immunodeficiencies, however, they proliferate to the point that they produce pathology. The clinical syndromes relative to the form of demodicosis present in dogs are localized demodicosis and generalized demodicosis.

The predominant clinical sign of the *localized* form of demodicosis is a patchy alopecia, especially of the muzzle, face, and forelimbs. It is thought that *Demodex* mites are acquired during the close, intimate contact that develops as the dam nurses the puppy. As a result of that contact,

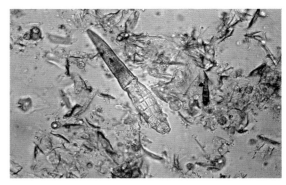

Figure 13-57   Adult *Demodex canis. Demodex* mites resemble eight-legged alligators; they are elongated, with very short, stubby legs. Adult and nymphal stages have eight legs; larvae have six legs.

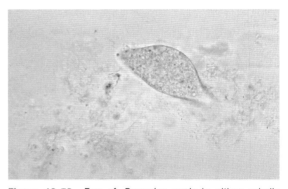

Figure 13-58   Egg of *Demodex canis* is either spindle shaped or tapered at each end.

localized demodicosis often develops in the region of the face or forelimbs.

Generalized demodicosis is characterized by diffuse alopecia, erythema, and secondary bacterial contamination over the entire body surface of the dog. An inherited defect in the dog's immune system is thought to be an important factor in the development and the pathogenesis of generalized demodicosis. Generalized demodicosis can affect the entire skin surface, and on occasion, demodectic mites have been known to infect internal organs.

Cats are infested by two species of demodectic mites, *Demodex canis* and an unnamed species of *Demodex*. *Demodex cati* is an elongated mite similar to *D. canis*. The unnamed species has a broad, blunted abdomen, unlike the elongated abdomen of *D. cati*. The presence of either species in the skin of cats is rare. In localized feline demodicosis, patchy areas of alopecia, erythema, and occasionally crusting occur on the head (especially around the eyes), ears, and neck. In generalized feline demodicosis, the alopecia, erythema, and crusting usually involve the entire body. Demodicosis also has been associated with ceruminous otitis externa.

Demodectic mites reside in the hair follicles of other species of domestic animals but rarely produce clinical disease. Cattle and goats are those most often infested, and then only rarely.

In cattle, *Demodex bovis* causes large nodules or abscesses on the shoulders, trunk, and lateral aspects of the neck. In goats, *Demodex caprae* occurs in small, papular or nodular lesions on the shoulders, trunk, and lateral aspect of the neck. Rarely, in sheep, *Demodex ovis* causes pustules and crusting around the coronet, nose, ear tips, and periorbital areas. Rarely, in pigs, *Demodex phylloides* produces pustules and nodules on the face, abdomen, and ventral neck. In horses, *Demodex equi* occurs around the face and eyes and rarely produces clinical disease.

Demodex aurati (Figure 13-59) and *Demodex criceti* (Figure 13-60) infest hamsters. As with other *Demodex* species, they live in hair follicles and adjacent sebaceous glands. Deep skin scrapings at the edges of the lesions are necessary to detect the mites. Lesions are most often seen on the dorsum of the hamster, near the rump.

Clinical signs that may indicate demodicosis in the hamster include alopecia and dry scaly skin or scabby dermatitis, particularly over the rump and on the back of the hamster. Demodicosis is most often observed in aged or otherwise stressed hamsters. The mite population in hamsters is usually greater in males than in females. As with *D. canis* in dogs, *D. aurati* and *D. criceti* may be present without producing clinical signs.

Gerbils have been reported to carry two species of *Demodex*, *D. aurati* and *D. criceti* (see

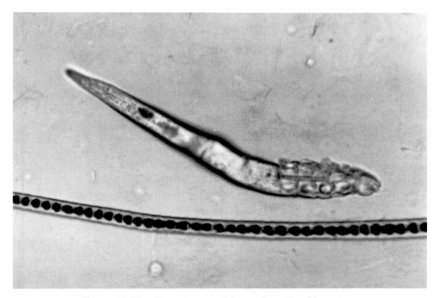

Figure 13-59 *Demodex aurati*, burrowing mite of hamsters.

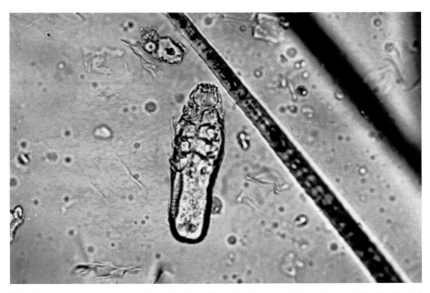

Figure 13-60   *Demodex criceti*, a hamster mite, is distinguishable from *Demodex aurati* by its blunt body shape.

Figures 13-59 and 13-60). These mites are similar in size and shape to the demodectic mites of hamsters. Demodectic mites also have been recovered from gerbils with facial dermatitis. As in other species with demodectic acariasis, infested gerbils have other concomitant disease. Lesions are similar to those described in the hamster.

Demodicosis may be detected on postmortem examination by histopathologic examination of skin sections. Transmission is by direct contact, with the primary route thought to be from mother to suckling young. *Demodex* species of hamsters are considered to be species specific, with the possible exception of the gerbil, and thus are not likely to cross-contaminate other species or pose a zoonotic problem to humans.

Skin with altered pigmentation, obstructed hair follicles, erythema, or alopecia should always be scraped. In localized demodicosis, the areas most often affected are the forelegs, the perioral region, and the periorbital regions. In generalized demodicosis of dogs, the entire body may be affected; however, the face and feet usually are the most severely involved. In dogs,

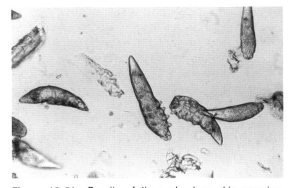

Figure 13-61   Results of thorough, deep skin scraping, revealing numerous mites of *Demodex canis.*

normal skin should also be scraped to determine if the disease is generalized. The areas should be clipped and a fold of skin gently squeezed to express any mites from the hair follicles. Scraping should be continued until capillary blood is observed oozing, because these mites live deep in the hair follicles and sebaceous glands (Figure 13-61).

Nodular lesions in large animals should be incised with a scalpel and the caseous material within smeared on a microscope slide with mineral oil, covered with a coverslip, and examined for mites.

The veterinary diagnostician should count the mites on the glass slide and determine the live:dead ratio. The presence of larval or nymphal stages or eggs should be noted. Treatment for demodicosis involves dipping the affected animal in an amitraz (not used on horses) or trichlorfon dip. During therapy for *Demodex* species, a decrease in the number of eggs and the number of live or moving mites is a good prognostic indicator.

TROMBICULA *SPECIES (CHIGGERS)*. The **chigger,** *Trombicula* species, is yellow to red, has six legs, and ranges in size from 200 to 400 μm in diameter (Figure 13-62). The larval stage is the only developmental stage that parasitizes humans, domestic animals, and wild animals. The larvae are most common during the late summer and early fall and are transmitted by direct contact of the host with the ground or by brushing against foliage in fields or heavy underbrush. The nymphal and adult stages of chiggers are nonparasitic and are free-living in nature.

Larval chiggers do *not* burrow into the skin, as commonly believed, nor do they feed primarily on host blood. Their food consists of the serous components of tissues. Chiggers attach firmly to the host and inject a digestive fluid that produces liquefaction of host cells. The host's skin becomes hardened, and a tube called a **stylostome** forms at the chigger's attachment site. Chiggers suck up liquefied host tissues. When the mite has finished feeding, it loosens its grip and falls to the ground. The injected digestive fluid causes the attachment site to itch intensely. In animals, cutaneous lesions tend to be restricted to areas of the body that come in contact with the ground or underbrush, that is, the head, ears, limbs, interdigital areas, and ventrum.

The most common chigger mite affecting animals and humans is *Trombicula alfreddugesi*, the **North American chigger.** Lesions caused by *T. alfreddugesi* consist of an erythematous, often pruritic, papular rash on the ventrum, face, feet, and legs.

The diagnosis of chiggers is based on the presence of an orange crusting dermatosis, a history of exposure (roaming outdoors), and identification of the typical six-legged larval stage on skin scraping or on collection from the host. The larval chigger remains attached to the skin only for several hours. Consequently, **trombiculosis** may be difficult to diagnose, because the pruritus persists after the larva has dropped off the host.

PNEUMONYSSOIDES (PNEUMONYSSUS) CANINUM *(NASAL MITES OF DOGS)*. *Pneumonyssoides (Pneumonyssus) caninum* is a rare species of mite that lives in the nasal passages and associated paranasal sinuses of dogs. Generally, nasal mites are considered to be nonpathogenic; however, reddening of the nasal mucosa, sneezing, shaking of the head, and rubbing of the nose often accompany infestation. Fainting, labored breathing, asthmalike attacks, and orbital disease have been associated with this mite. Sinusitis caused by these mites may lead to disorders of the central nervous system. Owners will observe these mites exiting the nostrils.

The life cycle of *P. caninum* is unknown, but it apparently takes place entirely within the host. Adult males, females, and larvae have been identified, but no nymphal stages have been

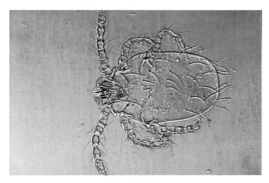

Figure 13-62 The chigger, *Trombicula* species, is yellow to red, has six legs, and ranges in size from 200 to 400 μm in diameter.

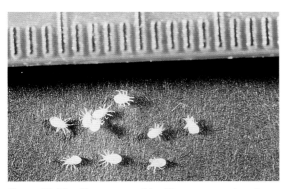

Figure 13-63 *Pneumonyssoides (Pneumonyssus) caninum,* a rare mite that lives in nasal passages and associated paranasal sinuses of dogs.

observed. Transmission probably occurs through direct contact with an infested animal.

Nasal mites are oval and pale yellow. They are 1 to 1.5 mm by 0.6 to 0.9 mm and possess a smooth cuticle with very few hairs. Larvae have six legs, and adults have eight legs. All legs are located on the anterior half of the body (Figure 13-63).

ORNITHONYSSUS SYLVIARUM *(NORTHERN MITE OF POULTRY) AND* DERMANYSSUS GALLINAE *(RED MITE OF POULTRY).* *Ornithonyssus sylviarum* and *Dermanyssus gallinae* both parasitize poultry but differ in the sites where they are collected. *O. sylviarum* is a 1-mm, elongate-to-oval mite usually found on birds; it also may be found on nests or within poultry houses. This species, the **northern mite of poultry,** feeds intermittently on birds, producing irritation, weight loss, decreased egg production, anemia, and even death. These mites have been known to bite humans.

D. gallinae is similar in appearance to *O. sylviarum* and is approximately 1 mm in length; elongate to oval; whitish, grayish, or black; and feeds on birds. This mite has a distinct red color when it has recently fed on its host's blood, thus its common name the **red mite of poultry.** *D. gallinae* lays its eggs in the cracks in the walls of poultry houses. Both the nymphal stage and the adults are periodic parasites, hiding in cracks and crevices of the poultry houses and making

frequent visits to the host to feed. Because of their blood-feeding activity, these mites may produce significant anemia and much irritation to the host. Birds are listless, and egg production may decrease. Loss of blood may result in death. These mites also occur in bird nests in the eaves of houses or in air conditioners. They migrate into homes and attack humans. *D. gallinae* can be treated with pyrethrin sprays or ivermectin. If a flock is infected with *D. gallinae*, dichlorvos strips may be used to treat the flock.

Because of their similar morphology, these mites are difficult to differentiate. *O. sylviarum* is usually found on the avian host, whereas *D. gallinae* is a periodic parasite, usually found in the host's environment. If specimens are recovered, they should be cleared in lactophenol and the ventral anal plates examined under a compound microscope. The anus of *O. sylviarum* is on the anterior half of the ventral anal plate, whereas that of *D. gallinae* is on the posterior half of the ventral anal plate.

ORNITHONYSSUS (LIPONYSSUS) BACOTI. *Ornithonyssus (Liponyssus) bacoti* is commonly called the **tropical rat mite.** This bloodsucking mite can cause severe problems in rats and mice and can also infect hamsters and guinea pigs. It is especially common in tropical and subtropical climates. *O. bacoti* has a wide host range beyond rodents and can also infect hamsters and guinea pigs.

Oddly, even though *O. bacoti* is a bloodsucking mite, it is more closely related to ticks than mites. This mite is unusual in that it spends most of its life cycle off the host animal, in the host's environment. Both male and female mites are bloodsuckers. The females are larger than the males. These mites may be filled with blood, which produces a reddish-brown color, or, if they have not fed, they may be white. The mites can measure up to 750 µm in length (Figure 13-64).

O. bacoti mites intermittently feed on rodent blood, dropping into nests or surrounding cracks and crevices between feedings. These mites can gain access to other pet animals by dropping

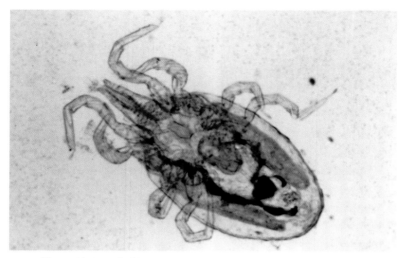

Figure 13-64 *Ornithonyssus (Liponyssus) bacoti,* the tropical rat mite.

from wild or feral animals; days later, when the original host is no longer in the area, they may attack a pet animal for a blood meal.

Infestation with *O. bacoti* is usually diagnosed by observing the blood-filled mites in the bedding, nests, or cracks and crevices near the cages of pet animals. Animals in an environment infested with *O. bacoti* may be anemic and may exhibit a marked reproductive decline. The mite can transmit rickettsial organisms and cause allergic dermatitis in humans. In the absence of a suitable rodent host, *O. bacoti* will readily attack humans for a blood meal.

O. bacoti has a wide host range beyond rodents and is especially common in tropical and subtropical climates.

Fur Mites

CHEYLETIELLA *SPECIES (WALKING DANDRUFF).* Mites of the genus *Cheyletiella* are surface-dwelling (nonburrowing) mites that reside in the keratin layer of the skin and in the hair coat of various definitive hosts, which may be dogs, cats, or rabbits. These mites ingest keratin debris and tissue fluids and are often referred to as *walking dandruff,* because the motile mites

resemble large, moving flakes of dandruff. Cheylettid mites have unique morphologic features. They are large mites (386 by 266 µm), visible to the naked eye. The compound microscope allows easy visualization of this mite's most characteristic morphologic feature, enormous hooklike accessory mouthparts *(palpi)* on the anterior end. These palpi assist the mite in attaching to the host as it feeds on tissue fluids. The mite also has comblike structures at the tip of each of its legs. Members of the genus are also known for their characteristic body shape, a silhouette that has been reported as resembling a shield, a bell pepper, the acorn of an oak tree, or a western horse saddle when viewed from above (Figure 13-65). Eggs are 235 to 245 µm long by 115 to 135 µm wide (smaller than louse nits) and supported by cocoonlike structures bound to the hair shaft by strands of fibers. Two or three eggs may be bound together on one hair shaft.

The key feature of active infestation by *Cheyletiella* species is often the moving, white, dandrufflike flakes along the dorsal midline and head of the host. A hand-held magnifying lens or a binocular headband magnifier (e.g., Optivisor) may be used to view questionable dandruff

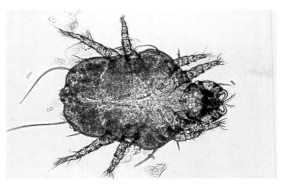

Figure 13-65 Adult mite, *Cheyletiella parasitivorax.* *Cheyletiella* species have hooklike accessory mouthparts (palpi) on the anterior end and comblike structures at the tip of legs. These mites have characteristic body shape described as a shield, bell pepper, acorn, or western horse saddle, when viewed from above.

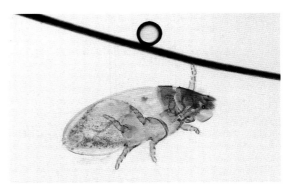

Figure 13-66 *Lynxacarus radovskyi,* the feline fur mite, attaches to hair shafts on back, neck, thorax, and hind limbs of cats.

flakes or hairs; these are perhaps the quickest methods of diagnosing **cheyletiellosis.** A fine-toothed flea comb may be used to collect mites; combing dandrufflike debris onto black paper often facilitates visualization of these highly motile mites. Using clear cellophane tape to entrap mites collected from the hair coat often simplifies localization and viewing under the compound microscope.

Cheyletiella species can be treated with iver-mectin (not approved for rabbits) and malathion dips.

LYNXACARUS RADOVSKYI *(FELINE FUR MITE).* *Lynx-acarus radovskyi,* the feline fur mite, is found attached to the shafts of individual hairs on the back, neck, thorax, and hind limbs of cats resid-ing in tropical or warm areas of the United States, such as Florida, Puerto Rico, and Hawaii. These fur mites are laterally compressed. The adults are approximately 500 µm long (Figure 13-66). Pru-ritus is not always associated with infestations of *L. radovskyi* in cats. These mites are diagnosed by observing the mites attached to hair shafts and examining the dander and other debris after combing. This mite may also affect humans who handle infested cats, producing a papular dermatitis.

MYOBIA MUSCULI, MYOCOPTES MUSCULINUS, *AND* RADFORDIA AFFINIS *(MOUSE FUR MITES).* The three most common fur mites of the mouse are *Myobia musculi, Myocoptes musculinus,* and *Radfordia affinis.* Mice housed in close association with rats may become infested with *Radfordia ensifera,* a fur mite of rats (see next discussion). Rodent mites have life cycles similar to those of mites of other animal species, with larval and nymphal stages. Larval mites have only six legs, whereas nymphal stages (Figure 13-67, *A*) and adult spec-imens have eight legs (Figure 13-67, *B*).

The first pair of legs of *M. musculi* and *R. affinis* is distinctly short and adapted for clasping the hair of the host, with the first two pairs of legs being somewhat clublike at the ends (Figure 13-67, *C*). This feature distinguishes *M. musculi-nus* from both *M. musculi* and *R. affinis.*

The second pair of legs of *M. musculi* and *R. affinis* end with clawlike features referred to as **empodia.** The empodia of *M. musculi* are long and single (Figure 13-68, *left*), whereas *R. affinis* has a shorter pair of empodia of unequal length on the second set of legs (Figure 13-68, *right*).

Adult females of *M. musculi* are about 400 to 500 µm long and 200 µm wide. Males are simi-larly shaped but proportionately smaller. *R. affinis* is similar in size and shape to *M. musculi.* Adult females of *M. musculinus* are smaller than

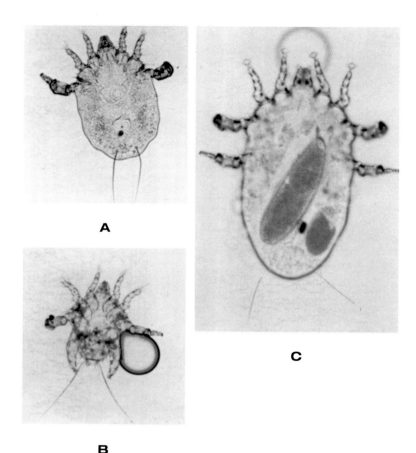

Figure 13-67   *Myocoptes musculinus,* fur mite of mice. **A,** Nymphal female. Note absence of adult's hind legs. **B,** Adult female. Oval shape within is an egg. **C,** Adult male with air bubble artifact.

other fur mites of mice, measuring 300 by 130 μm. The male is 190 by 135 μm.

Fur mite eggs can be found attached near the base of the host's hairs. The eggs are oval and about 200 μm long (Figure 13-69).

To detect fur mites on a live mouse, fur can be obtained by plucking with forceps or by pressing the adhesive side of cellophane tape on the pelt of the mouse. The plucked fur can be placed in a drop of mineral oil on a glass slide and examined microscopically for mites or eggs. The cellophane tape can be placed adhesive side down on a drop of mineral oil on a glass slide and similarly examined. Fur samples should be taken from the neck or shoulder area, because that is

where the mites most often reside and produce lesions.

Postmortem detection of fur-inhabiting mites of mice may be approached as in the antemortem method, or the dead mouse may be placed under a warm lamp for a few minutes. The heat attracts the mites in the pelt, causing them to migrate to the tips of the hairs. A hand-held magnifying glass, a head loupe, or a dissecting microscope aids in the detection of the mites. The mites may be collected on the tip of a metal probe or similar instrument that has been dipped in mineral oil, then placed in a drop of mineral oil on a glass slide and under a coverslip, and examined microscopically.

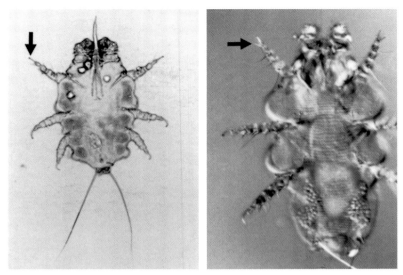

Figure 13-68   *Left*, Eight-legged nymphal form of *Myobia musculi*, showing single long empodial claw on second pair of legs *(arrow)*. Extended mouthpart is typical of nymphal form. *Right, Radfordia affinis*, showing paired empodial claws on second leg pair.

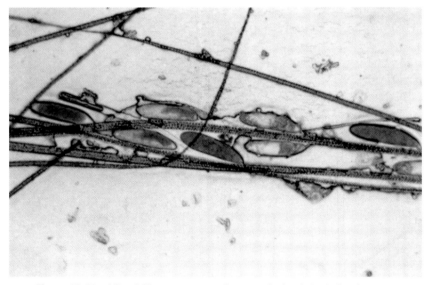

Figure 13-69   Nits of *Myocoptes musculinus* attached to hair shafts of mouse.

The pathogenicity of mouse fur mites varies greatly with the host and the degree of infestation, similar to demodectic acariasis in dogs. Clinical signs may be absent or may include alopecia, pruritus, and ulceration. More severe lesions may be the result of host sensitivity to the mites, in which case few if any mites are observed.

Transmission of mouse fur mites is by direct contact. Although mites are generally host spe-

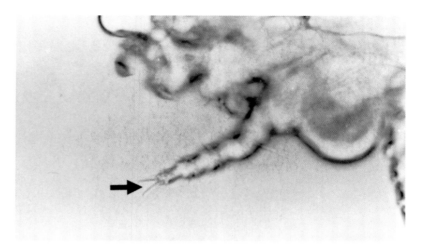

Figure 13-70 Second leg of *Radfordia ensifera*, showing equal length of empodial claws *(arrow).*

cific, the owner of multiple species of rodents should be advised that *M. musculi* and *R. affinis* may infest rats and guinea pigs housed in the same area with mice infested with *M. musculi* and *R. affinis*. The three species of mouse fur mites are not known to infest humans.

M. musculi and *M. musculinus* are treated with ivermectin.

RADFORDIA ENSIFERA *(RAT FUR MITE). Radfordia ensifera*, a fur mite of rats, is similar to *Myobia musculi* and *Radfordia affinis* (see Figure 13-68). *R. ensifera* is distinguished from *M. musculi* and *R. affinis* by the empodial claws of the second pair of legs. *M. musculi* has a single, long empodial claw (see Figure 13-68, *left*), whereas *R. ensifera* and *R. affinis* both have a pair of short claws. The two empodial claws of *R. ensifera* are of equal length (Figure 13-70), whereas those of *R. affinis* are of unequal length (see Figure 13-68, *right*).

Antemortem or postmortem, *R. ensifera* is detected using methods described for mouse fur mites. Light infestation of *R. ensifera* usually causes no clinical signs; however, self-inflicted trauma may be seen in heavy infestations. Transmission is by direct contact. *R. ensifera* is not known to infest humans.

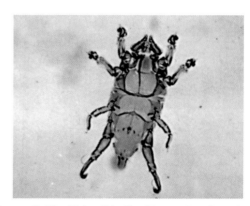

Figure 13-71 Male *Chirodiscoides caviae*, fur mite of guinea pig.

CHIRODISCOIDES CAVIAE *(GUINEA PIG FUR MITE)*. The fur mite that typically infests guinea pigs is *Chirodiscoides caviae. C. caviae* is an elongated mite, with a triangular cranial portion that appears similar to the head of the mite. All eight legs are adapted for grasping onto the hair. There are no empodial claws on the first two pairs of legs. The male is about 363 by 138 μm (Figure 13-71), and the female is 515 by 164 μm (Figure 13-72).

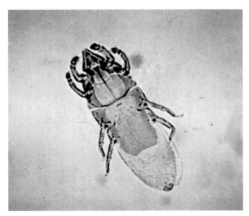

Figure 13-72 Female *Chirodiscoides caviae*, fur mite of guinea pig.

C. caviae is somewhat difficult to observe antemortem with the unaided eye. It may be detected by pulling hairs, either with forceps or by the cellophane tape method, then examining the specimen microscopically. *C. caviae* is found in the pelt and occurs in the greatest numbers in the area over the rump. Postmortem, a piece of the pelt from the rump of the dead animal may be placed in a Petri dish to cool and then examined with a hand-held magnifying glass or dissecting microscope for mites at the tip of the hairs.

Usually there are no clinical signs unless infestation is severe, when alopecia and pruritus may be seen. Although *C. caviae* is not considered transmissible to humans, transient infestation causing a pruritic, papular urticarial skin condition has been reported.

Myocoptes musculinus and *Radfordia affinis* are also transmissible to guinea pigs (see previous discussion).

LISTROPHORUS GIBBUS *(RABBIT FUR MITE).* Similar to *Cheyletiella parasitivorax* (see Figure 13-65), *Listrophorus gibbus* is a small, nonburrowing fur mite of rabbits. *L. gibbus* females are about 435 μm and males 340 μm long. Both species have a dorsal hoodlike projection covering the mouthparts. Males are further characterized by the clasping organs at their caudal end.

In the same manner as for *C. parasitivorax,* *L. gibbus* may be detected by pulling fur with forceps or cellophane tape and then examining the hairs under a dissecting microscope. Combing or brushing the fur may also be used to obtain mites for identification. *L. gibbus* mites are most likely located on the back and abdomen of rabbits. This mite appears to produce no clinical signs, even in heavy infestations.

L. gibbus is transmitted by direct contact. Infestation with *L. gibbus* is treated with malathion dips or ivermectin (not approved for rabbits). This mite is more often associated with wild rabbits than with domestic species, so owners should be aware that control of this parasite depends on controlling the rabbit's environment. *L. gibbus* is not a known vector of disease and has no zoonotic significance in humans.

TICKS OF VETERINARY IMPORTANCE

Ticks are small to medium-sized acarines with dorsoventrally flattened, leathery bodies. The tick's head, the capitulum, has two cutting, or lacerating, organs called *chelicerae;* a penetrating, anchorlike sucking organ, the *hypostome;* and two leglike accessory appendages, the *pedipalps,* that act as sensors or supports when the tick fastens to the host's body. The tick's body may be partially or entirely covered by a hard, chitinous plate, the *scutum.* Mouthparts may be concealed under the tick's body or may extend from the anterior border of the body. Most ticks are *inornate;* that is, they have a reddish or mahogany color. Some species are *ornate;* that is, they demonstrate distinctive white patterns on the dark reddish or mahogany background of the scutum. Larval ticks have six legs, and nymphal and adult ticks have eight legs with strong claws on the ends.

Ticks are important parasites because of their voracious blood-feeding activity. They are also important because they are capable of transmitting many parasitic, bacterial, viral, rickettsial, and other pathogenic diseases, such as *borreliosis* (Lyme disease), among animals and from animals to humans. These pathogenic organisms may be transmitted passively, or the tick may serve as an obligatory intermediate host for certain protozoan parasites.

Ticks are also important because the salivary secretions of some female ticks are toxic and can produce a syndrome known as **tick paralysis** in humans and domestic and wild animals. Tick species associated with tick paralysis are *Dermacentor andersoni,* the Rocky Mountain spotted fever tick; *Dermacentor occidentalis,* the Pacific Coast tick; *Ixodes holocyclus,* the paralysis tick of Australia; and *Dermacentor variabilis,* the wood tick.

The ticks of veterinary importance can be divided into two families, the **argasid,** or soft, ticks and the **ixodid,** or hard, ticks. Argasid ticks lack a scutum, the hard, chitinous plate that covers the body of the tick. The mouthparts of the adult soft tick cannot be seen when viewed from the dorsal aspect. Ixodid ticks, on the other hand, have a hard, chitinous scutum that covers all the male tick's dorsum and about a third or less of the female tick's dorsum, depending on the degree of engorgement. As a rule of thumb, male ticks are much smaller than female ticks.

Among the argasid ticks, two species are important: *Otobius megnini,* the spinose ear tick, and *Argas persicus,* the fowl tick. In the ixodid tick family, there are 13 economically important tick species. These include *Rhipicephalus sanguineus, Ixodes scapularis, Dermacentor* species, and *Amblyomma* species. Of these species, *R. sanguineus* infests buildings such as dwellings and kennels; the other ticks attack their hosts in outdoor environments.

Specific identification of ticks is difficult and should be performed by a veterinary parasitologist or trained acarologist or arthropodologist. Ticks are usually identified by the shape and length of the capitulum or mouthparts, the shape and color of the body, and the shape and markings on the scutum. Male and unengorged female ticks are easier to identify than engorged female ticks. It is most difficult to speciate larval or nymphal ticks. The common species can be identified by their size, shape, color, body markings, host, and location on the host.

There are four major stages in the life cycle of ticks: egg, larva, nymph, and adult. Following their engorgement on the host, female ticks drop off the host and seek protected places, such as in cracks and crevices or under leaves and branches, to lay their eggs (Figure 13-73). The six-legged larvae, or **seed ticks,** hatch from the eggs and feed on the host (Figure 13-74). The larva molts to the eight-legged nymphal stage, which resembles the adult stage but lacks the functioning reproductive organs of adult ticks. After one or two blood meals, the nymph becomes mature and molts to the adult stage. During the larval, nymphal, and adult stages, ticks may infest one,

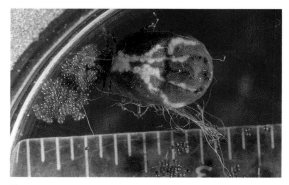

Figure 13-73 Adult female *Dermacentor variabilis* laying hundreds of eggs.

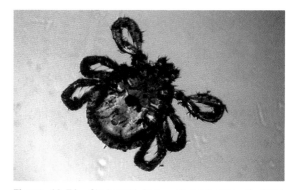

Figure 13-74 Six-legged larva, or seed tick, of *Rhipicephalus sanguineus* hatches from egg and feeds on host.

two, three, or even many different host species (Figure 13-75). This ability to feed on several hosts during the life cycle plays an important role in the transmission of disease pathogens among hosts. It is important to remember that any infestation of domestic animals by either mites or ticks is referred to as *acariasis.*

Most ticks do not tolerate direct sunlight, dryness, or excessive rainfall. They can survive as long as 2 to 3 years without a blood meal,

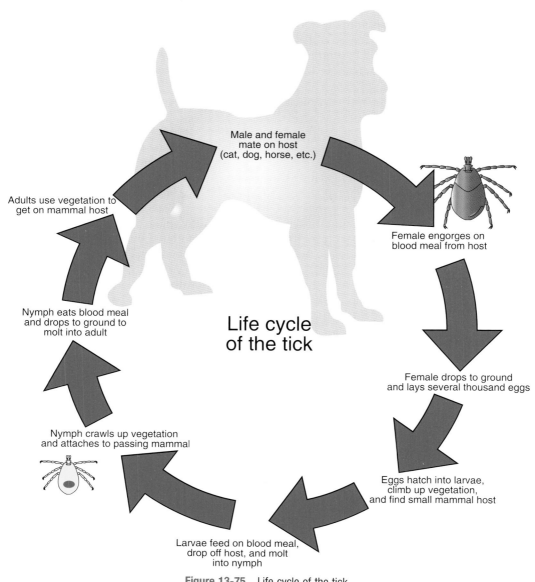

Male and female
mate on host
(cat, dog, horse, etc.)

Adults use vegetation to
get on mammal host

Female engorges on
blood meal from host

Nymph eats blood meal
and drops to ground to
molt into adult

Life cycle
of the tick

Female drops to ground
and lays several thousand eggs

Nymph crawls up vegetation
and attaches to passing mammal

Eggs hatch into larvae,
climb up vegetation,
and find small mammal host

Larvae feed on blood meal,
drop off host, and molt
into nymph

Figure 13-75   Life cycle of the tick.

but female ticks require a blood meal before fertilization and subsequent egg deposition. Tick activity is restricted during the cold winter months but increases dramatically during the spring, summer, and fall seasons.

Tick prevention is the best way to avoid acariasis by ticks. Prevention includes inspecting the animal for ticks each time the animal is outside and removing the ticks as soon as possible. Tick products, such as Frontline* or Frontline Plus* and Advantix,[†] will kill some species of ticks and are applied once a month. Amitraz is an effective dip for ticks, although there is no long-term residual effect. Amitraz may also be purchased as a tick collar and is effective against ticks.

Argasid (Soft) Ticks

OTOBIUS MEGNINI *(SPINOSE EAR TICK). Otobius megnini,* the **spinose ear tick,** is an unusual soft tick in that only the larval and nymphal stages are parasitic. The adult stages are not parasitic, but instead are free-living and are found in the environment of the definitive host, usually in dry protected places, in cracks and crevices, and under logs and fence posts. The larval and nymphal stages feed on horses, cattle, sheep, goats, and dogs. These ticks are associated with the semiarid or arid areas of the southwestern United States; with widespread interstate transportation of animals, however, this soft tick may occur throughout North America. As with most soft ticks, the mouthparts may not be visible when viewed from the dorsal aspect (Figure 13-76). The nymphal stage of *O. megnini* is widest in the middle and is almost violin shaped. It is covered with tiny, backward-projecting spines, thus the name *spinose.* The larval and nymphal forms are usually found within the ears of the definitive host, thus the name *ear tick.*

Spinose ear ticks are extremely irritating to the definitive host. They often occur in large

*Merial, 1-888-637-4251.
†Bayer Animal Health Corporation, Bedford, NH.

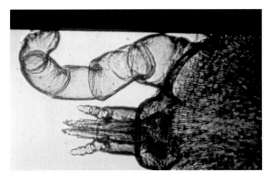

Figure 13-76 Only larval and nymphal stages of *Otobius megnini,* the spinose ear tick, are parasitic. Mouthparts of this soft tick may not be visible when viewed from dorsal aspect.

numbers deep within the external ear canal. These ticks imbibe large amounts of host blood; however, because they are soft ticks, they do not engorge or swell. Large numbers of these ticks may produce ulceration deep within the external ear. The ears become highly sensitive, and the animals may shake their heads. The pinnae may become excoriated by the constant shaking and rubbing of the animal's head.

The ticks may be visualized in situ with an otoscope. Any waxy exudate should be examined for the presence of larval and nymphal stages of the spinose ear tick.

ARGAS PERSICUS *(FOWL TICK). Argas persicus,* the **fowl tick,** is a soft tick of chickens, turkeys, and wild birds. These ticks are periodic parasites, hiding in cracks and crevices during the day and becoming active during the evening hours, when they feed intermittently on the avian host. The adults are 7 mm long and 5 mm wide. In the unengorged state, they are reddish brown, but after engorgement, they take on a slate-blue color. These ticks are flat and leathery, and the tegument is covered with tiny bumps. Because they are soft ticks, they lack a scutum. The mouthparts are not visible when the adult tick is viewed from the dorsal aspect.

Birds heavily infested with *A. persicus* may develop significant anemias. These ticks are worrisome to birds, particularly during the evening hours. The feeding activity of these ticks may cause the birds' egg laying to decrease or even cease.

All stages of *A. persicus* may be collected from infested birds but most often are found in cracks, crevices, and contaminated bedding in poultry houses.

Ixodid (Hard) Ticks

RHIPICEPHALUS SANGUINEUS *(BROWN DOG TICK)*. *Rhipicephalus sanguineus,* the brown dog tick, is an unusual hard tick in that it invades both kennel and household environments. This tick is widely distributed throughout North America. It has an inornate, uniformly reddish brown scutum and feeds almost exclusively on dogs, thus the common name **brown dog tick.** *R. sanguineus* also has a distinguishing key morphologic feature: its basis capitulum (or head) has prominent lateral extensions that give the structure a decidedly hexagonal appearance (Figure 13-77). The engorged female is often slate gray. In southern climates the tick is found outdoors, but in northern climates it becomes a serious household pest, breeding indoors in both home and kennel environments.

The bites of this tick can be very irritating to the dog. In severe infestations, heavy blood loss

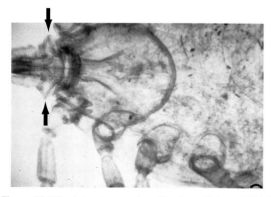

Figure 13-77 Lateral expansion of basis capitulum of *Rhipicephalus sanguineus*, the brown dog tick. This key morphologic feature is used to identify this tick, which can breed in host's environment.

may occur. This tick is also an intermediate host for *Babesia canis,* the etiologic agent that causes canine piroplasmosis.

R. sanguineus can be identified by its inornate brown color and characteristic lateral projections of the basis capitulum. These ticks are unique in that they can be found in indoor or kennel environments. Treatment can be accomplished by foggers that will kill ticks or a house spray labeled for use against ticks. This treatment will kill ticks indoors or in the kennel.

DERMACENTOR VARIABILIS *(AMERICAN DOG TICK, WOOD TICK)*. *Dermacentor variabilis,* the **American dog tick** or **wood tick,** is found primarily in the eastern two thirds of the United States; however, with the increased mobility of American households, the tick may become distributed throughout the country. Unlike *R. sanguineus,* the *D. variabilis* tick only inhabits grassy, scrub-brush areas, especially roadsides and pathways. This three-host tick initially feeds on small mammals, such as field mice and other rodents. However, dogs and humans can serve as preferred hosts for this ubiquitous tick. *D. variabilis* can serve as a vector of Rocky Mountain spotted fever, tularemia, and other microbes. It has also been associated with tick paralysis in domestic and wild animals and in humans. This tick has an ornate scutum that is dark brown with white striping. Unfed adult ticks are approximately 6 mm long; the adult engorged female is about 12 mm and is blue-gray (Figure 13-78). *D. variabilis* is a seasonal annoyance to humans and domestic animals.

D. variabilis can be diagnosed by its key morphologic features and the rectangular base of the capitulum and characteristic white markings on the dorsal shield.

AMBLYOMMA AMERICANUM *(LONE STAR TICK)*. *Amblyomma americanum* demonstrates a characteristic white spot on the apex of its scutum, thus its common name the **lone star tick.** The spot is more conspicuous on male than female ticks. This tick is distributed throughout the southern United States but is also found in the Midwest and on the Atlantic coast.

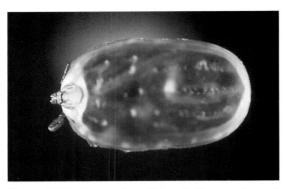

Figure 13-78 Engorged, adult female *Dermacentor variabilis.* Unfed adults are approximately 6 mm long; engorged adult females are about 12 mm long and blue-gray.

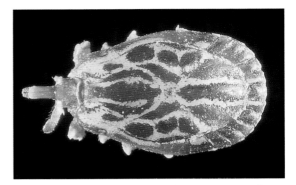

Figure 13-79 Ornate adult male *Amblyomma maculatum. A. maculatum* is easily diagnosed by silvery markings on its scutum.

This three-host tick is found most often in the spring and summer months, parasitizing the head, belly, and flanks of the wild and domestic animal hosts. It also will feed on humans and is said to have a painful bite. It can produce anemia and has been incriminated as a vector of tularemia and Rocky Mountain spotted fever.

A. americanum is easily diagnosed by the white spot on its scutum.

AMBLYOMMA MACULATUM *(GULF COAST TICK)*. *Amblyomma maculatum,* the **Gulf Coast tick,** is a three-host tick found in the ears of cattle, horses, sheep, dogs, and humans. It occurs in areas of high humidity on the Atlantic and Gulf Coast seaboards. It produces severe bites and painful swellings and is associated with tick paralysis. This tick has silvery markings on its scutum. Larval and nymphal stages occur on ground birds throughout the year. The numbers of adult ticks on cattle decreases during the winter and spring and increases in the summer and fall. When the ear canals of cattle and horses are infested, the pinna may droop and become deformed.

A. maculatum is easily diagnosed by the silvery markings on its ornate scutum (Figure 13-79).

BOOPHILUS ANNULATUS *(TEXAS CATTLE FEVER TICK)*. *Boophilus annulatus,* the **Texas cattle fever tick** or **North American tick,** uses only one host. This tick has historical significance in that it was the first arthropod shown to serve as an intermediate host for a protozoan parasite, *Babesia bigemina,* of cattle. This tick therefore marks a milestone in veterinary parasitology. *B. annulatus* has been completely eradicated from the United States; however, if it is ever diagnosed by a veterinary diagnostician, that fact **must** be reported to the proper regulatory agencies. The tick should be identified by a specialist and the appropriate control methods applied. *B. annulatus* frequently enters the United States from Mexico.

The engorged *B. annulatus* female is 10 to 12 mm in length, and the male is 3 to 4 mm. The mouthparts are very short, and there are no festoons on the posterior aspect of the abdomen.

Because this is a one-host tick, larvae, nymphs, and adult ticks may be found on cattle. They do not leave the host to complete the life cycle. Animals with heavy infestations are restless and irritated. To rid themselves of ticks, they rub, lick, bite, and scratch. Irritated areas may become raw and secondarily infested. If ticks are numerous, anemia may occur.

The veterinary diagnostician must use a key to identify adults of *B. annulatus.* Again, ticks identified as such must be reported to both state and federal authorities. Determining the origin of suspect ticks is of paramount importance.

Most often these ticks may be collected from within an enzootic area in the United States or from animals originating from Mexico.

HAEMAPHYSALIS LEPORISPALUSTRIS *(CONTINENTAL RABBIT TICK).* Although numerous kinds of ticks may infest rabbits, most have a limited geographic distribution and are generally recognized by veterinarians in each geographic area. This discussion centers on *Haemaphysalis leporispalustris,* the **continental rabbit tick.** This tick has the widest geographic distribution of rabbit ticks in the Western Hemisphere. *H. leporispalustris* is a three-host tick, meaning that each developmental stage (larva, nymph, and adult) requires a separate host for a blood meal. Although rabbits may serve as the host for each stage, they seem to be the definitive host for only the adult stage. Larval and nymphal stages also feed on birds, occasionally on dogs and cats, and rarely on humans. Feeding on birds is thought to account for much of the wide geographic distri-

bution of *H. leporispalustris,* because these birds are often migratory.

H. leporispalustris is a small, eyeless tick and is distinguished in all stages of the life cycle by the laterally pointed angles formed at the base of the mouthparts, the basis capitulum. The basis capitulum causes the mouthparts to resemble a triangular head. Males are 2.2 mm long and females 2.6 to 10 mm long, depending on whether they are engorged with blood. The ticks may be found in the external ear canal and on the pinnae but are more frequently seen on the head and neck.

In extreme cases, large numbers of these ticks may produce emaciation and death. These rabbit ticks may spread diseases such as Rocky Mountain spotted fever, Q fever, and tularemia. In general, *H. leporispalustris* occurs more frequently on wild than domestic rabbits, so owners should be warned of the disease potential for domestic rabbits that are not kept safely away from wild rabbits and birds.

14

Introduction to the Phylum Arthropoda, Subphylum Pentastomida

PENTASTOMES (PARASITES OF REPTILES)

Reptiles have served as hosts to protozoan and metazoan parasites for eons. One of the oldest continuing host-parasite relationships is that between snakes and pentastomes. Pentastomes are almost exclusively parasites of the reptilian respiratory system. According to theory, the pentastomes' ancestors were once land animals that invaded the respiratory passages of reptiles. These rare parasites hold serious zoonotic consequences for humans, who can unwittingly serve as incidental hosts.

Pentastomes have lost most of their morphologic similarity to other major phyla; they are a taxonomist's dilemma. During their life cycle, pentastomes are *pleomorphic* (demonstrating a variety of morphologic forms). They resemble *acarines* (mites) during their larval stage, but look like *annelids* (earthworms) during their nymphal and adult stages. It is difficult to assign them to either phylum, which probably means that they possess a common ancestor with the annelids and the arthropods. Therefore these creatures have been assigned to the subphylum Pentastomida.

MORPHOLOGY

The name *pentastome* (*penta* meaning "five" and *stome* meaning "mouth," thus five mouths) was chosen because these parasites, as adults, have a mouth on the anterior end that is surrounded by four hooked claws. Early investigators erroneously believed these claws to be four additional mouths; "one mouth" plus "four mouths" equals "five mouths." Pentastomes have also been called *tongue worms* and *linguatulids* because of their distinct tongue-shaped appearance, being wider anteriorly than posteriorly (Figure 14-1). Infection with pentastomes is referred to as *pentastomiasis, linguatuliasis, linguatulosis,* or rarely, porocephalosis or porocephaliasis (after Porocephalida, one of two orders composing the subphylum Pentastomida).

Grossly, pentastomes resemble helminths; however, they are often grouped with the phylum Arthropoda because of the mitelike larval stage that appears during their life cycle.

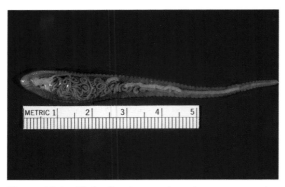

Figure 14-1 Distinctive tongue-shaped appearance of a pentastome. Because these strange parasites are flattened and wider anteriorly than posteriorly, they are often referred to as "tongue worms." The canine pentastome, *Linguatula serrata*, has transversely striated cuticle. The female is 8 to 13 cm long, and the male is 1.8 by 2 cm.

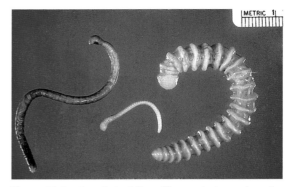

Figure 14-2 Assorted adult reptilian pentastomes from the respiratory tract of snakes. *Left to right,* Mature *Kiricephalus* species, immature *Kiricephalus* species, and mature *Armillifer* species.

Pentastomes are almost always parasites of reptiles; the exceptions to this rule are species of *Linguatula serrata* from carnivores and *Reighardia sternae* from seagulls and terns. Within the phylum are nine genera that parasitize snakes, three in lizards, four in crocodiles, and two in turtles. Among snakes, the most common genera are *Armillifer* species from pythons and vipers, *Kiricephalus* from cobras, and *Porocephalus* from boas and rattlesnakes (Figure 14-2).

LIFE CYCLE

Adult reptilian pentastomes are *dioecious* parasites; they have separate sexes, and there are both male and female pentastomes. Pentastomes are parasites that occur almost exclusively within the lungs, trachea, and nasal passages of the reptilian definitive host, feeding on tissue fluids and blood cells. Female pentastomes produce several million fully embryonated eggs, each containing a single larva with two or three pairs of rudimentary clawed legs. Eggs are "coughed up," swallowed, and passed to the outside environment within the host feces. Oval, tailed larvae with four to six stumpy legs, each with one or

two retractable, pincerlike claws, hatch from the eggs and are infective for the intermediate host. Figure 14-3 shows the life cycle of a reptilian pentastome.

Intermediate hosts include rodents, herbivores, carnivores, nonhuman primates, and humans. The larva bores through the intestinal wall of the intermediate host and passes with the blood to the mesenteric lymph nodes, the liver, the lungs, the omentum, or other internal organ, where it becomes encysted. The larva becomes "quiescent" and changes into the annelid (wormlike) nymphal stage, which can pass through as many as five molts. The reptilian definitive host becomes infected by ingesting the intermediate host with its encysted nymphal pentastomes. The infective nymphs penetrate the host's intestine and bore into the lungs, where they become sexually mature, adult parasites. The life cycle of the typical pentastome is an oddity in that the organism serving as the intermediate host (e.g., a mammal) is *higher* in the phylogenetic classification scheme than the definitive host (the reptile); this situation is uncommon among the life cycles of parasites. With most parasites, the organism serving as the intermediate host is

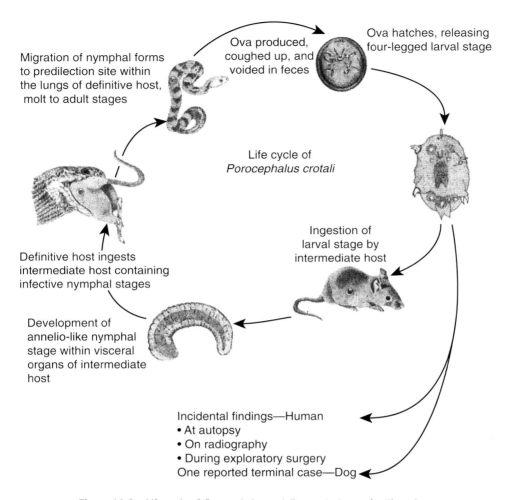

Migration of nymphal forms to predilection site within the lungs of definitive host, molt to adult stages

Ova produced, coughed up, and voided in feces

Ova hatches, releasing four-legged larval stage

Life cycle of *Porocephalus crotali*

Definitive host ingests intermediate host containing infective nymphal stages

Ingestion of larval stage by intermediate host

Development of annelio-like nymphal stage within visceral organs of intermediate host

Incidental findings—Human
• At autopsy
• On radiography
• During exploratory surgery
One reported terminal case—Dog

Figure 14-3   Life cycle of *Porocephalus crotali,* a pentastome of rattlesnakes.

lower in the phylogenetic classification scheme than the host that serves as definitive host.

DIAGNOSIS

Definitive Host

Clinical signs of reptilian pentastomiasis include lethargy, anorexia, dyspnea, and production of blood-tinged sputum or mucus within the pharynx or the trachea. The sputum can contain eggs that microscopically appear to contain four-legged to six-legged larvae with retractable claws. These pentastome eggs also can be found in the feces of the definitive host. Hematologic studies might demonstrate leukocytosis and eosinophilia. Radiographic examination might reveal adult worms or remnants of calcified cysts.

Adult reptilian pentastomes are not confined to the lungs. Adult and juvenile pentastomes might attempt to exit the host through the reptile's nostrils or the mouth or through the body wall and skin whenever the reptile is stressed. Reptilian pentastomiasis also can be diagnosed by biopsy of infected tissues or recovery of the parasite at necropsy.

Incidental Host

In contrast to pentastomid infections in natural intermediate hosts, infections in incidental hosts are striking. An incidental host is usually asymptomatic to nymphal invasion; nymphs are often found during radiographic examination, during surgery, or at necropsy. Nymphs can affect vital structures and produce pathology that leads to demonstration of related clinical signs. Death can result.

A case of incidental nymphal pentastomiasis has been reported in the dog. Eosinophilic inflammatory responses were noted in the thoracic and abdominal cavities. These responses were presumably caused by extensive migratory paths of the pentastomes. During exploratory surgery, it was noted that all peritoneal and visceral surfaces were covered with 3-mm to 5-mm, C-shaped, cystic structures, each of which contained an elongated, coiled nymph. The nymphs were identified as those of *Porocephalus crotali,* a pentastome of rattlesnakes.

Humans also are incidental mammalian hosts of pentastomids. The fact that humans can serve as intermediate hosts for reptilian pentastomes is sufficient need for veterinarians to recognize the zoonotic potential of these parasites. Human infections with reptilian pentastomes have been reported from all continents but are most common in Africa and Malaysia. Almost all recorded infections in humans have been incidental findings during radiographic examination (pentastomes often die in tissue locations and become calcified), exploratory surgery, or autopsy. Those pentastomes recovered during autopsy are usually not related to the cause of death; however, under certain circumstances, nymphs may cause significant pathology because of the organ location, the large number of nymphs involved, or their extensive tissue migrations.

On histopathologic examination of tissue, the characteristic **C** shape of the nymph can be seen. Pentastomid nymphs have a pseudosegmented body with a prominent body cavity, striated musculature, a digestive tract with numerous villi, and acidophilic glands surrounding the intestine. The nymphal pentastome's cuticle may be spiny, smooth, or annulated and may possess numerous acidophilic skin glands that communicate with the cuticle through sclerotized openings. Most of these morphologic features can be identified by either a trained pathologist or a parasitologist.

Antemortem diagnosis of pentastomiasis in the intermediate host can be accomplished by radiographic examination. In these hosts, pentastomes may die in their tissue sites and become calcified; these calcified pentastomes may be visible on radiography.

ADULT PENTASTOME THAT INFECTS NASAL PASSAGES AND TURBINATES OF A MAMMALIAN HOST

Linguatula serrata, the canine pentastome, is found in the nasal passages and sinuses of dogs and other canids. Intermediate hosts are cats, rats, porcupines, guinea pigs, rabbits, hedgehogs, pigs, and wild and domestic ruminants. In North America, rabbits are the most common intermediate hosts. Both adult and nymphal stages of this parasite may infect humans. Humans harbor nymphal stages after ingesting eggs from contaminated feces. Nymphs may be found in a variety of organs—the spleen, liver, and mesenteric lymph nodes. Humans become definitive hosts by eating raw or undercooked meat or meat by-products that contain the nymphal stages.

DIAGNOSIS
Definitive Host

Usually there are no signs of infection; however, the dog may exhibit catarrhal or suppurative rhinitis and bleeding of the nose. Restlessness, sneezing, difficulty breathing, and a reduced sense of smell have been observed. The adult parasite may be observed in its predilection site or may be sneezed out or coughed up. The adult parasite resembles a helminth (worm), but as with all pentastomes, it is an arthropod. The parasite is tongue shaped and flattened and has a transversely striated cuticle. The female is 8 to 13 cm long, and the male is 1.8 by 2 cm in size (see Figure 14-1).

Eggs may be observed on fecal flotation or nasal swabs. Eggs are yellow-brown, oval, 70 by 90 μm, and have a thick chitinous shell. An embryo with two pairs of irregularly arranged, chitinous claws may be observed on the inside of the egg. Each egg is initially enclosed in a thin, bladderlike envelope containing a clear fluid. This envelope is usually removed during passage through the gastrointestinal tract (Figure 14-4).

Intermediate Host

Nymphs of *L. serrata* in the intermediate host are detected by biopsy, exploratory laparotomy, postmortem examination, and subsequent histopathology.

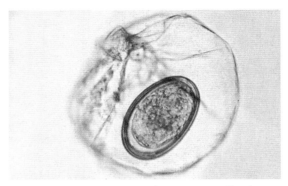

Figure 14-4 Eggs of *Linguatula serrata* are yellow-brown, oval, 70 by 90 μm, and have a thick chitinous shell. An embryo with two pairs of irregularly arranged chitinous claws may be observed on inside of egg. Each egg is initially enclosed in a thin, bladderlike envelope containing clear fluid. This envelope is usually removed during passage through the gastrointestinal tract.

The veterinarian must remember that pentastomes are rare, unusual parasites of snakes and dogs. It is important to note that the hands should *always* be washed after handling snake feces. Humans can serve as an intermediate host for this strange parasite.

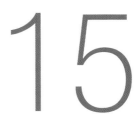

The Phylum Annelida

Kingdom: Animalia
 Phylum: Annelida
  Class: Hirudinea

Leeches and earthworms are *annelids.* Leeches are not considered to be true helminths but are often described as *parasitic worms.* As external parasites of humans and domesticated and wild animals, leeches are members of the phylum Annelida and the class Hirudinea.

HIRUDINEA (LEECHES)

Leeches can be predatory or scavenging. Most often they are parasitic on a wide variety of vertebrates and invertebrates. The ectoparasitic leeches feed on blood from fish, crustaceans, frogs, turtles, mollusks, and birds and land animals such as cattle, horses, assorted primates, and humans. These ectoparasites range in size from tiny species that are 5 mm long to varieties such as *Haemopis sanguisuga*, the horse leech, which has been reported to be as long as 45 cm when extended and swimming.

MORPHOLOGY

Leeches have slender, leaf-shaped bodies that lack bristles. The typical leech has two suckers, a large, adhesive posterior sucker and a smaller anterior sucker. The anterior sucker is actually a *pseudosucker* and surrounds the mouth. As a member of the phylum Annelida, the leech is segmented and lacks a hard exoskeleton; in its place the leech has a thin, flexible cuticle. Because of this thin cuticle, leeches dry out quickly and must always be closely associated with water. A few leeches are found in saltwater; a few terrestrial (land) leeches are found in moist, damp locations. For the most part, leeches should be considered aquatic animals.

As a result of these different habitats, leeches have developed two widely different locomotory habits, swimming and stepping. *Swimming* is the method of locomotion used when the leech is in water. The leech's body becomes flattened dorsoventrally as waves of muscular contraction pass down its length. The result is an undulating motion that propels the leech forward.

Stepping is the method of locomotion used when the leech is on solid ground. While in this mode, the leech moves in an "inchworm-like" manner, using its cranial and caudal suckers as organs of attachment to move along the substrate (surface). The layer of circular muscle just beneath the epidermis contracts, and the leech becomes long and thin. The cranial sucker then attaches to the substrate, the caudal sucker releases, and the longitudinal muscle layer beneath the circular muscle brings the caudal sucker up to the vicinity of the cranial sucker, where it attaches. The overall effect is "stepping."

While the leech is attached to the host with its caudal sucker, it uses the cranial sucker to explore the host's skin to locate a suitable feeding site and to attach tightly. Three rows of jaws with approximately 100 teeth are found in the cranial sucker. These teeth operate similar to a circular saw, penetrating through the skin to a depth of 1.5 mm. The wound produced by the leech bite is a characteristic Y-shaped skin incision. When the incision is made, the host feels very little pain.

In the past, analgesia was thought to be caused by the release of an anesthetic in the leech saliva, but it is now believed that leech saliva does *not* contain an anesthetic. The ability of a leech to feed is made easier by the secretion of powerful anticoagulants into the site of attachment. A histamine-like substance is added to the wound to prevent the collapse of adjacent capillaries. As blood passes through the mouth, the anticoagulant hirudin is added to it. *Hirudin* is a 64–amino acid peptide that functions similar to antithrombokinase. It has been described as the most powerful anticoagulant known. Active agents in the saliva of various species of leeches include a hyaluronidase, a collagenase, and two fibrinases.

When engorged with blood, the leech is dark and bloated; some leeches can ingest blood meals that are 900% of their body weight. True bloodsucking leeches require a blood meal only occasionally; consumed blood is used very slowly, so slowly that some leeches have been kept in captivity for more than 2 years without being fed. The mouth leads to a pharynx with salivary glands that secrete hirudin, a crop where ingested blood is stored, a stomach, an intestine, a rectum, and an anal pore near the caudal sucker.

LIFE CYCLE OF THE LEECH

As with the flatworms (flukes and tapeworms), leeches are hermaphroditic. Because male and female organs are located on adjacent body segments, self-fertilization is impossible, and cross-fertilization must take place. After copulation, both partners are fertilized. Eggs are laid in cocoons. The cocoon of each species of leech has a characteristic shape and design. *Hirudo medicinalis,* the medicinal leech, produces from one to seven cocoons, each of which may contain 5 to 15 eggs. Depending on the species of leech, cocoons may be attached to the parent's body or adhere to solid surfaces within the aquatic environment. Young leeches hatch from the eggs, feed for a few days on the yolk, and develop to the adult bloodsucking mode. Adult leeches can live for as long as 18 to 27 years.

The term *hirudiniasis* is derived from the classic Linnaean nomenclature and can be defined as invasion of the nose, mouth, pharynx, or larynx by leeches or the attachment of leeches to the skin. The terrestrial, or land, varieties of leeches are found in the tropical regions of the world, particularly Southeast Asia, the Pacific islands, the Indian subcontinent, and South America. Land leeches are found on the surfaces of trees and grasses and under stones in damp places. One terrestrial leech, *Haemopis terrestris,* has been plowed up in fields in the Midwestern United States.

Punctures made in the skin by land leeches are painless and remain open and continue to bleed long after the leech has detached. Land leeches in Southeast Asia and India congregate in such large numbers on the legs of cattle, horses, and other native animals that they interfere with the ambulation of the host. Another result of the attachment of numerous land leeches is that they can ingest so much blood that the host becomes anemic and may die from blood loss.

Terrestrial leeches that attach to the skin should never be pulled off but instead must be induced to detach. If pulled off, these leeches may leave their jaws embedded in the skin; such remnants can induce ulceration and serve as a site of infection. Drops of concentrated salt solution, alcohol, or strong vinegar applied around the mouth of the leech or heat with a lighted match or cigarette applied to the leech's body will cause land leeches to release their hold. The open wound should be treated with a styptic and an antiseptic.

Aquatic leeches can be external or internal parasites. Two genera of aquatic leeches (*Limnatis* and *Dinobdella*) have veterinary significance because they parasitize monkeys and domestic animals. *Theromyzon tessulatum* parasitizes wild and domestic aquatic birds. These genera reside in freshwater, where they come in contact with the vertebrate host.

Leeches entering the mouth or nostrils of the host can pass to the nasopharynx, epiglottis, esophagus, trachea, and bronchi. After attaching itself to the mucous membranes, the leech secretes its anticoagulant and engorges. Depending on the site of attachment, leeches may cause the host to exhibit nosebleeds, cough up blood, or vomit blood. A leech attached in the laryngeal region may produce a cough with a bloody discharge, difficulty in breathing, pain, and even suffocation. A leech localized in the region of the epiglottis may cause difficulty in swallowing. In severe breathing disturbances, the host's neck may be extended, and the animal may exhibit open-mouth breathing.

Several species of leeches have proved to be beneficial to humans. Perhaps the best known leech used for bloodletting is *Hirudo medicinalis*, the European medicinal leech. This leech is a native of Europe, parts of Asia, and (after its introduction) South America. It possesses a distinct green pattern of pigmentation with brown stripes and ranges in size from less than 1 cm to more than 20 cm in length (Figures 15-1 and 15-2). On its anterior end is a muscular sucker that contains three sharp chitinous jaws armed with

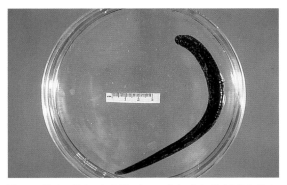

Figure 15-1   Extended *Hirudo medicinalis* in Petri dish. Note that narrow end is cranial end and has an oral sucker. Wide end is caudal end with sucker.

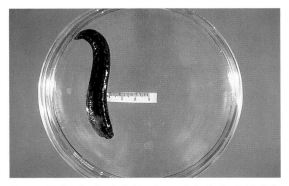

Figure 15-2   Contracted *Hirudo medicinalis* in Petri dish. Note external segmentation on body.

saw-shaped teeth; its caudal end has a characteristic suckerlike disk. This species can ingest an amount of blood up to five times its own weight. When the leech has taken a blood meal from the host, it may take as long as 200 days for digestion. This leech is reported to have gone without food for as long as 18 months.

H. medicinalis has been the leech used most often for bloodletting purposes throughout history. Its present use in reconstructive and microvascular surgery in humans is gaining impetus. Medicinal leeches have also been used in applications in both veterinary surgery and medicine. Recently there has been revived interest in these unique ectoparasites.

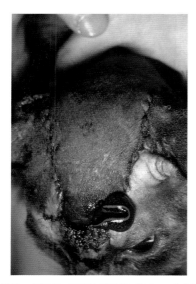

Figure 15-3 *Hirudo medicinalis* feeding on full-thickness skin graft in a cat 24 hours after surgery. Surgical techniques used were a single-pedicle advancement flap and full-thickness mesh with graft bed. Note congested area in rostral portion of pedicle flap.

H. medicinalis serves as an important medical tool because it can produce a small, bleeding wound that mimics venous outflow in tissues with impaired venous circulation (Figure 15-3). Leeches are indicated only for tissues with such impairment. The leech's main benefit is not the average 5 mL of blood removed during attachment but rather the volume of blood (reportedly as much as 50 mL) that continues to ooze for 24 to 48 hours after the leech has detached. This local bleeding is related to pharmacologically active anticoagulants and vasodilator substances introduced by the leech bite. Each bite can be encouraged to bleed further by gently removing clots that form. Research has demonstrated that new vessels begin to grow around the flap margins after approximately 72 to 120 hours.

Thus the leeches can demonstrate both pathogenic and beneficial effects on humans and wild and domesticated animals.

16

Parasites of Public Health Importance in Veterinary Parasitology

Chapter 1 defined a *zoonosis* as any disease or parasite that is transmissible from animals to humans. In veterinary clinical practice, it is important for veterinarians to inform their clients concerning zoonotic diseases or parasites that may be transmitted from their domestic animals. Such zoonotic parasites include *Toxoplasma gondii*, *Trichinella spiralis*, *Ancylostoma caninum*, and *Toxocara canis*. This chapter discusses the major parasitic diseases that are of public health importance in veterinary clinical practice.

It is often the veterinarian's role (and also the role of the veterinary diagnostician) to diagnose a parasite in a domestic animal. The veterinary diagnostician must also communicate to the public and often to medical personnel, such as physicians, laboratory personnel, and other public health workers, the significance of many of the zoonotic parasites. It is important for veterinary personnel to understand that in suspected cases of zoonotic parasites or conditions, the client should *always* be referred to a physician, family practitioner, obstetrician, or public health worker, as appropriate, for diagnosis or treatment. In no instance should a veterinarian or veterinary technician attempt to diagnose or treat any of these zoonotic parasites in humans. The veterinarian's role is to inform, not to treat. Attempting to diagnose or treat a human is a violation of state veterinary practice acts across the United States. Treatments are included in this chapter for veterinarians in an advisory capacity for communicating with human health care workers and not as direct treatment for a human patient.

For each zoonotic parasite discussed here, the following areas are addressed:

- The symptoms of infection with the particular parasite in humans and the way in which it is diagnosed.
- Treatment of the condition in humans.
- Ways in which transmission of this zoonotic parasite, condition, or syndrome from animals to humans can be prevented.

Just as the parasites are broken down in the previous chapters into the major groups, the important zoonotic parasites are divided into zoonotic protozoans, zoonotic trematodes, zoonotic cestodes, zoonotic nematodes, zoonotic arthropods, and zoonotic pentastomes. The acanthocephalans and the leeches have no zoonotic significance.

PROTOZOANS OF PUBLIC HEALTH IMPORTANCE

TOXOPLASMA GONDII (TOXOPLASMOSIS)

Toxoplasmosis in humans is an extremely rare protozoan disease with which humans (particularly a pregnant woman and her developing fetus) can become infected. It is an important zoonotic parasite because a very popular domestic pet, the cat, is the only definitive host for this parasite. The cat can serve as a source of infection for the pregnant woman and her unborn child. Toxoplasmosis can infect the fetus in the womb and produce serious birth defects. This parasite can also wreak havoc in individuals with acquired immunodeficiency syndrome (AIDS).

Although this is a very rare parasite, several precautions must be taken to prevent infection. To sell papers, the "sensational press" often exploits this parasite in its headlines, alarming the general public. As a result, the veterinary clinical practice may receive phone calls regarding this parasite. Also, uninformed clients may request that veterinarians find a new home for (or even euthanize) the family's cat. It is important for the veterinarian to alleviate the client's concerns and to work in conjunction with the obstetrician-gynecologist to answer questions, thwart this parasite, and prevent toxoplasmosis. It is important to note that almost every warm-blooded animal can become infected with *Toxoplasma gondii.*

Human Infection with Toxoplasmosis

Humans become infected with toxoplasmosis in one of two ways: congenital or acquired. *Congenital toxoplasmosis* occurs when a woman becomes infected during her pregnancy; the woman ingests sporulated oocysts of *T. gondii*

found in the feces of the cat. The domestic house cat with access to the outdoors (and predation) serves as the definitive host for *T. gondii* and will shed unsporulated oocysts in its feces. These unsporulated oocysts will sporulate (or become infective) in 1 to 5 days. If a pregnant woman accidentally ingests the sporulated oocyst, the parasite's *tachyzoites* (rapidly multiplying stages) can infect the developing fetus.

Acquired toxoplasmosis occurs when a human ingests the sporulated oocyst containing tachyzoites or ingests infected meat or tissue stages containing bradyzoites. Many domesticated animals (e.g., cattle, pigs, sheep) serve as intermediate hosts for *T. gondii*. Within their muscle, these intermediate hosts harbor *bradyzoites* (slowly multiplying stages) that can infect various tissue sites, including lymph nodes, meninges, eyes, and the heart, of humans. The infected human ingests the bradyzoites, which then infect a variety of tissue sites.

Symptoms and Diagnosis

If congenital infection occurs early in the pregnancy, abortion is common. If this infection occurs late in the pregnancy, the central nervous system may become infected, and a variety of neurologic abnormalities may result. These include cerebral calcification, chorioretinitis, hydrocephaly, microcephaly, and psychomotor irregularities. The child may be born dead or alive. If alive, the child may be mentally retarded.

Infected humans with acquired toxoplasmosis exhibit lymphadenopathy, malaise, fever, lymphocytosis, and myocarditis. Most cases, however, are characterized by mild fever and slight enlargement of the lymph nodes.

Diagnosis of clinical toxoplasmosis in humans is quite difficult. Diagnosis relies on the demonstration of organisms or antibodies against it. The best diagnostic test is the inoculation of suspected material into mice and demonstration of the organism multiplying in the mice. Serologic tests are also available. The veterinary diagnostician must remember that these tests need to be delegated to a more sophisticated diagnostic laboratory.

Treatment

There is no completely satisfactory treatment for toxoplasmosis in humans, although pyrimethamine has been found effective. This drug, in conjunction with triple sulfa drugs, has given good results in ocular toxoplasmosis. Remember that suspected cases of toxoplasmosis in humans should *always* be referred to a neonatologist, pediatrician, gynecologist, obstetrician, or family practitioner. The Centers for Disease Control and Prevention (CDC) has many specialists who are qualified to answer the most complex issues of toxoplasmosis in humans.

Prevention of Transmission to Humans

Transmission of *T. gondii* to pregnant women is prevented by having someone else (preferably a man) empty the cat's litter box daily. This step eliminates the woman's potential exposure to the sporulated oocysts of *T. gondii.* A person should always wash the hands after handling the cat and before eating. Litter boxes should never be placed in the kitchen or dining area. Gloves should be worn while gardening because feral cats often defecate in flower beds. If children's sandboxes are present in the backyard, they should remain covered when not in use. After gardening, hands should be thoroughly washed. Cats should never be allowed to roam freely and hunt. Likewise, uncooked meat should never be fed to cats. Rodent prey or uncooked meat may contain the tissue stages of *T. gondii,* which will set the life cycle in motion in the cat. Likewise, to avoid acquired infection with *T. gondii* (and a variety of pathogenic bacteria), humans should be wary of undercooked infected meat.

CRYPTOSPORIDIUM PARVUM (CRYPTOSPORIDIOSIS)

Cryptosporidiosis is a rare protozoan disease that produces a prolific, painful, watery diarrhea in humans. This protozoan parasite has been reported in the news because it has contaminated the drinking water supplies of several major metropolitan areas throughout North America and the world. As with toxoplasmosis, cryptosporidiosis is especially harmful in individuals with AIDS. For this reason, it is also an important parasite. Cryptosporidiosis was first reported in farmworkers and individuals who worked around very young calves. This organism is spread by ingestion of infective oocysts in calf feces.

Human Infection with Cryptosporidiosis

Humans become infected with cryptosporidiosis by ingestion of oocysts from feces of young calves or from contaminated supplies of drinking water.

Symptoms and Diagnosis

Cryptosporidiosis produces a transient, painful, watery diarrhea in humans, and all ages are susceptible. The duration of clinical signs in affected individuals varies considerably. Acute cases last from 3 to 7 days, and chronic wasting syndromes can persist for weeks to a few months. The development of natural immunity against the parasite determines the duration of clinical signs. Most humans infected with *Cryptosporidium* species develop immunity and recover from the infection.

Infections with *Cryptosporidium* species may persist indefinitely in people with immunodeficiencies, particularly AIDS. The prognosis for immunologically compromised individuals with cryptosporidiosis is poor.

Fecal flotation and concentrating solutions, such as zinc sulfate and Sheather's sugar solution, may be used to identify oocysts of *Cryptosporidium* species. These parasites are extremely tiny, less than 5 μm in diameter, and thus may be easily overlooked. Acid-fast stains such as Ziehl-Neelsen or Kinyoun can be used, as well as auramine-rhodamine, Giemsa, and methylene blue. All these stains may be used to improve the identification of the parasite in fecal flotation.

There are several commercially available enzyme-linked immunosorbent assay (ELISA) tests. These tests have a higher degree of sensitivity and specificity in diagnosing infections with *Cryptosporidium* species than can be obtained from stained fecal flotation smears. A commercially available indirect fluorescent antibody (IFA) test has been shown to be quite effective in diagnosing infection with *Cryptosporidium* species.

Treatment

Although cryptosporidiosis is caused by a protozoan parasite with a life cycle similar to that of coccidia, **coccidiostats** have shown minimal to no efficacy when used to treat infected cattle. An effective chemotherapeutic means of eliminating the parasite is not available.

Human cryptosporidiosis is treated symptomatically. Individuals who become dehydrated should be given appropriate fluids either intravenously or orally. Clinical improvement has been demonstrated in patients treated with dialyzable leukocyte extract from calves immunized with *Cryptosporidium* species.

Prevention of Transmission to Humans

Infection with *Cryptosporidium* species can be prevented by good sanitation and hygiene practices when handling young animals, particularly calves. Infants, young children, or immunologically compromised individuals should not handle animals with diarrhea. Immunocompromised individuals should be advised to wash their hands after handling pets, especially before eating, and should avoid contact with their pet's feces. Many of the agents and processes used to sanitize public drinking water have little effect on *Cryptosporidium* species.

TREMATODES OF PUBLIC HEALTH IMPORTANCE

SCHISTOSOMES OF WILD MIGRATORY BIRDS (SCHISTOSOME CERCARIAL DERMATITIS, SWIMMER'S ITCH)

Swimmer's itch is a highly pruritic skin condition in humans caused by repeated penetration of the cercariae of the schistosomes (blood flukes) of wild migratory aquatic birds and small

mammals native to the water's edge. On first exposure of the cercariae, there is mild redness and edema in the skin; with repeated exposure, however, there is severe pruritus (itching) and a papular or pustular dermatitis (a pus-filled pimple). This dermatitis may persist for several days or even weeks and can become secondarily infected.

Human Infection with Swimmer's Itch

Migratory waterfowl frequently harbor schistosomes (blood flukes) in their blood vasculature. These schistosomes produce eggs that pass in the bird's feces to the watery environment. The eggs hatch, producing miracidia, which in turn penetrate aquatic snails. Within the snail, the miracidia undergo asexual reproduction and produce thousands of cercariae. These cercariae exit the snail to penetrate the definitive host, the migratory waterfowl.

Humans serve as incidental hosts for these avian schistosomes. During the summer months, people swim or wade in the lakes, ponds, rivers, and even ocean waters frequented by the wild birds. These waters are home to aquatic snails. The cercariae produced within the snails penetrate the skin of the humans instead of the skin of the migratory birds. The cercariae cannot complete the migration in the human host, and the host's immune system kills the cercariae. At the same time, the cercariae release allergenic substances that cause severe dermatitis. Repeated exposure produces the highly pruritic, papular or pustular dermatitis, or **schistosome cercarial dermatitis** ("swimmer's itch"). This condition may have many other regional or colloquial descriptive names.

Symptoms and Diagnosis

After the cercaria penetrates the skin, a reddened spot appears at the point of entry. The diameter of this spot increases, and the itching commences. If the area becomes raised, it is called a *papule* and will reach its maximum size in about 24 hours. In severe cases the affected individual may develop a fever, become nauseated, and spend several sleepless nights. The papule itches for several days before subsiding, but in a week or so the symptoms disappear.

Swimmer's itch can be diagnosed by the observation of typical lesions in skin that has come in contact with pond, lake, stream, or ocean water containing infective cercariae from the snail intermediate host. A history of swimming in infested waters also aids in diagnosis. Laboratory findings usually have no role in establishing a diagnosis of swimmer's itch.

Treatment

Suspected cases of swimmer's itch in humans should *always* be referred to a dermatologist or family practitioner. Antihistamines are prescribed to relieve the itch and topical steroid creams to reduce the swelling. Remember that these are prescription drugs and must be prescribed by a physician or dermatologist.

Prevention of Transmission to Humans

During the seasonal occurrence of swimmer's itch, many public health agencies post warnings about swimmer's itch on beaches adjacent to ponds, lakes, streams, or the ocean. The public should heed these warnings and comply with the ban on swimming in infested waters. Swimming in water away from the shore will reduce the chance of contact with the cercariae; cercariae tend to congregate close to the shoreline. If contact is suspected, the swimmer should towel down immediately after leaving the water.

For those who must work in such waters, protective waterproof clothing is available. Repellents, such as benzyl benzoate and dibutylphthalate, are available. *Molluscicides* (snail-killing compounds) are available; however, they may have adverse effects on plants and other animals in the environment.

CESTODES OF PUBLIC HEALTH IMPORTANCE

TAENIA SAGINATA (BEEF TAPEWORM)

Taenia saginata, the beef tapeworm, parasitizes the small intestine of humans. Its larval or metacestode stage, *Cysticercus bovis,* is found in the musculature of beef cattle, the intermediate host.

Human Infection with Beef Tapeworm

Humans become infected with the beef tapeworm by ingesting the musculature of beef cattle that contains the cysticercus, or bladder worm, the larval (metacestode) stage for this tapeworm. This cysticercus stage has a scientific name, *Cysticercus bovis,* and may be found in a variety of sites in the bovine musculature: skeletal and heart muscle, masseters, diaphragm, and tongue. Humans are infected by ingesting raw or undercooked, cysticercus-infected beef. This meat is often referred to as **measly beef** or **beef measles.** The covering of the cysticercus is digested away, and the young tapeworm is released and attaches to the wall of the small intestine. This young tapeworm begins to grow its proglottids. The gravid (most mature) proglottids are released to the outside environment. Each gravid proglottid contains about 80,000 eggs. In the outside environment the gravid proglottids rupture, and the released eggs may be ingested by a beef cow. The eggs hatch, and the embryos penetrate the intestinal mucosa and reach the general circulation; they are then distributed throughout the musculature of the beef cow.

Symptoms and Diagnosis

Adult *Taenia saginata* in the small intestine of humans may cause a variety of nonspecific abdominal signs, such as diarrhea, constipation, and cramps. About 10 gravid proglottids are passed in the feces each day; this fact is quite evident to the infected individual. These proglottids are quite motile and will migrate a few centimeters over the human host's body, clothes, or bedding.

The gravid proglottids from human feces are unusual in appearance. Each proglottid has a prominent uterus with 14 to 32 lateral branches. The uterus contains approximately 80,000 eggs. Perianal swabs may be used to detect these eggs. Diagnosis of cysticerci in cattle is usually made by meat inspection procedures.

Treatment

Suspected cases of the beef tapeworm in humans should *always* be referred to a family practitioner or internist. The treatment of choice is praziquantel or niclosamide.

Prevention of Transmission to Humans

All infected humans should be treated by a physician. Feedlot employees should be educated concerning transmission of bovine cysticercosis and personal hygiene practices. Adequate and accessible toilet facilities must be provided for all workers. Meat inspection should be thorough. Infected carcasses may be condemned for human consumption or treated by freezing for 10 days to 2 weeks at −10° C or by cooking at 50° to 60° C. Likewise, humans should be wary of undercooked meat, to avoid acquired infection with *T. saginata* (and a variety of pathogenic bacteria).

TAENIA SOLIUM (PORK TAPEWORM)

Taenia solium, the pork tapeworm, parasitizes the small intestine of humans. The larval, or metacestode, stage of this tapeworm, *Cysticercus cellulosae,* is found in the musculature of pigs, the intermediate host. This is an unusual parasite in that humans can also harbor the larval stage, which may occur not only in the musculature, but also within the eye and the brain. Therefore, humans can serve as both the definitive and the intermediate host for this parasite.

Human Infection with Pork Tapeworm

Humans become infected with the pork tapeworm by ingesting the musculature of pigs that contains the cysticercus, or bladder worm, the larval (metacestode) stage. This cysticercus stage has a scientific name, *Cysticercus cellulosae,* and may be found in a variety of muscle sites: skeletal and heart muscle, masseters, diaphragm, and tongue. Humans are infected by ingesting raw or undercooked, cysticercus-infected pork. This meat is often referred to as *measly pork* or *pork measles.* The covering of the cysticercus is

digested away, and the young tapeworm is released and attaches to the wall of the small intestine. This young tapeworm begins to grow proglottids. The gravid (most mature) proglottids are released to the outside environment. Each gravid proglottid contains about 40,000 eggs. In the outside environment the gravid proglottid ruptures; the released eggs must be ingested by a pig. The eggs hatch, and the embryos penetrate the intestinal mucosa and reach the general circulation, to be distributed throughout the musculature of the pig.

If a human ingests one of the eggs, the egg hatches in the human intestine. This embryo penetrates the intestinal mucosa and reaches the general circulation, to be distributed not only throughout the musculature of the human, but also in subcutaneous sites and within the brain and the eye. In such sites, tremendous damage can result.

When the metacestode stage develops in the brain, the condition is known as **neurocysticercosis.** The parasite usually develops in the ventricles and is proliferative in nature.

Symptoms and Diagnosis

Adult *Taenia solium* in the small intestine of humans may cause a variety of nonspecific abdominal signs, such as diarrhea, constipation, and cramps. Chains of gravid proglottids do not leave the host spontaneously but are passed in the feces each day; this fact is quite evident to the infected individual. These proglottids are quite motile and will migrate a few centimeters over the human host's body, clothes, or bedding.

Neurologic symptoms vary with the site of the offending cysticercus in the nervous tissue. Pain, paralysis, and epileptic seizures have been associated with neurocysticercosis. Ocular lesions may result in blindness.

The gravid proglottids from human feces are unusual in appearance. Each proglottid has a prominent uterus with fewer than 16 lateral branches. The uterus contains approximately

40,000 eggs. Diagnosis of cysticerci in pigs is usually made by meat inspection procedures.

Sophisticated radiographic imaging techniques, such as computed tomography (CT) and magnetic resonance imaging (MRI), may reveal the presence of cysticerci within the brain and other sites in the central nervous system (CNS).

Treatment

Suspected cases of pork tapeworm in humans should *always* be referred to a family practitioner, neurologist, surgeon, or internist. The treatment of choice is praziquantel. Because of the infectivity of the eggs for humans and the resulting CNS involvement, these cases must be handled with great care. Treatment of human cysticercosis is by surgical removal of the offending lesion.

Prevention of Transmission to Humans

All infected humans should be treated by a physician. Feedlot employees should be educated concerning transmission of porcine cysticercosis and personal hygiene practices. Household workers such as maids and cooks should be educated regarding proper hygiene, such as handwashing before preparing a meal. Adequate and convenient toilet facilities must be provided for all workers. Meat inspection should be thorough. Infected carcasses may be condemned for human consumption or treated by freezing for 10 days to 2 weeks at −10° C or by cooking at 50° to 60° C. Likewise, humans should be wary of undercooked meat to avoid acquired infection with *T. solium* (and a variety of pathogenic bacteria).

ECHINOCOCCUS GRANULOSUS AND *ECHINOCOCCUS MULTILOCULARIS* (UNILOCULAR AND MULTILOCULAR HYDATID DISEASE)

Hydatid disease is a syndrome characterized by the development of the larval, or metacestode, stage of a genus of tapeworm, *Echinococcus* species, found in the small intestine of dogs and cats, the definitive hosts. Hydatid disease is characterized by the formation of large, fluid-filled cysts in the internal organs of the intermediate host. There are two species of importance in veterinary parasitology: *E. granulosus,* a tapeworm that produces a **unilocular** (large, singular, thick-walled, fluid-filled) hydatid cyst, and *E. multilocularis,* a tapeworm that produces a **multilocular** (multiple, extremely invasive, thin-walled, fluid-filled) hydatid cyst. These hydatid cysts may occur in a variety of internal organs in the human intermediate host: the liver, lungs, kidney, spleen, bone, and brain.

Human Infection with Hydatid Disease

Humans become infected with hydatid disease by ingesting the egg of *Echinococcus* species. Once ingested, the egg hatches in the intestine of the human intermediate host. The released *oncosphere* ("growth ball") penetrates an intestinal venule or lymphatic lacteal and reaches the liver, lungs, or other internal organs. Once in these extraintestinal sites, the oncosphere develops into the hydatid cyst. *E. granulosus* produces a unilocular hydatid cyst. This cyst has a thick, multilayered cyst wall that keeps the developing cyst restricted to a single compartment. The hydatid cyst may grow up to 50 cm in diameter; however, it will not invade the surrounding tissues of the parasitized organ. *E. multilocularis* produces a multilocular hydatid cyst. In contrast to the unilocular hydatid cyst of *E. granulosus,* this hydatid cyst lacks the thick, multilayered cyst wall. Without this cyst wall, the developing cyst is capable of "budding off," or producing additional compartments, which in turn, bud off other compartments. As a result, this type of hydatid cyst readily invades the surrounding tissues. This multilocular hydatid cyst takes on a "malignant," invasive role.

Symptoms and Diagnosis

The symptoms of infection with hydatid disease depend on the site where the organism develops; these sites include the liver, lungs, kidney, spleen, bone, and brain. Neurologic symptoms vary with the site of the offending cysticercus in the nervous tissue. Pain, paralysis, and epileptic seizures have also been associated with *echinococcosis.*

In humans, examination of histopathologic sections of unilocular hydatid cysts reveal the unique structure of the germinal membrane supported by a thicker, acellular, laminated membrane. Protoscolices are contained in the saclike brood capsules. When viewed macroscopically, these brood capsules look like sand. Humans with *E. multilocularis* develop tumorlike masses, or nodules, in their livers. When sectioned, these masses reveal the alveolar-like microvesicles containing protoscolices.

Sophisticated radiographic imaging techniques, such as CT and MRI, may reveal the presence of hydatid cysts within the brain and other organ sites throughout the body.

Treatment

Suspected cases of echinococcosis in humans should always be referred to a surgeon, internist, or neurologist. Surgical intervention is recommended for the disease syndromes caused by *E. granulosus* and *E. multilocularis.* For patients in whom the hydatid cyst cannot be removed or those for whom surgery is not an option, there may be new therapeutic alternatives. Treatment with mebendazole has shown varied success, although albendazole has been more promising.

State public health officials should be notified when canine or feline echinococcosis is diagnosed. Additionally, the CDC should be notified. The CDC has many specialists who are qualified to answer the most complex questions regarding both unilocular and multilocular hydatid disease in humans.

Prevention of Transmission to Humans

Handwashing, particularly for children, should be emphasized. It is important to prevent exposure to eggs of *Echinococcus* species. Dogs should never be fed raw livestock viscera or allowed to roam freely to feed on wild rodents.

DIPYLIDIUM CANINUM (HUMAN DIPYLIDIASIS)
Human Infection with *Dipylidium*

Children become infected with the common *tapeworm* of dogs and cats, *Dipylidium caninum,* by ingesting dog or cat fleas containing cysticercoids of this common canine and feline tapeworm.

Symptoms and Diagnosis

As in the canine or feline host, proglottids are passed in the feces or are found around the anus (if the child is an infant and is still wearing diapers). Most infections occur in children under 8 years of age. Most patients are asymptomatic, but diarrhea, abdominal pain, and anal pruritus may occur. The child may have moderate eosinophilia.

Treatment

Suspected cases of *D. caninum* in humans should *always* be referred to a family practitioner or internist. This human disease occurs rarely; humans appear to be highly resistant to the infection, given the high frequency of flea infestation on dogs and cats. Suspected cases of *dipylidiasis* in children should always be referred to a pediatrician or general practitioner. The drugs of choice for human dipylidiasis are praziquantel and niclosamide. For treating *D. caninum,* the adult dose of praziquantel is 10 to 20 mg/kg given once; the pediatric dose is the same. The adult dose of niclosamide is 2 g given once. For children from 11 to 34 kg, the dose is 1 g given once; for children greater than 34 kg, the one-time dose is 1.5 g. Since the method of transmission is by ingestion of dog or cat fleas containing the infected cysticercoids, the child probably is the only family member infected with this canine parasite. It would not be necessary to treat other family members for infection with this canine and feline cestode. All household pets should be treated with anthelmintics; a rigorous flea control program should be instituted for all dogs and cats.

Prevention of Transmission to Humans

Infection in humans or animals by *D. caninum* requires ingestion of the intermediate host, the dog or cat flea containing the larva (cysticercoids) of the tapeworm. Many cases in humans are asymptomatic. Dipylidiasis affects mainly infants and young children, who may swallow a flea that hops up while the infant is crawling on the floor or cuddling the family pet. Again, humans appear to be highly resistant to the infection, given the high frequency of flea infestation on dogs and cats and the relative rarity of human disease.

HYMENOLEPIS NANA (HYMENOLEPIASIS)
Human Infection with *Hymenolepis*

Hymenolepis nana, the **dwarf tapeworm**, is usually found in rodents, primates, and humans. It is common in children under 3 years of age throughout the world and can be passed from human to human. The tapeworms are usually regarded as hand-to-mouth parasites. *Hymenolepis diminuta*, the **rat tapeworm**, is primarily a parasite of rodents and humans. Children become infected with *Hymenolepis* species by ingesting insects (e.g., rat fleas, mealworms, cockroaches) containing cysticercoids of these tapeworms.

Symptoms and Diagnosis

Large numbers of tapeworms can cause necrosis and desquamation of the intestinal epithelial cells. Light infections cause no significant damage to the mucosa and are either asymptomatic or cause vague abdominal complaints. Young children frequently have loose bowel movements or frank diarrhea with mucus. Bloody diarrhea is rare; diffuse, persistent abdominal pain is the more common complaint. A pruritic anus is another common complaint among infected individuals. Many children also have headaches, dizziness, and sleep and behavioral disturbances, which resolve after therapy. Serious neurologic disturbances have been reported. A moderate eosinophilia (5% to 10%) may be associated with **hymenolepiasis.**

Diagnosis is by finding the characteristic eggs in fecal flotation. Proglottids are usually not found because they degenerate before passage in the stool.

Treatment

In suspected cases of *H. diminuta*, humans should *always* be referred to a family practitioner or internist. Praziquantel is the drug of choice. For treating *H. diminuta*, the dose of praziquantel (for both adults and children) is 25 mg/kg given once.

Prevention of Transmission to Humans

Control depends on improved personal and environmental hygiene. Within institutions, all children should be treated.

DIPHYLLOBOTHRIUM LATUM (DIPHYLLOBOTHRIASIS)
Human Infection with *Diphyllobothrium*

The **broad fish tapeworm**, or *Diphyllobothrium latum,* is often found in many areas of the world where raw, insufficiently cooked, or lightly pickled freshwater fish are consumed. Infected fish contain the plerocercoid, or **sparganum,** stage; this is the stage eaten by the human. These parasites are often found in northern temperate and subarctic regions. The adult tapeworms are found within the small intestine of the host; humans may also become infected with the plerocercoid (sparganum) stage. When a homeopathic doctor uses an infected piece of fish as a poultice, the sparganum moves into the wound and sets up an infection in the subcutis, the connective tissue of the muscles, or in other sites within the body.

Symptoms and Diagnosis

Intestinal infections in humans are often asymptomatic. Often the diagnosis is made during routine fecal examination when eggs or chains of proglottids are observed in the feces. Infection in humans may also cause nonspecific abdominal symptoms. Some individuals may complain of abdominal pain, bloating, allergic reactions, hunger pains, loss of appetite, or increased appetite. On rare occasions, mechanical intestinal obstruction may result from tapeworms becoming entangled; intussusception may result. Diarrhea may occur, and infected individuals may pass long sections of spent proglottids in the stool.

Adult tapeworms in the small intestine may successfully absorb vitamin B_{12} from the gut; this loss of vitamin B_{12} produces *megaloblastic anemia* or *pernicious anemia.* This condition manifests itself as a macrocytic, hypochromic anemia.

Infection with the sparganum, or *sparganosis,* produces a severe inflammatory reaction and fibrosis of infected tissues. Clinical signs include urticaria, painful edema, and irregular nodules containing the plerocercoids. If spargana infect the eye, the infection may lead to exophthalmos, swelling of the eyelids, lagophthalmos, and corneal ulcers.

Treatment

Suspected cases of the intestinal form of the broad fish tapeworm in humans should *always* be referred to a family practitioner or internist. Praziquantel and niclosamide are the drugs of choice. For treating *Diphyllobothrium latum,* the adult dose of praziquantel is 10 to 20 mg/kg given once; the pediatric dose is the same. The adult dose of niclosamide is 2 g given once. For children from 11 to 34 kg, the dose is 1 g given once; for children greater than 34 kg, the one-time dose is 1.5 g.

Suspected cases of the sparganum (plerocercoid) form of the broad fish tapeworm in humans should *always* be referred to a surgeon. Spargana within tissue sites in humans must be surgically removed.

Prevention of Transmission to Humans

Proper cooking of freshwater fish eliminates all possibility of human infection. Likewise, domestic animals such as dogs, cats, and pigs should not be fed raw fish. Freezing at $-10°$ C will kill the infective plerocercoid (sparganum) stage. In the United States, smoked salmon is brined before hot smoking; this process eliminates salmon as a source of infection. Food handlers should never taste raw fish while preparing it for cooking. Practitioners of natural medicine should be discouraged from applying poultices made of fish to openings in the skin or to the eye.

NEMATODES OF PUBLIC HEALTH IMPORTANCE

TOXOCARA CANIS AND TOXOCARA CATI (TOXOCARAL LARVA MIGRANS, VISCERAL LARVA MIGRANS, OCULAR LARVA MIGRANS)

Toxocaral larva migrans is a disease of humans caused by the migration of certain parasitic larvae in the organs and tissues. The most incriminated nematodes are the common ascarids of dogs and cats, *Toxocara canis* and *Toxocara cati,* respectively. *Baylisascaris procyonis,* an ascarid of raccoons, causes a similar syndrome.

Human Infection with Toxocaral Larva Migrans

Humans become infected with toxocaral larva migrans when they ingest eggs of *Toxocara* species from the soil or on contaminated hands or other objects. Eggs of *Toxocara* species require 2 or more weeks before infective larvae develop within the eggs. Persons should also take precautions when handling young puppies still being nursed by their dams. The entire litter area (and their hair coats) may often become extremely contaminated with their aged feces, which may contain infective eggs.

Symptoms and Diagnosis

Infection by a few larvae is usually asymptomatic. Two distinct syndromes are produced by *Toxocara* species: *visceral larva migrans* (VLM) and *ocular larva migrans* (OLM). VLM results from the migration of larvae though the human's somatic tissues and organs, including the liver, lungs, heart, and brain. VLM is characterized by fever, leukocytosis, persistent eosinophilia, hypergammaglobulinemia, and hepatomegaly. Pulmonary involvement, with symptoms that include bronchiolitis, asthma, or pneumonitis, may be common. Fatalities may result when the myocardium or CNS becomes involved.

OLM results when larval *Toxocara* species invade the eye. Ocular disease may be seen in the absence of VLM and is often seen in young children. Faulty vision may result; blindness may also occur.

VLM may be diagnosed based on the demonstration of lesions and the larvae in biopsy material. Serum samples may be sent to the CDC for serodiagnostic confirmation of toxocariasis. With OLM, the larvae may be observed during an ophthalmic examination.

Treatment

Suspected cases of toxocaral larva migrans in humans, particularly young children, should always be referred to a family practitioner, pediatrician, internist, or ophthalmologist. No proven treatment is available. Suggested drugs of choice include mebendazole and diethylcarbamazine. Prednisone helps to control symptoms.

Prevention of Transmission to Humans

Three major methods are used to prevent transmission of *Toxocara* species from dogs and cats to humans. First, it is important to prevent the fouling of backyard and public places, especially playgrounds, with dog and cat feces. All fecal material should be disposed of properly. Second, pet owners should be educated regarding the potential health hazards of roundworms in cats and dogs. Pet owners should be informed of the methods of transmission and of the special risks associated with puppies and their nursing mothers. After handling any young puppy, hands should be thoroughly washed in soap and warm water. Third, it is important that all cats and dogs be routinely tested for intestinal parasites, such as ascarids. If infected, pets should be treated with an appropriate anthelmintic.

BAYLISASCARIS PROCYONIS (NEURAL LARVA MIGRANS, CEREBROSPINAL NEMATODIASIS)

Neural larva migrans, a variation of visceral larva migrans, is the prolonged migration and persistence of parasite larvae of *Baylisascaris procyonis* (an ascarid that normally resides in the small intestine of the raccoon) in the brain and spinal cord of humans and animals. In this case, the human or other animal is serving as a *paratenic* host. This syndrome is similar to that of VLM and OLM of *Toxocara* species of both dogs and cats.

Human Infection with Larvae of *Baylisascaris procyonis*

Humans become infected with the larvae of *B. procyonis* by accidentally ingesting eggs that contain its infective second-stage larvae. The eggs are ingested from the environment, from raccoon feces, or from contaminated soil, water, fomites, or hands. The source of these ascarid eggs is the raccoon, a feral animal that should *never* be maintained in any interior or exterior household environment. These eggs are extremely resistant and can remain viable in the environment for several months to years. This resistance increases the likelihood of transmission from animals to humans.

Symptoms and Diagnosis

As mentioned, *B. procyonis* can produce visceral and ocular larva migrans in humans, similar to that produced by *Toxocara* species of both dogs and cats. However, these larvae tend to be more pathogenic because they can migrate through the CNS. Typically, the extent of the infection depends on the number of infective larvae ingested and their locations and behavior in the body. When only a few larvae are ingested, individuals probably are asymptomatic; visceral damage is minor, and most larvae become encapsulated (walled off) in noncritical sites such as skeletal muscle or connective tissue. If larger numbers of larvae are ingested, however, the host may exhibit nonspecific clinical signs or more classic signs attributable to those of classic VLM: fever, leukocytosis, persistent eosinophilia, hepatomegaly, and pneumonitis. These larvae also have an affinity for migration in neurologic tissues, and depending on the location and extent of migration, neurologic signs vary. If enough larvae are ingested, progressive CNS disease can develop rapidly, producing signs such as sudden lethargy, loss of muscle coordination, decreased head control, torticollis, ataxia, and nystagmus. These signs progress to stupor; extensor rigidity, or hypotonia; coma; and finally, death. Clinical signs of OLM include unilateral loss of vision and photophobia.

Because neither eggs nor larvae of *B. procyonis* are found on fecal flotation or in blood samples from humans, diagnosis of *B. procyonis* in humans must be made based on history, clinical findings, and serologic testing. A history of exposure to raccoons or their feces is important. Clinical findings of VLM include leukocytosis, persistent eosinophilia, hypergammaglobulinemia, hepatomegaly, and pneumonitis. CNS disease may present suddenly and develop progressively. Eosinophilia may be present in both the peripheral blood and the cerebrospinal fluid. OLM may be diagnosed by ophthalmologic examination that reveals inflammatory tracks in the retina and inflammation of the vitreum and choroid. A specific diagnosis may be made by identification of characteristic morphologic features of larval *B. procyonis* in histopathologic section. Serologic tests, such as indirect immunofluorescence, protein immunoblotting, and ELISA, are being evaluated.

Treatment

Any person who has contact with raccoons or raccoon feces and develops visual or CNS disturbances should be examined by a physician, who should be alerted to the possibility of infection with *B. procyonis*. Suspected cases of *cerebrospinal nematodiasis* in humans should *always* be referred to a neurologist, ophthalmologist, internist, or family practitioner. It is unfortunate that effective anthelmintic treatments do not exist for visceral or ocular larva migrans or for cerebrospinal nematodiasis. Patients with the ocular form of this syndrome can be treated with a laser, if the larvae can be localized and visualized with the eye.

Prevention of Transmission to Humans

B. procyonis is more prevalent in raccoons from northern states than in raccoons from southern states, especially those states in the deep South. Nevertheless, precautions should be taken around raccoons in all areas of the United States.

First in regard to prevention, raccoons are *not* suitable pets. Wild raccoons should not be encouraged to visit or frequent urban, suburban, or rural dwellings or environments.

For those who rehabilitate raccoons and return them to nature, it is important to prevent shedding of the eggs and to limit the exposure of humans and other animals with contaminated areas. Raccoons should be quarantined away from other animals, in cages or enclosures that could be decontaminated if needed. All raccoons should be on a strict anthelmintic program to eliminate adult *B. procyonis* from the small intestine.

Access by humans, especially children, to known or potentially contaminated areas should be restricted. Raccoon feces should be removed and disposed of daily, in a manner that prevents contact with humans and animals. The feces should be destroyed. Contaminated areas, cages, or traps that have held infected raccoons should be decontaminated. Gloves and rubber boots should be worn by individuals who clean these cages, and hot, soapy water should be used. Protective coveralls should be used, and these should be washed in near-boiling water and bleach.

ANCYLOSTOMA CANINUM, ANCYLOSTOMA BRAZILIENSE, ANCYLOSTOMA TUBAEFORME, AND *UNCINARIA STENOCEPHALA* (CUTANEOUS LARVA MIGRANS, CREEPING ERUPTION, PLUMBER'S ITCH)

Cutaneous larva migrans is a skin condition caused by the migration of hookworm larvae in the skin of humans (Figure 16-1). It is also known as *creeping eruption, dermal larval migrans, ground itch, plumber's itch, sandworms,* and many other regional or colloquial names. It is a serpentine, reddened, elevated pruritic skin lesion usually caused by the larvae of *Ancylostoma braziliense,* a hookworm of both dogs and cats. Other nematode parasites of domestic and wild animals have been implicated in causing similar lesions in humans. These nematodes include *Ancylostoma caninum,* the canine hookworm; *Uncinaria stenocephala,* the northern hookworm of dogs; *Bunostomum phlebotomum,* the cattle hookworm; *Gnathostoma spinigerum; Dirofilaria* species; *Strongyloides procyonis,* a parasite of raccoons; and *Strongyloides westeri,* an equine parasite. Even the larvae of some of the myiasis-inducing flies (*Gasterophilus* and *Hypoderma* spp.) have been associated with the condition. However, hookworm larvae (*Ancylostoma* spp., particularly *A. braziliense*) are the pathogens most often incriminated.

Human Infection with Cutaneous Larva Migrans

Humans become infected with larvae of canine and feline hookworms when these larvae penetrate unprotected skin. This usually happens when human skin (usually of the bare feet) contacts moist, sandy soil contaminated with larval hookworms. Larval hookworms penetrate and migrate within the skin; in most cases they do not complete their life cycle or mature to adults in the small intestine.

Three scenarios have been developed regarding cutaneous hookworm infections in humans. The first scenario involves young children and adults who go barefoot in areas frequented by hookworm-infected pets. Children may also become exposed to contaminated sand or soil for extended periods (i.e., by playing in sandboxes or dirt containing larvae).

The second scenario involves travelers returning from exotic vacation sites throughout the world; while on holiday, these individuals usually have walked barefooted in the sand or were nude in the sand for an extended time. Third-stage hookworm larvae developing from eggs passed from parasitized pets or stray dogs and cats penetrate the naked skin and cause cutaneous larva migrans. This dermatitis usually occurs in individuals who frequent beaches; therefore the persons infected are said to be "parasitized with sandworms."

The third scenario concerns plumbers, electricians, masons, and technicians working in the crawl space beneath houses and horticulturists tending flower beds and vegetable gardens. If hookworm-infected dogs or cats have been allowed access to these moist sites and have defecated there, infective larvae may penetrate the laborer's skin. These workers are most often infected on their knees, elbows, buttocks, and

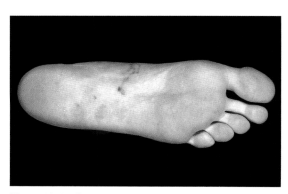

Figure 16-1   Cutaneous larva migrans in sole of man's foot. This skin condition is caused by migration of hookworm larvae in skin of humans. It is also known as creeping eruption, dermal larval migrans, ground itch, plumber's itch, and sandworms.

shoulders. Cutaneous larva migrans acquired in this manner is also known as "plumber's itch."

Symptoms and Diagnosis

The skin-penetrating larval hookworms migrate in the dermis of humans and cause distinct symptoms. The human is an abnormal, or incidental, host. The severity of skin lesions is directly related to the degree of exposure to infective larvae. Symptoms are characterized by red, tunnel-like migration tracks, with severe pruritus; therefore the common name for the condition is "creeping eruption." After skin penetration, the larvae reside in the superficial layers of the skin, actively producing and secreting hyaluronidase, an enzyme that aids their tunneling activity. Hookworm dermatitis is characterized by blisters, red bumps, and red tracts within a few days of initial penetration. The reddened site is usually 3 to 4 cm away from the penetration site, with the larva itself 1 to 2 cm ahead of the lesion. Within weeks to months after the initial infection, the larva dies and is resorbed by the host.

The skin condition is diagnosed by the observation of typical lesions in skin that has come in contact with moist soil containing infective hookworm larvae. A history of contact with the soil also aids in diagnosis. Laboratory findings usually have no role in the establishment of a diagnosis of cutaneous larva migrans.

Treatment

Suspected cases of cutaneous larva migrans in humans should *always* be referred to a dermatologist or family practitioner. Patients often receive both oral and topical treatment with thiabendazole. Pruritus often ceases rapidly for all patients after treatment with this anthelmintic. Surgical treatment to extract migrating larvae is often unsuccessful. Because the larva is situated 1 to 2 cm ahead of the visible track, it cannot be localized and removed surgically. The application of liquid nitrogen has been advocated; however, the larvae may continue to migrate. Hookworm larvae are capable of surviving temperatures as low as −21° C for more than 5 minutes.

Prevention of Transmission to Humans

Pets should be routinely examined for the presence of parasites and treated appropriately with anthelmintics. Pet owners should not allow their pet's feces to accumulate in the lawn or garden environment. Children's sandboxes should remain covered when not in use.

The seaside resort, with its moist, sandy environment, is an excellent locale for propagating larval hookworms. Pet owners should not allow dogs or cats infected with intestinal parasites to frequent beaches, either at home or abroad. Infected pets residing in seaside communities are most likely to transmit cutaneous larva migrans to humans. Seaside communities should also have leash laws, and well-trained animal control officers should regularly patrol beaches and remove free-roaming dogs and cats.

If an infected pet on a leash defecates in a public area, the feces should be promptly removed from the area, preferably by use of a disposable plastic bag. Burial of feces on the beach is not sufficient because tides and shifting sands are capable of exposing feces at a later time.

Travelers to exotic (or even local) beaches without enforced leash laws are at increased risk of contracting infective hookworm larvae if sandals or appropriate attire are not worn. Likewise, a person should never sit directly in the sand on beaches where infected animals have been allowed to roam and defecate freely.

ANCYLOSTOMA CANINUM (ENTERIC HOOKWORM DISEASE)

Infective larvae of the canine and feline hookworms that penetrate the skin usually produce a cutaneous manifestation. Recently, *Ancylostoma caninum* has been found to grow to the adult stage within the intestine of humans. Human enteric infections with *A. caninum* have been reported in Australia and, more recently, in the United States. Pulmonary involvement and corneal opacities also have been reported in humans infected with *A. caninum,* and an *Ancylostoma* larva has been recovered from the muscle fiber of a patient with cutaneous larva migrans.

Human Infection with Enteric Hookworm Disease

Humans become infected with hookworm when the larval hookworms penetrate unprotected skin. This usually happens when skin (usually of the bare feet) contacts moist, sandy soil contaminated with larval hookworms. Larval hookworms penetrate and migrate within the skin; in most cases they do not complete their life cycle or mature to adults in the small intestine. In the case of enteric hookworm disease, however, they do complete the life cycle and mature to adults in the small intestine.

Symptoms and Diagnosis

It is interesting that *A. caninum* has caused enteric infections in humans residing in developed, urban communities in northeastern Australia. Although the infections may be subclinical, the chief symptom is abdominal pain, which is frequently severe with sudden onset. After biopsy the chief pathologic finding is focal or diffuse eosinophilic inflammation resulting from a type 1 hypersensitivity response to secreted antigens. Additionally, two cases of eosinophilic enterocolitis attributable to canine hookworms have been reported in the United States. Canine hookworms adapt poorly in the human host; the infection is scant, and the worms do not produce eggs. Therefore, fecal flotation will not reveal the presence of hookworm eggs.

A. caninum also has been reported to occur sporadically in the human intestine in several locales throughout the world, such as the Philippines, South America, and Israel. In these instances, *A. caninum* did not produce clinically evident disease, was not fully developed, or was not capable of producing eggs. The three cases of infection with a single adult *A. caninum* were reported in eastern Australia, with results confirmed by ELISA and Western blot testing. Not all the recent cases of canine hookworm infection

in humans have been restricted to Australia. Cases of eosinophilic enterocolitis in two female children were reported in the United States in Louisiana.

Treatment

Suspected cases of enteric hookworm infection in humans should *always* be referred to a family practitioner or gastroenterologist. In the Australian study, canine hookworms were extracted using biopsy forceps, during either laparotomy or colonoscopy. After removal of the worms, all patients recovered and remained well. Both patients in the United States were treated with mebendazole (100 mg twice a day for 3 days), with repeat treatment in 2 to 6 weeks.

Prevention of Transmission to Humans

Human exposure to infective third-stage larvae of hookworms is directly related to prevalence of the parasite in the local canine population. The same precautions as listed for cutaneous larva migrans should be observed. Because most of the world's population shares the environment with dogs infected with *A. caninum,* hookworms could be encountered widely as a human enteric pathogen. As more physicians and human pathologists become aware of this condition, enteric infections with hookworms acquired from pets will become recognized as a major zoonosis. This zoonosis also stresses the need for awareness among public health workers, veterinarians, and pet owners.

TRICHINELLA SPIRALIS (TRICHINOSIS, TRICHINELLOSIS)

Trichinosis (also known as **trichinellosis**) is a disease caused by parasitic nematodes of the genus *Trichinella.* The most common cause of clinical trichinosis in humans is *Trichinella spiralis,* a parasite acquired from domestic pigs.

Human Infection with Trichinosis

Humans become infected with trichinosis by eating pork products containing infective larvae of *T. spiralis.* Pork products have been found to be the cause of approximately two thirds of the reported cases and disease episodes of trichinosis. These products usually are obtained through commercial outlets. Humans become infected by eating lightly processed, partially cooked or raw pork sausage or spiced pork. Home-raised or locally purchased swine also serve as an important source for human infection. Another important source of infection in humans is the consumption of wild game, particularly bear and boar.

Symptoms and Diagnosis

The severity and clinical outcome of the disease are related to the number of larvae ingested, the species of *Trichinella,* and a variety of host factors, such as age, gender, ethnic group, and immune status. Most cases of trichinosis in humans are subclinical, related to the low infection level. Mild, moderate, and severe cases also occur. These clinical manifestations increase in severity and may be life-threatening. The clinical manifestation can be classified into two types: the early abdominal syndrome and the later general trichinosis syndrome. In the *early abdominal syndrome,* clinical signs may commence 2 to 7 days after infection and may last for many weeks. This syndrome is typified by an enteritis, caused by the development and maturity of the worms parasitizing the small intestine and by the penetration of the newborn larvae into the intestinal wall. Infected humans may exhibit malaise, nausea, vomiting, anorexia, mild fever, abdominal pain, or diarrhea. Diarrhea may become persistent.

The *later general trichinosis syndrome* may appear weeks to months after the abdominal syndrome. On penetration of the intestine, the larvae have migrated throughout the body via the circulatory system. Although these larvae invade various tissues, the encysts are found only in striated skeletal muscle cells. Infected individuals develop an allergic vasculitis. This appears as vascular leakage and hemorrhage and may be observed as periorbital edema and fingernail-bed and conjunctival hemorrhages. Myalgia (muscle pain) and muscle weakness are common signs, related to invasion of the skeletal muscle, inflammation, and related damage. In severe cases, patients may also develop immune-mediated myocarditis, pneumonitis, encephalitis, and other, even more serious complications.

Human trichinosis is usually diagnosed during the muscle phase of the disease. Cases of trichinosis may be diagnosed by blood hemograms and serum chemistries. Persistent eosinophilia is a characteristic sign of trichinosis in humans. Patients may also exhibit a leukocytosis. Serum chemistries may reveal increased immunoglobulin E (IgE), creatine kinase (CK), and lactate dehydrogenase (LDH) values.

Treatment

Suspected cases of trichinosis in swine should *always* be reported by the veterinarian to both state and federal authorities. Humans infected with trichinosis should *always* be referred to a physician. The benzimidazole anthelmintics, particularly mebendazole, flubendazole, and cambendazole, are highly effective against the muscle larvae. The CDC has many specialists who are qualified to answer the most complex issues regarding trichinosis in humans.

Prevention of Transmission to Humans

Trichinosis can be contracted only by eating infected meat containing live *Trichinella.* People must assume that pork and wild game may be infected and should prepare the meat accordingly. Pork should be cooked at a uniform temperature of 140° F (60° C) throughout for at least 1 minute. Consumers at home are encouraged to cook pork at a temperature of 160° F (71° C), which ensures that all larval *Trichinella* are killed. Because microwave cooking often may produce "cold spots" in the meat, it is considered least effective for killing the larvae. People must take care to ensure uniform heating of pork products in microwave ovens.

Larval *Trichinella* also may be killed by freezing. Meat less than 15.25 cm (6 inches) thick should be frozen to 5° F (−15° C) for 20 days,

−10° F (−23° C) for 10 days, and −22° F (−30° C) for 6 days. Gamma irradiation of pork by the packing industry may also safeguard consumers from infection with this parasite.

DIROFILARIA IMMITIS (PULMONARY DIROFILARIASIS)

Only *Dirofilaria immitis,* the **canine heartworm,** causes pulmonary dirofilariasis in humans. *Pulmonary dirofilariasis* has been reported in more than 20 instances outside the United States and more than 90 times within the borders of the United States. Because humans are an incidental host for this parasite, most of the cases of pulmonary dirofilariasis result in the formation of a single, isolated nodule containing one necrotic (rotting) heartworm at its center.

Human Infection with Dirofilariasis

Mosquitoes are the intermediate host for *D. immitis,* the canine heartworm. Infected mosquitoes must readily attack both the canine definitive host and the human incidental host. The infective third-stage larvae emerge from the proboscis of the mosquito and are contained in a small drop of the mosquito's body fluid. These moist larvae must be close to the puncture wound made by the mosquito; the larvae enter this wound. After passage through the puncture wound made by the mosquito, the larva continues to develop in the subcutaneous tissues. It begins its wandering migration. Rather than residing in the right ventricle and pulmonary arteries, the larva finds its way to the lungs. In the lungs, the single larval *D. immitis* produces an infarction that results in a solitary pulmonary nodule. This infarction is caused by the occlusion (blockage) of an arteriole when a thrombus (blood clot) forms around an impacted worm. The nodule assumes a spherical shape from the secondary granuloma and the fibrotic reaction that occurs when the antigen from the degenerating worm diffuses into the surrounding pulmonary tissues. These nodules have been reported to occur in every lobe of the lung.

Symptoms and Diagnosis

Most cases of pulmonary dirofilariasis in humans are asymptomatic. Infected patients usually are found by radiographic detection of a density or an opacity in the lung field after routine radiography of the chest. The patient is scheduled for exploratory thoracic surgery, and the nodule is excised. Histopathology usually reveals the presence of a single, necrotic worm at the center of the fibrotic nodule. Special stains are available for identification of necrotic worm fragments. Tissue samples from suspected cases should be sent to a pathologist who is familiar with the appearance of these parasites in histopathologic section.

Eosinophil counts vary considerably among humans with pulmonary dirofilariasis and consequently are of little value. Both IgM and IgG ELISA for *D. immitis* antibodies have been used in studies of human populations. An ELISA has also been used to detect *D. immitis*–specific IgE in human sera.

Treatment

Suspected cases of pulmonary dirofilariasis in humans should *always* be referred to a thoracic surgeon or human histopathologist. Additionally, the CDC has many specialists who are qualified to answer the most complex issues of pulmonary dirofilariasis in humans.

Prevention of Transmission to Humans

The transmission cycle of dirofilariasis can be interrupted in several different ways. Veterinarians play an important role in the prevention of dirofilariasis in humans by encouraging pet owners to provide their dogs with preventive medicine. The daily or monthly administration of larvicidal drugs is an effective means of controlling the disease in dogs and preventing "spillover" infection in humans. These drugs are safe and effective. Because the weather in many southern states in the United States is mild, preventive medication should be given throughout the year. Control of stray and feral dogs also is an important consideration for the control of dirofilariasis. These animals represent a major reservoir for this disease.

Control of mosquitoes can reduce the exposure of humans and dogs and cats to these parasites. The removal of mosquito breeding sites and proper drainage of low-lying areas can be helpful. Mosquito larvicides may be used in some cases; however, resistance to these compounds can occur, and such compounds also disrupt the normal ecologic balance in the area. Recently, the biologic control of mosquitoes has been attempted in some areas, and the use of various species of fish to reduce larval populations has been successful.

A final line of defense is the prevention of mosquito bites in both humans and animals. People can prevent mosquito bites by the application of repellents and by wearing protective clothing. All effective mosquito repellents contain *deet* (diethyltoluamide). Walking dogs in the early evening hours when mosquitoes are most abundant should be avoided to reduce exposure in both humans and animals. Mosquitoes are not attracted to light, so electrocution devices are not helpful for their control; use of these devices may actually be detrimental because they destroy insects that may feed on adult mosquitoes.

ARTHROPODS OF PUBLIC HEALTH IMPORTANCE

SARCOPTES SCABEI VARIETY *CANIS* (CANINE SCABIES)

Canine scabies is a zoonotic skin condition caused by an ectoparasitic, tunneling sarcoptiform mite, *Sarcoptes scabei.* Both human and canine varieties of this mite are found; these varieties are classified as *Sarcoptes scabei* variety *hominis* and *Sarcoptes scabei* variety *canis,* respectively. Although these varieties are morphologically identical, they are different in their primary definitive host and in the characteristic lesions they produce.

Human Infection with Canine Scabies

Humans become infected with canine scabies by coming into direct contact with infested dogs. During most of their life cycle, these mites tunnel in the cornified layer of the epidermis (the outermost layer of the skin). During a short period, however, they reside on the surface of the skin and are capable of transferring from one host to another. If the infested dog comes in direct contact with another uninfested dog, the mite can be transferred. If the infested dog comes in direct contact with a human, the mite also can be transferred. It is important to remember that this mite is a transitory mite and does not establish itself in the skin of humans.

Symptoms and Diagnosis

Canine scabies in humans, particularly children, is characterized by the presence of characteristic lesions on the trunk, arms, abdomen, and rarely the face and genitalia. These lesions have been described as *papules* (red bumps) or *vesicles* (tiny blisters). Although these mites tunnel in the canine definitive host, they do not tunnel in human skin. The lesions caused by these mites are extremely pruritic; the onset of the pruritus commences with the appearance of the lesions.

Skin scrapings of the infested human's papular or vesicular lesions are rarely positive. The skin condition is diagnosed by the observation of typical lesions in skin that has come in contact with infested dogs. A history of contact with such dogs also aids in the diagnosis. Laboratory findings usually have no role in the establishment of a diagnosis of canine scabies.

Treatment

Suspected cases of canine scabies in humans should *always* be referred to a dermatologist or family practitioner. Antihistamines are prescribed to relieve the itch and topical steroid creams to reduce the papules and vesicles. Antibiotics may be administered to prevent secondary bacterial infection. Remember that these are prescription drugs and must be prescribed by a dermatologist or physician.

Prevention of Transmission to Humans

Transmission of this mite to humans can be prevented by avoiding contact with infested dogs harboring *S. scabei* variety *canis*. Naturally, when one dog is diagnosed with this parasitic mite, all dogs in the household must be treated to kill the offending ectoparasite.

PENTASTOMES OF PUBLIC HEALTH IMPORTANCE

REPTILIAN PENTASTOMIASIS

Reptilian pentastomiasis is the presence of encysted, wormlike nymphal stages of snake pentastomes within the mesenteric lymph nodes, liver, lungs, omentum, and other visceral organs of humans. One mammalian pentastome, *Linguatula serrata*, the tongue worm of dogs, behaves similarly and should be handled with precautionary measures as thorough as those for the reptilian pentastomes.

Human Infection with Reptilian Pentastomes

Adult reptilian pentastomes occur within the lungs, trachea, and nasal passages of the reptilian definitive host, feeding on tissue fluids and blood cells. Female pentastomes can produce several million fully embryonated eggs, each containing a single larval stage with two or three pairs of rudimentary, jointed legs that are clawed. These eggs are "coughed" up by the host, swallowed, and passed to the outside environment in snake feces. An oval-tailed larva with four (or six) stumpy legs, each of which has two retractable pincerlike claws, hatches from the egg and is infective for the intermediate host. Intermediate hosts include rodents, herbivores, carnivores, nonhuman primates, and in this case, humans. The larva bores into the intestinal wall of the intermediate host and passes with the blood to the mesenteric lymph nodes, liver, lungs, omentum, or other visceral organ, where it becomes encysted. The larva becomes quiescent and metamorphoses into a wormlike, nym-phal stage. The reptilian definitive host is infected by ingesting the intermediate host with its encysted nymphal pentastomes. The infective nymphs penetrate the snake's intestine, bore to the lungs, and become sexually mature adult parasites. It is important to note that humans serve as incidental intermediate hosts.

Symptoms and Diagnosis

Most cases of nymphal pentastomiasis in humans are asymptomatic; the patient is unaware of the infection. *Incidental nymphal pentastomiasis* in humans is diagnosed during exploratory surgery on radiographic examination and by histopathologic examination of autopsy specimens. The nymphal pentastome may assume a characteristic C shape during its development in the intermediate host. On histopathologic examination, certain morphologic features of the nymphal pentastome can be used for definitive diagnosis.

Antemortem diagnosis of pentastomiasis in humans can be accomplished by radiographic examination. Nymphal pentastomes often die in the human incidental intermediate host. In response, the human host will calcify the dead parasite. These dead, calcified parasites may be visible on radiographic examination. There are no satisfactory laboratory tests for antemortem diagnosis of nymphal pentastomiasis in humans.

Treatment

Persons having contact with snakes or snake feces and who suspect that they may be serving as an incidental host for reptilian pentastomes should be examined by an internist, who should be alerted to the possibility of pentastomiasis. In cases of limited infection in humans, free or encysted nymphs can be surgically removed. If tissues are removed for biopsy or autopsy purposes, a histopathologist should be alerted to the suspicion. Additionally, the CDC has many specialists who are qualified to answer the most complex issues of nymphal pentastomiasis in humans.

Prevention of Transmission to Humans

It is now "trendy" or "fashionable" to keep snakes and other reptiles as pets. Many individuals believe erroneously that reptiles are easier to maintain than either cats or dogs; reptiles do not require daily feeding. Many drawbacks await the unsuspecting owner, including the zoonotic potential of reptilian pentastomes.

In the United States, snakes and other reptiles can be easily obtained in pet stores in almost any mall or shopping center. The initial sources of these snakes often are unknown to the proprietor and owner. Snakes and other reptiles can originate from across town, across the continent, or from the other side of the globe. The public is largely unaware of the potential risks involved in caring for snakes. It is the veterinarian's duty to educate the client regarding the severity of incidental nymphal pentastomiasis and to instruct the owner in the proper care and husbandry of captive snakes and other reptiles.

A newly acquired reptile, whether purchased or collected from the wild, should be presented to the veterinarian for physical examination. This visit should include a routine fecal flotation. If this initial fecal examination is negative, examinations should be performed on at least two successive fecal specimens to reduce the possibility of false-negative results. If pentastome eggs are present in the feces, the client should be warned of the zoonotic potential of these parasites and advised to select another reptile. Anthelmintic drugs are probably ineffective against pentastomes because of the location of the adult parasites within the lungs of snakes. Clients who insist on maintaining poisonous reptiles as pets should be referred to zoos or herpetaria. Snake owners should be instructed regarding proper hygienic procedures and good husbandry techniques. Owners and veterinarians should wash their hands after handling snakes, snake feces, or cage and aquarium items. Water bowls and cages must be cleaned regularly.

Snake owners should be instructed about the intricate life cycle of the pentastomes. Because rodent intermediate hosts cannot be identified antemortem, the one practical preventive measure is to feed only clean, laboratory-reared rodents to captive snakes, lizards, crocodilians, and tuataras. Feeding wild, potentially pentastome-infected rodents to reptiles should be avoided.

CONCLUSION

Because of the public health significance of the parasites discussed in this chapter, it is the veterinarian's responsibility to inform and protect the general public in regard to pathogenic zoonoses.

17

Common Laboratory Procedures for Diagnosing Parasitism

The term *parasite* represents many different types of organisms that live within or on animals, feeding on tissues or body fluids or competing directly for the animal's food. These parasites demonstrate an amazing variety in size and appearance. Although none of the bacteria or viruses are visible to the naked eye, parasites include organisms that range in size from those that must be observed with the most powerful microscopes up to organisms that measure more than a meter in length. Parasites also show great variety in the locations in which they live in animals and the ways in which they are transmitted from one animal to another. Because of the wide variations in sizes and life cycles, there is no one particular diagnostic procedure to identify all parasites.

This chapter describes many of the procedures that a veterinary diagnostician may perform to diagnose both internal and external parasites. Generally, these procedures are used to detect the presence of parasites or their offspring, their eggs or larval stages, on the skin or in the animal's excretions or blood. Additionally, serologic tests are being used more frequently in veterinary clinical practice. Many of the diagnostic procedures described in this chapter, however, are not in common use in most veterinary practices but are mentioned because they may be useful to technicians employed in diagnostic or research laboratories.

It is important to note that these tests are not by themselves totally reliable. Sometimes an animal may be infected with parasites, but because the infection is slight, no detectable stages can be observed. If the wrong test is used, no parasite will be detected. For this reason, veterinary practitioners use not only these tests but also the animal's history, clinical signs, and other laboratory tests, such as blood values, to arrive at a specific diagnosis of internal parasites.

DIAGNOSIS OF PARASITES OF THE DIGESTIVE TRACT

The following procedures can be used as aids in diagnosis of parasitism of the esophagus, stomach, liver, bile ducts, and large and small intestines. They can also be used for diagnosis of parasitic infections in other parts of the body, when the eggs or the larval stages are passed by way of the digestive tract (e.g., "coughed up and swallowed" eggs of lung parasites).

COLLECTION OF THE FECAL SAMPLE

Veterinary diagnosticians usually do not have the opportunity to collect fecal samples and must rely on samples brought in by clients or samples collected during farm calls. Regardless of how the samples are obtained, it is important to have fresh feces for testing; this fact must be emphasized to clients. Feces collected from the yard, pen, or litter box may be old, and as a result, parasite eggs may have embryonated or larvated, oocysts may have sporulated, or pseudoparasites may be present. Some protozoans are recognized by their distinctive movements, and in old feces, these parasites may have died. The need for fresh feces stems from the rapid development and changes that occur in some common parasites' eggs or larvae once they are passed from the animal. If fresh feces cannot be promptly submitted, clients should be advised to refrigerate the sample for no more than 24 hours.

Feces should be submitted in a sealed glass or plastic container, clearly marked with the time and date of collection, species of animal, animal's name, owner's name, and any other information relevant to the case. The condition of the stool should be noted for color, consistency, and presence of parasites. Adult nematodes or tapeworm segments observed by the client may be overlooked by the veterinary practitioner.

Clients are often confused about the amount of feces needed to perform a fecal examination. An excellent rule of thumb is that the amount of feces submitted should be approximately the size of an adult man's thumb.

Small Animal Samples

For small animal samples, it is best that the client actually witness the animal defecating to be sure of the source of the sample and to note any straining, blood in the feces, or other problems. Again, all samples should be properly identified. In laboratories that process a large number of fecal samples, it is sometimes convenient to assign each sample an "accession number" to ensure that samples are processed in the order in which they are received and to aid in thorough recordkeeping.

Large Animal Samples

Large animal fecal samples should be collected directly from the animal's rectum, if possible. While wearing a disposable plastic glove, the veterinarian performing the rectal examination of cattle or horses can grasp a handful of feces and retrieve it from the rectum. This feces can then be placed in a sealed container and the container appropriately marked with the owner's name, animal's name or number, and date and time of collection.

The practice of turning the disposable palpation glove inside out while removing it and tying the open end with a knot, thus containing the feces, should be discouraged. These makeshift containers are difficult to label, and the process of removing collected feces from such a flexible container can be quite difficult and distasteful.

Samples from pigs, feedlot cattle, or other grouped animals are often "pooled" samples; that is, several fecal samples are collected from a pen without the specific animal of origin being known. Again, these samples should be as fresh as possible, and each sample should represent only one group of animals in direct contact with one another. Disposable, zipper-locking plastic bags make good containers for pooled, large animal fecal samples. These samples should be labeled with the owner's name, specific location of the pen, number of animals, and date and time of collection. The basic rule of thumb is to always have clean containers that can be tightly sealed to prevent spillage or loss of samples. Any fecal sample that cannot be examined within an hour after collection should be refrigerated to slow down or stop the parasite's development and reduce unpleasant odors.

EXAMINATION OF THE FECAL SAMPLE

Several procedures commonly used to examine feces for internal parasites are described in this section. Before attempting to apply these procedures, the following rules should be remembered:

- *Always handle fecal samples carefully.* Some parasites, bacteria, and viruses in animal feces are a threat to human health. When examining the samples, the diagnostician should always wear appropriate outer clothing (e.g., clean laboratory coat) and rubber or plastic gloves. If gloves are not available, hands should be washed thoroughly with a disinfectant soap when the diagnostic tests have been completed. Under no circumstances should food or drink be consumed or tobacco products used in the area where these tests are performed. Likewise, makeup or contact lenses should never be applied in the diagnostic laboratory.
- *Always clean up immediately after the tests have been performed.* Leaving spilled fecal material or dirty glassware or equipment lying about creates a source of contamination and could lead to serious infections in both animals and humans. The surface top of the area should be thoroughly cleaned with Roccal-D or Nolvasan solution.*
- *Always keep good records.* A central record book should be kept in the laboratory area, and every sample should be listed by the date, owner's name, and animal's name or number. Any observations about the appearance of the fecal sample, as well as any parasites found, should be written down immediately. If no parasites are recovered, that fact should be reported; otherwise it will appear that a particular diagnostic test has not been performed. In recording negative results, the phrase "No Parasites Observed" should be written in the results column. It is always important to transfer the results from the central record book to the animal's permanent veterinary medical record and to the clinic's central computer file.

The record book serves as a backup for veterinary medical records and provides a catalogue of parasites that are prevalent in the pet and livestock population of that geographic area. An accurate diagnosis of parasitism is based primarily on the diagnostician's awareness of parasites prevalent within the geographic region. Because twenty-first century humans are extremely mobile, however, the movement of pets and livestock to and from other geographic regions should also be considered when parasitism is suspected.

Gross Examination of Feces

The following characteristics of feces should be recorded and relayed to the attending veterinarians:

- *Consistency.* The condition of the feces, that is, soft, watery (diarrheic), or very hard (constipation), should be noted. This description will vary with the animal species. For example, cattle feces are normally softer than those of horses or sheep.
- *Color.* Unusual fecal colors should always be reported. For example, light-gray feces may indicate excessive fat in the feces, a sign of poor intestinal absorption.
- *Blood.* In fresh feces, blood may appear dark brown to black and tarlike (a melanous stool) or demonstrate the red color associated with fresh blood. Blood may indicate severe parasitism, as well as other intestinal disease. It is important to record the presence of blood because this will assist the veterinary practitioner in identifying certain diseases.
- *Mucus.* Mucus on the surface of fresh feces may be associated with intestinal parasitism or some other metabolic disease.
- *Age of the feces.* If the feces appear old and dry, this should be noted. In aged samples, as noted earlier, parasite eggs may have embryonated or larvated, oocysts may have sporulated, or pseudoparasites may be present. Some protozoan parasites are recognized by their distinctive movements. In old feces, these parasites may have died.

---

*Roccal-D manufactured by Pharmacia & Upjohn Company, Kalamazoo, MI; Nolvasan solution manufactured by Wyeth, Madison NJ.

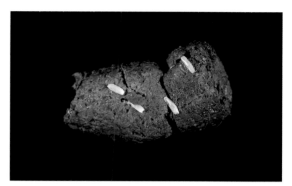

Figure 17-1 Fresh dog feces containing tapeworm proglottids (segments). Proglottids may be motile and will exit from feces into surrounding environment.

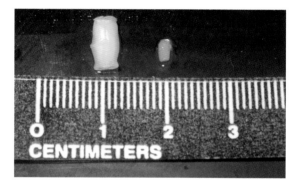

Figure 17-2 Segments of two common tapeworms (*Dipylidium caninum* and *Taenia pisiformis*) found in feces of dogs and cats. Morphology, shape, size, and movement of these common small animal tapeworms may aid in identification.

- *Gross parasites.* Some parasites, portions of parasites, or larvae are large enough to observe with the naked eye. Probably the most common are the proglottids of tapeworms, entire roundworms, or even larval arthropods (horse bot fly larvae).

Figure 17-1 shows tapeworm segments **(proglottids)** in fresh feces. These should be gently removed from the feces with thumb forceps and examined with a hand-held lens or dissecting microscope. Figure 17-2 shows segments of two common tapeworms (*Dipylidium caninum* and *Taenia pisiformis*) found in the feces of dogs and cats; their morphology, shape, size,

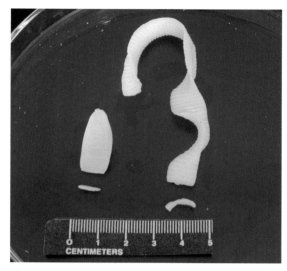

Figure 17-3 Chains and individual mature proglottids of tapeworms of ruminants, *Moniezia* species *(left)*, and horses, *Anoplocephala* species *(right)*.

and movement may aid in identification. Short segments of ruminant and equine tapeworms may also be recovered from feces (Figure 17-3). Of interest, swine in the United States do not demonstrate adult tapeworm segments in their feces.

Occasionally, clients will bring in dried tapeworm segments that they have found in their pet's bedding or hair coat. For identification, these segments must be rehydrated by soaking for 1 to 4 hours in a Petri dish or small container of water or physiologic saline. These segments will resume their natural state and can then be identified by their morphologic features. Alternatively, they may be "teased" open in a small amount of water on a glass microscope slide. If they are *gravid* (egg-containing) proglottids, they may release their eggs and be easily identified.

The diagnostician should always attempt to identify the parasite in terms of genus and species so that the veterinarian can use this information in the control and treatment of the tapeworm infection. The morphology of the segment can assist in the identification of the tapeworms. For example, with *D. caninum,* the tapeworm of dogs and cats that is transmitted by fleas, the diagnostician can observe with a hand-held magnifying lens the "double-pored effect," the presence of a genital pore on both sides of every segment. Segments of tapeworms of the genus *Taenia,* which uses rodents and mammals as intermediate hosts, have a single pore on each segment. These pores are irregularly alternating. Again, tapeworm segments can also be definitively identified by teasing them open and demonstrating the characteristic eggs they contain.

Segments of some uncommon tapeworm species may be "spent" proglottids; that is, the proglottids have dispelled their eggs and the uteri are empty. If the diagnostician is confused as to whether these are tapeworms, the suspect material can be macerated between two microscope slides and examined microscopically to determine if the tissue has small mineral deposits (called *calcareous bodies,* or *calcareous corpuscles*) that are unique to tapeworms (Figure 17-4).

Other types of parasites are large enough to be observed in animal feces. These include adult worms expelled from their host by drug treatments or overcrowding by fellow parasites (Figure 17-5). Horse feces may contain *bots,*

which are the larvae of a certain type of fly, *Gasterophilus* species. The larval flies are parasitic in the stomach of horses and are passed in the feces to complete their life cycle outside the body of the equine host (Figure 17-6).

Aged feces may also contain nonparasitic fly larvae called *maggots* (Figure 17-7). The maggots do not live within the animal's intestines but instead develop from eggs laid by free-living adult flies after the feces have been passed. Flesh flies of the genus *Sarcophaga* deposit larvae (rather than eggs) on the feces of many domestic

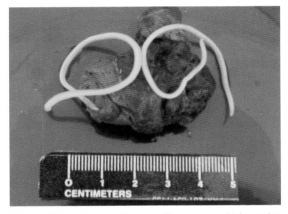

Figure 17-5 Two roundworms *(Toxocara canis)* in canine feces after treatment with a nematocide.

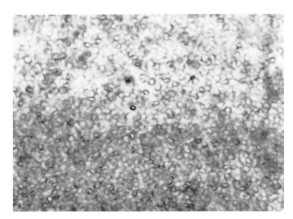

Figure 17-4 Microscopic calcium deposits (calcareous bodies, or calcareous corpuscles) are unique to tapeworm tissue. (140× magnification.)

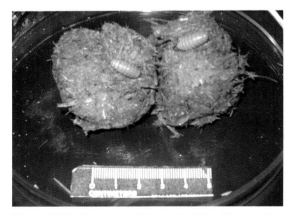

Figure 17-6 Two larvae (bots) of bot flies (*Gasterophilus* spp.) in equine feces.

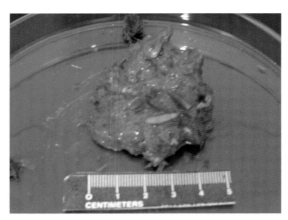

Figure 17-7 Free-living fly larvae (maggots) in 2-day-old bovine feces.

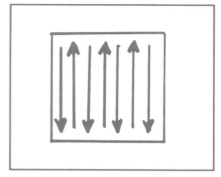

Figure 17-8 Pattern of movement of microscopic field for thorough examination of area under coverslip.

animals. Usually, fly maggots seen in feces voided more than 12 hours previously should not be mistaken for internal parasites; they should be considered *pseudoparasites.* There is one exception to this rule: *Gasterophilus* species, or horse bot fly larvae, may be found in fresh horse feces.

In general, when the veterinary diagnostician cannot identify parasite-like material (whether parasite or pseudoparasite) found within feces, the unidentified specimen should be sent to a diagnostic facility (a university or state diagnostic laboratory) for proper identification. These specimens should be preserved in 70% alcohol or 10% formalin and shipped as described later in this chapter. An up-to-date history should accompany each specimen.

Microscopic Examination of Feces

Compound microscopes used in a veterinary diagnostic setting vary widely in features and in the magnifications they provide. For parasitologic diagnostic examinations, objective lenses with magnification powers of 4×, 10×, and 40× are most often used. Oil-immersion objectives (e.g., 100× magnification) are occasionally used in veterinary practice, particularly in blood smear preparations. A mechanical stage is preferable and convenient for parasitologic work be-

cause it allows for smooth, uniform movement in a thorough search of the microscope slide. Regardless of how the slide is moved, the area under the coverslip must be thoroughly and uniformly searched (Figure 17-8).

To search the slide thoroughly, the diagnostician must begin using an objective lens that magnifies at least 10× and, with experience, should be able to scan the slides more rapidly at 4×. The edge of the coverslip can be used for adjusting the coarse focus and any debris under the coverslip used for fine focus adjustment. Each circular area of the slide seen through the coverslip is called a *field.* The slide should be moved so that the field follows either of the patterns of arrows shown in Figure 17-8. Each time the edge of the coverslip is reached, a piece of debris or other object at the edge of the field (in the direction of the search) should be identified. The slide is then moved until the piece of debris or other object is at the edge of the field. In this manner, every field scanned slightly overlaps the previous field, and every area beneath the coverslip is examined. When the slide is being scanned in this manner, it is important to move the fine focus knob continually back and forth slightly to aid in visualization of parasite eggs or cysts not in a single plane of focus. When a parasite egg or cyst is observed at low magnification, higher-power objectives (10× or 40×) may be used to more closely examine it.

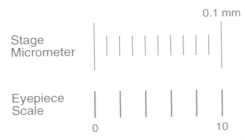

0.1 mm

Stage Micrometer

Eyepiece Scale

0   10

Figure 17-9 Stage micrometer *(upper scale)* and eyepiece scale *(lower scale)* used to calibrate microscope.

CALIBRATING THE MICROSCOPE. The size of various stages of many parasites is often important for correct identification. Some examples are eggs of *Trichuris vulpis* versus eggs of *Capillaria* species and microfilariae of *Acanthocheilonema recinditum* versus microfilariae of *Dirofilaria immitis*. Accurate measurements are easily obtained by using a calibrated eyepiece on the microscope. Calibration must be performed on every microscope to be used in the laboratory. Each objective lens (4×, 10×, 40×) of the microscope must be individually calibrated.

INSTRUMENTS. The stage micrometer is a microscope slide etched with a 2-mm line marked in 0.01-mm (10-µm) divisions (Figure 17-9). Note that 1 micron (micrometer, µm) equals 0.001 mm. Also note that the stage micrometer is used only once to calibrate the objectives of the microscope. Once the ocular micrometer within the compound microscope has been calibrated at 4×, 10×, and 40×, it is calibrated for the service life of the microscope; the stage micrometer will never be used again. Therefore it is a good idea not to purchase a stage micrometer, but instead borrow one from a university or some other diagnostic laboratory and return it following calibration.*

The eyepiece scale (or ocular micrometer) is a glass disc that fits into and remains in one of the microscope eyepieces. The disc is etched with 30

hatch marks spaced at equal intervals (see Figure 17-9). The number of hatch marks on the disc may vary, but the calibration procedure does not change.†

The stage micrometer is used to determine the distance in microns between the hatch marks on the ocular micrometer for each objective lens of the microscope being calibrated. This information is recorded and firmly affixed to the base of the microscope for future reference.

PROCEDURE. Start at low power (10×) and focus on the 2-mm line of the stage micrometer. Note that 2 mm equals 2000 µm. Rotate the ocular micrometer within the eyepiece so that its hatch-mark scale is horizontal and parallel to the stage micrometer (see Figure 17-9). Align the *0* points on both scales.

Determine the point on the stage micrometer aligned with the *10* hatch mark on the ocular micrometer. In Figure 17-9, this point is at 0.1 mm on the stage micrometer.

Multiply this number by 100. In this example, $0.1 \times 100 = 10$ µm. This means that at this power (10×), the distance between each hatch mark on the ocular micrometer is 10 µm. Any object may be measured with the ocular micrometer scale, and that distance is measured by multiplying the number of ocular units by a factor of 10. For example, if an object is 10 ocular units long, its true length is 100 µm (10 ocular units × 10 µm = 100 µm).

This procedure should be repeated at each magnification (4× and 40×). For each magnification, this information is recorded and labeled on the base of the microscope for future reference.

Objective Distance between Hatch Marks (Microns)
    4×–25 µm
    10×–10 µm
    40×–2.5 µm

Direct Smear

The simplest method of microscopic fecal examination for parasites is the direct smear, which consists of a small amount of feces placed directly on the microscope slide (Box 17-1). The

*Item number 59-1430; Carolina Biological Supply Company, Burlington, NC.

†Item number 59-1423 or 59-1425; Carolina Biological Supply Company, Burlington, NC.

BOX 17·1 Direct Fecal Smear Procedure

1. Place several drops of saline or fecal flotation solution on a slide with an equal amount of feces.
2. Mix the solution and feces together with a wooden applicator until the solution is homogenous.
3. Smear the solution over the slide into a thin film. The film should be thin enough to read print through.
4. Remove any large pieces of feces.
5. Place a coverslip over the smear.
6. Examine the area of the slide under the coverslip with the compound microscope (see text), and record any protozoan cysts, eggs, larvae, or gross parasites seen.

advantages of the direct smear are the short procedure time and minimal equipment needed. Some veterinary practitioners make direct smears with only the amount of feces that clings to a rectal thermometer after the animal's temperature has been recorded. The direct smear allows the diagnostician to observe eggs and larvae undistorted by the procedures discussed later.

A disadvantage to the direct smear technique is that the small amount of fecal material required for this procedure is not a good representative sample size; this procedure can be inaccurate. Such a small quantity of feces may not contain the larvae or eggs of the adult parasite the animal is harboring. The animal may be incorrectly assumed to be free of parasites. This procedure also leaves much fecal debris on the slide that may be confusing to the veterinary diagnostician.

CONCENTRATION METHODS FOR FECAL EXAMINATION

The greatest disadvantage to the direct smear procedure is the small amount of feces used, which greatly reduces the chance of finding parasite eggs or larvae or protozoan cysts. To overcome this problem, methods have been developed to concentrate parasitic material from a larger fecal sample into a smaller volume, which may be examined microscopically. Two primary types of concentration methods are used in veterinary practice: fecal flotation and fecal sedimentation.

Fecal Flotation

Fecal flotation procedures are based on differences in specific gravity of parasite eggs, cysts, and larvae and that of fecal debris. *Specific gravity* refers to the weight of an object (e.g., the parasite egg) compared with the weight of an equal volume of pure water. Most parasite eggs have a specific gravity between 1.1 and 1.2 (g/mL), whereas tap water is only slightly higher than 1 g/mL. Therefore, parasite eggs are too heavy to float in tap water. To make the eggs float, a liquid with a higher specific gravity than that of the eggs must be used. Such liquids are called *flotation solutions* and consist of concentrated sugar or various salts added to water to increase its specific gravity. Flotation solutions usually have specific gravities between 1.2 and 1.25. In this range, fecal material, much of which has a specific gravity of 1.3 or greater, does not float (Figure 17-10). The result of using flotation solutions is that parasite eggs float to the surface of the liquid and large particles of fecal material sink to the bottom, making eggs easier to observe (Box 17-2).

If the specific gravity is below the desired range (1.2-1.25), add more reagent until the hydrometer indicates this range. If the specific gravity is above 1.25, add water until the proper reading is obtained.

Sugar (Sheather's solution), saturated sodium chloride (table salt), magnesium sulfate (Epsom salt), zinc sulfate, and sodium nitrate solutions are the flotation solutions most often used in veterinary practices. Veterinarians may select from among these solutions based on personal preference, availability of reagents, and target parasites.

Sheather's solution is less efficient than sodium nitrate solution because it floats fewer eggs and is messy to work with (it is quite sticky). Sugar, however, is readily available and inexpensive, does not distort roundworm eggs, and floats an adequate percentage of the eggs.

17·2   Preparation of Flotation Solutions

SUGAR FLOTATION SOLUTION (SHEATHER'S SOLUTION)

Determine the amount of sugar solution required, and use about half that amount of water. Use an appropriate-size pot (e.g., cooking pot). Heat the water, but be careful not to let it boil. Add granulated pure cane sugar (table sugar) to the water while stirring. About 454 g (1 lb) are required for every 355 mL (12 oz) of water. Add 6 mL of 40% formaldehyde solution or 1 g of crystalline phenol for every 100 mL of solution; these chemicals serve as preservatives and prevent mold from growing in this sugar solution. The solution's specific gravity should always be checked with a hydrometer (Figure 17-10), an instrument available from scientific supply houses.*

SODIUM NITRATE FLOTATION SOLUTION

Add about 315 g of sodium nitrate for every liter of water, while stirring. Heating is not necessary but hastens the dissolution process. Adjust the solution to a specific gravity of 1.2 to 1.25, as discussed for the sugar solution.

ZINC SULFATE FLOTATION SOLUTION

Add 386 g of zinc sulfate for every liter of water, while stirring. Heating the water is not necessary but hastens the dissolution process. Using a hydrometer, adjust the solution to a specific gravity of 1.2 to 1.25, as discussed for the sugar solution.

MAGNESIUM SULFATE FLOTATION SOLUTION

Add about 350 g of magnesium sulfate (Epsom salt) for every liter of water, while stirring. Heating the water hastens the dissolution process. Using a hydrometer, adjust the solution to a specific gravity of 1.3, as discussed for the sugar solution.

SATURATED SODIUM CHLORIDE FLOTATION SOLUTION

Add sodium chloride (table salt) to boiling water until the salt no longer dissolves and settles to the bottom of the pot. There is no need to adjust the specific gravity because it cannot go above 1.2 with this solution.

*Scientific Products, McGaw Park, IL.

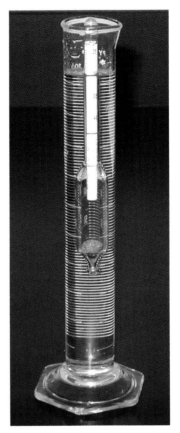

Figure 17-10   Measuring specific gravity of flotation solution with hydrometer.

Sodium nitrate solution is the most efficient flotation solution, but it forms crystals and distorts the eggs after a time. Sodium nitrate may be difficult to acquire, but it can be purchased through chemical supply houses. Sodium nitrate solution is used in commercial fecal diagnostic kits and may be purchased already prepared in the form of refill bottles for these kits. Sodium nitrate solution is more expensive than sugar solution.

Saturated sodium chloride solution is the least desirable flotation solution. Its main disadvantages are that it corrodes expensive laboratory equipment, such as compound microscopes and centrifuges; forms crystals on the microscope slide; and severely distorts the eggs.

Because it reaches a specific gravity of 1.2, some heavier eggs may not float in this solution. However, sodium chloride is inexpensive, easily prepared, and readily available.

Zinc sulfate solution is similar in efficiency to sugar solution and can be purchased through chemical supply houses. Cystic stages of intestinal protozoans such as *Giardia* are best concentrated with zinc sulfate solution. *Magnesium sulfate solution* (Epsom salt) also forms crystals on the microscope slide. It is an inexpensive solution and is easily prepared and readily available.

SIMPLE FLOTATION. The simple flotation method is probably the second most common parasitologic test performed in veterinary practices, after the direct smear (Box 17-3). A specimen of 2 to 5 g of feces is placed in a suitable container, such as a paper cup. Flotation solution is added directly to the feces, mixed thoroughly with a tongue depressor, and strained through a metal tea strainer (or cheesecloth) into a second paper cup. The contents of the second paper cup are poured into a test tube, and the flotation medium is added until a meniscus is formed (Figure 17-11). A glass coverslip is placed over the meniscus and allowed to remain for 10 to 15 minutes (depending on the flotation medium used), after which the coverslip is removed and placed on a glass microscope slide. The parasite eggs are lighter than the solution and float to the top of the tube (or vial) of flotation solution. The coverslip is removed from the liquid and examined with a microscope. This method is less efficient than the centrifugal flotations described next, but it does not require a centrifuge.

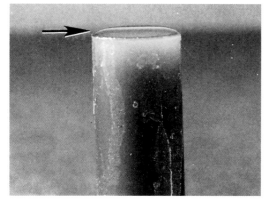

Figure 17-11 Shell vial filled with flotation medium, showing meniscus *(arrow).*

BOX **17-3** Simple Flotation Procedure

1. Place about 2 g (½ tsp) of the fecal sample in a 90- to 150-mL waxed paper cup. Add approximately 30 mL of flotation medium. Using a tongue depressor, make an emulsion by thoroughly mixing the solution with the feces until a fecal slurry has been made.

2. Bend the side of the wax paper cup into a spout, and cover the spout with a piece of cheesecloth. Pour the emulsion through the cheesecloth into a straight-sided shell vial. A tea strainer may be used rather than cheesecloth, pouring the contents of the cup through the strainer into a second wax paper cup, and the contents of that cup into the shell vial. Wash the tea strainer thoroughly in hot, soapy water before using it again.

3. Fill the shell vial to the top and slightly overfill it so that a meniscus forms above the lip of the vial (Figure 17-11). If there is not enough fluid in the cup to fill the shell vial, a small amount of fresh flotation medium may be added. Place a glass coverslip gently on top of the fluid, and allow it to settle on the meniscus.

4. Allow the coverslip to remain undisturbed on top of the vial for 10 to 20 minutes (sugar solution requires longer than sodium nitrate). If removed before this time, all the eggs may not have had time to float to the top. If left for more than 1 hour, some eggs may become waterlogged and begin to sink or become distorted.

5. Remove the coverslip carefully, picking it straight up, and immediately place it on the microscope slide. When placing the coverslip on the slide, be sure to hold the coverslip with one edge tilted slightly up, and allow it to gradually settle level on the slide. This reduces the number of air bubbles beneath the coverslip.

6. Examine the area of the slide under the coverslip with the compound microscope (see text), and record any protozoan cysts, eggs, larvae, or gross parasites seen.

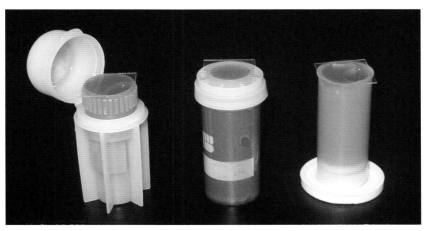

Figure 17-12   Three commercially available fecal flotation kits: Fecalyzer *(left),* Ovassay *(center),* and Ovatector *(right).* These kits are based on the principles of the simple flotation procedure.

Some veterinary diagnostics companies have packaged simple flotation kits consisting of pre-pared flotation solution, disposable plastic vials, and strainers; examples include the Ovassay, Fecalyzer, and Ovatector (Figure 17-12).* Instructions for use are included with these kits. The main disadvantages to these kits are the expense and the environmental contamination by the dis-posal of plastics.

CENTRIFUGAL FLOTATION. The centrifugal flota-tion procedure more efficiently recovers parasite eggs and cysts and requires less time than the simple flotation procedure (Box 17-4 and Figure 17-13). However, it does require a centrifuge capable of holding 15-mL test tubes and produc-ing a centrifugal force of 400× to 650× *g.* Most tabletop centrifuges are capable of producing this force. Centrifuges with a fixed-angle head piece are not suitable for such centrifugal flota-tion procedures.

Fecal Sedimentation

Sedimentation procedures concentrate both feces and eggs at the bottom of a liquid medium,

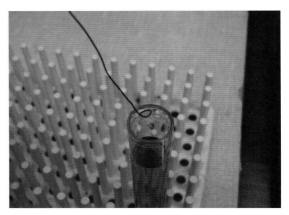

Figure 17-13   Use of bacteriologic loop to transfer drop from top of fecal flotation emulsion after centrifugation procedure. Note that loop is bent at 90-degree angle to wire handle.

usually water (Box 17-5). Sedimentation detects most parasite eggs but is not as good as flotation for providing a clear sample for microscopic examination. Sedimentation is primarily used to detect eggs or cysts that have too high a specific gravity to float or that would be severely dis-torted by flotation solution.

Sedimentation can be used for roundworm and tapeworm eggs, but there is usually too much fecal debris hiding the eggs to make it

*Ovassay manufactured by Synbiotics Corp., San Diego CA; Fecalyzer manufactured by EVSCO Pharmaceuticals, Buena, NJ; Ovatector manufactured by BGS Medical Products, Inc., Venice, FL.

BOX 17·4 Centrifugal Flotation Procedure

1. Using a paper cup and tongue depressor, mix approximately 1 tsp of feces with enough water to make a semisolid suspension.
2. Place a wire tea strainer (or piece of cheesecloth) over a second paper cup and empty the fecal suspension into it. Use the tongue depressor to press out most of the liquid; return the solid waste to the first cup and discard. Wash the strainer in hot running water; soak it in water containing dishwashing solution.
3. Pinch the rim of the second paper cup to form a pouring spout, and transfer the contents into a 15-mL centrifuge tube (a test tube). Place the tube into the centrifuge, remembering to counterbalance the tube with an identical tube filled to the same level with water. Be sure that all tubes are marked so they can be identified after centrifugation.
4. Centrifuge for 3 minutes at 400× to 650× g. For many centrifuges, this is about 1500 revolutions per minute (rpm). Decant the supernatant, which contains fats and dissolved pigments that interfere with the identification of parasite eggs, larvae, or cysts.
5. Add concentrated flotation solution to within ½ to ¾ inch of the top of the tube, and resuspend the sediment using a stirring action with a wooden applicator stick. Insert a rubber stopper and mix by four or more inversions so that the solution is thoroughly mixed with the sediment.

VARIATION A
Return the tube to the centrifuge, remembering to counterbalance the tube with an identical tube filled to the same level with the same flotation solution. Centrifuge for 5 minutes. Without removing the tube from the centrifuge, pick up the surface film containing eggs, larvae, or cysts by touching the surface gently with a wire loop (bent at a 90-degree angle) (see Figure 17-13) or a glass rod. Transfer the surface film to a glass microscope slide and add a coverslip. Examine under the compound microscope using the 10× objective (see text).

VARIATION B
Return the tube to the centrifuge and fill the centrifuge tube with the flotation solution until a meniscus is formed. Apply a coverslip to the top of the tube. Remember to counterbalance the tube with an identical tube filled to the same level with the same flotation solution and covered with a coverslip. Centrifuge for 5 minutes. After centrifugation, lift the coverslip straight up and place it on the glass slide. This modification will work only if a variable-angle (not a fixed-angle) centrifuge is used. Examine under the compound microscope, using the 10× objective (see text).

BOX 17·5 Sedimentation Procedure

1. Using a tongue depressor, mix about 2 g of feces with tap water in a cup or beaker. Strain the mixture through cheesecloth or a tea strainer into a centrifuge tube, as described for centrifugal flotation.
2. Balance the centrifuge tubes and centrifuge the sample at about 400× g (about 1500 rpm). If a centrifuge is unavailable, allow the mixture to sit undisturbed for 20 to 30 minutes.
3. Pour off the liquid in the top of the tube without disturbing the sediment at the bottom.
4. Using the pipette and bulb, transfer a small amount of the top layer of sediment to a microscope slide. If the drop is too thick, dilute it with a drop of water. Lugol's iodine solution (diluted 1:5 in water) may be used for dilution instead of water to aid in identification of protozoan cysts. Apply a coverslip to the drop. Repeat the procedure using a drop from the bottom layer of the sediment.
5. Examine both slides microscopically (see text).

worthwhile. Therefore, this procedure is not used routinely and has its greatest use in suspected trematode (fluke) infections. Fluke eggs are somewhat denser and sometimes larger than roundworm eggs. Some fluke eggs float in flotation solutions, and others do not. Some laboratories increase the specific gravity of their flotation solutions to 1.3 to ensure recovery of fluke eggs by the flotation technique. The problem with use of flotation methods for recovery of fluke eggs is that the eggs may be damaged by the high concentration of the solution and may become difficult to identify.

QUANTITATIVE FECAL EXAMINATION

All the procedures previously described are *qualitative*, which means they reveal the presence or absence of parasite ova. *Quantitative* procedures indicate the number of eggs or cysts present in each gram (g) of feces. The results of these procedures are a rough, or approximate, indication of the number of adult parasites present within the host (the severity of the infection). These procedures are not completely accurate, because different species of parasites produce different numbers of eggs. Also, the most severe signs of disease are produced by parasites that have not yet started to produce eggs or larvae.

Several procedures are used to estimate the numbers of parasite eggs or cysts per gram of feces, including the Stoll egg-counting technique, the modified Wisconsin sugar flotation method, and the McMaster technique. These techniques are used most often in research laboratories and are not usually performed in veterinary clinical practice. Of these tests, the modified Wisconsin sugar flotation method is used most often (Box 17-6).

BOX 17-6 Modified Wisconsin Sugar Flotation Method

1. Fill a 20-mm × 150-mm test tube with Sheather's solution 1 inch below the top of the tube.
2. Using scales, weigh exactly 3 g of the fecal sample into a paper cup.
3. Pour the Sheather's solution from the test tube into the paper cup containing the feces and mix well.
4. Place a tea strainer in a second paper cup and pour the Sheather's solution and feces mixture through the strainer. Using a tongue depressor, press all the liquid out of the fecal pat and through the tea strainer.
5. Return the Sheather's solution and strained feces mixture to the test tube originally containing the Sheather's solution and place in a test tube rack.
6. Add Sheather's solution to the test tube until a small meniscus forms. Carefully place a glass coverslip on top of the meniscus.
7. Allow the test tube with its coverslip to stand undisturbed for 4 hours.
8. Remove the coverslip, place it on a glass microscope slide, and examine the entire coverslip on low power (10×), counting parasite eggs, cysts, or oocysts. This count represents the number of eggs, cysts, or oocysts per 3 g of feces.

EXAMINATION OF FECES FOR PROTOZOA

All the procedures for microscopic fecal examination are useful for detection of cysts of intestinal protozoa. However, some protozoa do not form cysts and will be passed in the feces as *trophozoites* (motile forms). Cyst-forming protozoa may also pass trophozoites in the feces in large numbers when the host has diarrhea. Trophozoites lack the rigid wall of cysts, and they collapse and become difficult to recognize in flotation solutions.

To observe live trophozoites, a fecal smear should be prepared as previously described, but physiologic saline must be used to dilute the feces. Trophozoites are recognized by their movement, which varies among the different groups of protozoa. *Balantidium coli*, a parasite of humans, pigs, and dogs, moves in a slow, tumbling manner. *Giardia* species, which are found in several species of animals, swim in a jerky motion. Trichomonads, also found in several different types of hosts, appear to wobble and have a sail-like, undulating membrane that ripples as they swim. Amoebae, found in humans and dogs, move by extending part of their cell body (a pseudopod) and moving the rest of the body after it.

Many methods have been used to stain and preserve intestinal protozoa. The simplest method to stain cysts is a direct smear stained with an iodine solution (as described under the direct smear procedure). This method does not preserve the sample but highlights any protozoa in the smear, facilitating identification. Several iodine solutions are available for staining. Modified D'Antoni's iodine is often used in diagnostic laboratories to stain protozoan cysts (Box 17-7).

Fecal smears containing protozoal trophozoites may be allowed to dry and then are stained with Giemsa, Wright's, or Diff-Quik stain.* Once stained in this manner, the slides

---

*Diff-Quik, product number B4132-1; Baxter Diagnostics, Scientific Products Division, McGaw Park, IL.

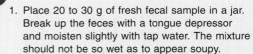

BOX 17-7 Preparation of Modified D'Antoni's Iodine Solution

1. Before preparing this solution, the technician should remove all jewelry because this iodine solution can permanently stain precious metals. Distilled water, 100 mL
   Potassium iodide (KI), 1 g
   Powdered iodine crystals, 1.5 g
2. The potassium iodide solution should be saturated with iodine, with some excess remaining in the bottle. It should be stored in brown, glass-stoppered bottles and kept in the dark. The solution is ready for use immediately and should be decanted into a brown, glass dropping bottle. When the solution lightens, it should be discarded and replaced with fresh stock. The stock solution is good as long as an excess of iodine remains in the bottom of the bottle.
3. When using this solution in the laboratory around the compound microscope, the technician should take great care not to spill the solution onto the metal parts of the microscope because it is extremely corrosive.

BOX 17-8 Fecal Culture of Roundworm Eggs

1. Place 20 to 30 g of fresh fecal sample in a jar. Break up the feces with a tongue depressor and moisten slightly with tap water. The mixture should not be so wet as to appear soupy.
2. Place the jar on a shelf, away from direct sunlight, and allow it to incubate at room temperature for 7 days. There should be enough moisture so that droplets of condensed water can be seen on the sides of the glass jar. If moisture does not form, add a few drops of water.
3. Some species of nematode larvae can migrate up the walls of the jar. These may be recovered by removing condensation drops from the glass with an artist's paintbrush and transferring them to a drop of water on a microscope slide. Other species must be recovered with the Baermann technique (see p. 243).
4. Apply a coverslip to the slide (a drop of modified D'Antoni's iodine may be added) and pass it over the open flame of a Bunsen burner once or twice to kill the larvae while they are in an extended position. Place the slide on the microscope slide stage and identify the larvae.

may be sent to a diagnostic laboratory for identification of the organism.

Other procedures for the concentration, staining, and preservation of intestinal protozoa include merthiolate-iodine-formaldehyde (MIF) solution, polyvinyl alcohol, and iron hematoxylin. These staining procedures are generally too complex and time-consuming for use in veterinary practice.

FECAL CULTURE

Fecal culture is used in diagnostic parasitology to differentiate parasites whose eggs and cysts cannot be distinguished by examination of a fresh fecal sample. For example, the eggs of large strongyles in horses are very similar to those of small strongyles. To distinguish between them, feces containing strongyle eggs are allowed to incubate at room temperature for several days while the larvae hatch from the eggs. The newly hatched larvae can then be identified.

Nematode (Roundworm) Eggs

The procedure for culture of nematode (roundworm) eggs in feces is simple; however, identifying the larvae once they are recovered is much more tedious (Box 17-8). Diagnosticians required to culture and identify nematode larvae are referred to state or private diagnostic laboratories.

Coccidial Oocysts

Another type of fecal culture that has some use in veterinary practices is sporulation of coccidial oocysts (Box 17-9). *Sporulation* is a process of development that takes place within the oocyst. In fresh feces, oocysts of various species of coccidia may appear similar to one another; however, once sporulation occurs, coccidia of the genus *Eimeria* can be easily distinguished from those of the genus *Isospora*. A fully sporulated oocyst of the genus *Eimeria* contains four sporo-

17-9 BOX Fecal Culture of Coccidial Oocysts

1. When coccidial oocysts are found in a fresh fecal sample, place 10 to 20 g of the sample in a beaker or a paper cup and cover with about 60 mL of 2.5% potassium dichromate solution. Mix this solution thoroughly with a tongue depressor.
2. Pour into a Petri dish and allow to incubate at room temperature for 3 to 5 days. Open the plate daily and swirl the contents gently to allow air to reach the developing oocysts.
3. After incubation, centrifuge the plate's contents as described under the sedimentation procedure (see p. 238).
4. Process the fecal sediment by the centrifugal flotation procedure to recover the oocysts, then examine microscopically.

17-10 BOX Decanting Method for Sample Collection at Necropsy

1. Using wrapping twine, tie off each portion of the digestive tract, that is, stomach, duodenum, small intestine, large intestine, and so on. Open each individual organ and pour its contents into a bucket marked with the animal's identification and the organ being examined. Scrape the interior lining of the organ with a spatula or blunt edge of a pair of scissors, and add the scraping into the bucket.
2. Add an equal volume of water to the contents in each labeled bucket and mix thoroughly with a stirring spoon or paddle.
3. Allow the heavier part of the contents to settle to the bottom of the bucket. This usually takes about 45 minutes. Carefully pour off the liquid on top, leaving the sediment.
4. Add an equal volume of water to the sediment and stir again. Allow this to resettle. Repeat this process until the water over the sediment becomes clear.
5. Pour off the clear water over the sediment, then transfer the sediment to the dissection pan.
6. Using the dissecting microscope, examine a small amount of the sediment at a time. Any parasite found should be gently removed from the sediment with thumb forceps and preserved (see text). Each parasite should be identified using a compound microscope.

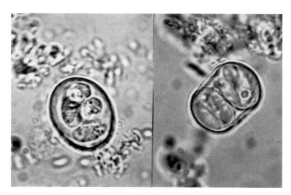

Figure 17-14 Fully sporulated oocysts of *Eimeria* species *(left)* and *Isospora* species *(right).* (1400×.)

cysts, whereas a fully sporulated oocyst of the genus *Isospora* has two sporocysts (Figure 17-14).

SAMPLE COLLECTION AT NECROPSY

Necropsy, or postmortem examination, is an important method for diagnosing parasitism of the digestive tract. Lesions of internal organs are often fairly indicative of the type of parasites that produce them. The veterinary technician is responsible for assisting during necropsy procedures and, in particular, helping with the preservation and processing of the samples collected. During necropsy and the processing of samples, all workers should wear gloves.

The contents of the digestive system may contain many types of parasites, some of which may be nematodes (roundworms). Trematodes (flukes) and cestodes (tapeworms) are easily seen and can be individually isolated. The two preferred methods for recovering roundworms are the decanting method (Box 17-10) and the sieving method (Box 17-11). With either method, the contents of the different parts of the digestive tract should be separated into individual containers.

It is not always necessary to examine all sediment or sievings. An estimate of the number of worms may be obtained by counting an *aliquot*

Sieving Method for Sample Collection at Necropsy

1. Using wrapping twine, tie off each portion of the digestive tract, that is, stomach, duodenum, small intestine, large intestine, and so on. Open each individual organ and pour its contents into a bucket marked with the animal's identification and the organ being examined. Scrape the interior lining of the organ with a spatula or blunt edge of a pair of scissors, and add the scraping into the bucket.
2. Add an equal volume of water to the contents in each labeled bucket and mix thoroughly with a stirring spoon or paddle.
3. Pour the mixture through a 1-mm mesh (no. 18) sieve and then through a 0.354-mm mesh (no. 45) sieve.* Reverse wash the sieves' contents with water.
4. Using the dissecting microscope, examine a small amount of the sieve contents at a time. Any parasite found should be gently removed from the contents with thumb forceps and preserved (see text). Each parasite should be identified using a compound microscope.

*Sieves available from Fisher Scientific, Pittsburgh, PA.

(a known percentage of the total volume) of the sediment.

When parasites are recovered from the digestive tract or other parts of the body, it may be necessary to preserve them for identification later. *Nematodes* (roundworms) should be briefly washed in water to remove any attached debris and then placed in hot 70% ethyl alcohol (ethanol). Isopropyl alcohol may be used but is not preferred. The alcohol is allowed to cool, after which the worms are examined. The worms may be stored in the alcohol after adding glycerine to make a 5% concentration. *Cestodes* (tapeworms), including the scolices (heads), should be placed in water at about 37° C (98.6° F) for about 1 hour and then stored in a mixture of 5% glycerine or 70% alcohol or 5% to 10% formalin. *Trematodes* (flukes) may be preserved in the same manner as tapeworms. If tapeworms and flukes are to be stained later, they should be "relaxed" in alternate changes of ice water and tap water for about 3 hours and then lightly pressed between sheets of glass immersed in 10% formalin.

Sometimes during necropsy of domestic animals, *cysticerci*, or bladder worms, may be seen in the abdomen, muscles, or other internal organs. These are the larval stages of certain species of tapeworms and appear as fluid-filled, balloonlike structures that vary from the size of a pea to the size of a basketball, depending on the species of tapeworm. Caution should be used in handling these parasites because the fluid inside could produce allergic reactions.

Also during necropsy of large animals, long filarial parasites of the genus *Setaria* may be observed in the abdominal cavity. These should be recorded and saved as part of the tissues collected and parasites recovered from the animal.

Government or private diagnostic laboratories are useful in assisting with identification when questions arise, but they must be supplied with well-preserved specimens and adequate histories from the animals on which the necropsies were performed.

Many diagnostic laboratories have the capability of identifying both protozoan and metazoan parasites in histopathologic section. Again, the laboratories must be provided with well-preserved tissue samples and adequate histories from the animals. These procedures are beyond the scope of this textbook; however, the diagnostician must remember that even tiny cross sections or longitudinal sections of parasites in histopathologic section may be used to diagnose both infections and infestations of all types of parasites.

SHIPPING PARASITOLOGIC SPECIMENS

Any parasitologic specimen shipped to a diagnostic laboratory by the United States Postal Service or other private carrier should be in a preservative, such as 70% ethyl alcohol or 10% formalin, to render it noninfectious. Specimen jars must be sealed well so that they do not leak, and a suitable packing material, such as Styrofoam "peanuts," added to cushion the contents from any rigorous handling during the shipping process. During the summer months or during any hot spell, cool packs should accompany any specimen.

Fecal materials should be mixed with 10% formalin at a ratio of 1 volume of feces to 3 volumes of formalin and placed in a screw-cap vial of 20- to 30-mL capacity. The vials should be sealed with tape and labeled with the practitioner's name, the client's name, and the species of animal and its name or number, gender, and age. The relevant clinical history or diagnostic questions should also accompany the specimen. It is always wise to place any pertinent papers detailing the case history in a separate plastic bag in case leakage occurs during the shipping process. Parasite specimens preserved in alcohol or formalin should be shipped in similar vials. The vials should be wrapped in absorbent material, such as soft tissue or paper towels, and placed in a Styrofoam mailing container or heavy cardboard mailing tubes. To ensure the greatest of care during shipping, specimens should be checked in at a postal window in a post office with instructions on the package requesting that postal workers "hand cancel" and "handle with care." For either private or postal carriers, it is important to consult with them regarding proper rules and regulations.

MISCELLANEOUS PROCEDURES FOR DETECTION OF DIGESTIVE TRACT PARASITES

Cellophane Tape Preparation

The cellophane tape preparation is used to detect the eggs of *pinworms* (Box 17-12). Female pinworms are nematodes (roundworms) that protrude from the anus and deposit their eggs on the skin around the anus. Pinworm eggs usually are not seen in routine fecal examinations. Of the major domesticated species, only horses are infected by pinworms (*Oxyuris equi*). Of animals used in laboratory research, primates, rodents, and rabbits serve as hosts for pinworms. It is important to remember that dogs and cats are never hosts for pinworms. Pinworms are para-

---

 BOX 17-12 **Cellophane Tape Presentation for Detection of Pinworms in the Horse**

1. Place transparent cellophane tape in a loop, adhesive (sticky) side out, on one end of a tongue depressor.
2. Stand to the side of the horse's hindquarters and raise the tail with one hand while using the other hand to press the tape on the tongue depressor firmly against the skin immediately around the anus.
3. Place a small drop of water on the slide, allowing the water to spread out under the tape.
4. Using a compound microscope, examine the tape for the presence of asymmetric pinworm eggs.

 BOX 17-13 **Baermann Technique**

1. Spread a piece of cheesecloth or a gauze square out on the support screen in the Baermann apparatus. Place 5 to 15 g of the fecal, soil, or tissue sample on the cheesecloth. Fold any excess cheesecloth over the top of the sample. Be sure that the sample is covered by the warm water or physiologic saline; add more if necessary.
2. Allow the apparatus to remain undisturbed overnight.
3. Hold a glass microscope slide under the cut-off pipette, and open the pinch clamp long enough to allow a large drop of fluid to fall on the slide. Apply a coverslip to the slide and examine it microscopically for the presence of larvae. Repeat by examining several slides before deciding that the sample is negative.

---

sites of herbivores (horses and rabbits) and omnivores (rodents, primates, and humans) but never parasites of carnivores (dogs and cats).

Baermann Technique

The Baermann technique is used to recover the larvae of roundworms from feces, soil, or animal tissues (Box 17-13). This method takes advantage of the fact that warm water stimulates nematode larvae in a sample to move about. Once the larvae move out of the sample, they relax in the

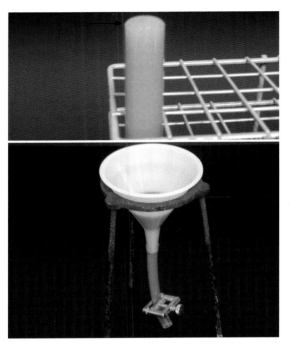

Figure 17-15 Baermann apparatus is used to recover larvae of roundworms from feces, soil, or animal tissues. This apparatus is most useful in recovering larvae of lungworms.

water and sink to the bottom of the container. A Baermann apparatus may be easily constructed to perform this function (Figure 17-15). The Baermann apparatus consists of a ring stand and a ring supporting a large glass funnel. The funnel's stem is connected by a piece of rubber tubing to a tapered tube (a cut of Pasteur pipette). The rubber tubing is clamped shut with a pinch clamp. A piece of metal screen is placed in the funnel to serve as a support for the sample. The funnel is then filled with water or physiologic saline at about 30° C (86° F) to a level 1 to 3 cm above the sample. Innovative alternative designs of this apparatus can be devised from similar materials, provided the same features are preserved.

Larvae recovered from fresh ruminant and equine feces are almost always lungworms. Larvae of *Strongyloides stercoralis*, the intestinal threadworm, also may be recovered from canine feces. Larvae of *Aelurostrongylus abstrusus* may be found in feline feces. Both larvae and adults of *Ollulanus tricuspis* may be found in feline vomitus.

BLOOD IN THE FECES

Some parasitic infections of the digestive tract cause extensive damage to the intestinal lining, resulting in bleeding. This blood may be visible in the fecal sample or may be present in such small quantities that it is only detectable by means of a chemical test. Blood present in such small amounts is termed **occult blood.** Numerous tests are available for the detection of blood in the feces. The simpler tests are based on detection of enzymelike activity of the red blood cell component, hemoglobin.*

These tests are easily performed by following the directions provided by the manufacturer. Blood is detected through an obvious color change. False-positive results may be obtained in fecal samples from animals on a meat diet, so dogs or cats to be tested should be maintained on a meat-free diet for 24 to 48 hours before testing. The presence of fecal blood may be the result of a condition other than parasitic infection, such as gastrointestinal ulcers, other infectious agents, or neoplasms.

GROSS EXAMINATION OF VOMITUS

Vomitus (the product of vomiting) may be grossly examined for adult parasites. These parasites are usually roundworms, which may be particularly common in the vomitus of puppies or kittens. In these young animals, infections with *Toxocara* species or *Toxascaris leonina* may be extensive. Some of the adult worms are expelled by vomiting.

MICROSCOPIC EXAMINATION OF VOMITUS

The microscopic examination of vomitus may reveal the presence of parasites of the stomach of

*Hematest reagent tablets, Ames Division, Miles Laboratories, Elkhart, IN.

dogs and cats. Parasites of the stomach may cause an inflammation of the stomach lining, producing a condition known as *gastritis*. One of the signs of this inflammation is chronic vomiting. *Physaloptera* species, a nematode that attaches to the lining of the stomach of both dogs and cats, is a voracious blood-feeder. A standard flotation procedure performed on the vomitus (as with feces) may reveal the presence of oval, thick-walled, larvated eggs. *Ollulanus tricuspis,* a tiny nematode found in the stomach of cats, produces chronic vomiting. Likewise, a standard flotation procedure performed on the cat's vomitus (as with feces) may reveal the presence of adult parasites and third-stage larvae of *O. tricuspis.* When confronted with chronic vomiting in a dog or cat, practitioners often overlook this important diagnostic procedure.

DIAGNOSIS OF PARASITES OF THE BLOOD AND BLOOD VASCULAR SYSTEM

Dirofilaria immitis, the canine heartworm, is the most important parasite of the vascular system of domestic animals in North America. For this reason, most of the blood examinations for parasites in veterinary practices are aimed specifically at heartworm identification, although other blood parasites occasionally may be diagnosed in the United States. This section describes general tests that may be used to detect some blood parasites, as well as some specific tests for *D. immitis.*

COLLECTION OF BLOOD SAMPLES

Any collection of blood from an animal should be performed *aseptically.* This includes swabbing the skin over the vein with isopropyl alcohol and using a sterile needle.

Blood may be drawn with a standard needle and syringe or a vacuum collection tube (e.g., Vacutainer, Becton Dickinson, Rutherford, NJ). No anticoagulant is required if the blood is to be used immediately for tests, such as the direct smear or filter test, or if it is to be allowed to clot

so that serum may be obtained. If the tests cannot be performed immediately or if some of the blood must be reserved for further testing, clotting must be prevented by addition of an anticoagulant.

Vacuum blood collection tubes are sold containing several different anticoagulants, with color-coded stoppers indicating the particular anticoagulant in each tube. Of these, ethylenediaminetetraacetic acid (EDTA), in tubes with lavender stoppers is among the best for collecting blood for parasite examination, because the amount of distortion it produces is minimal. If the blood is allowed to clot to obtain the clear serum, as for immunologic tests for canine heartworm, vacuum tubes with red stoppers, which contain no anticoagulant, should be used.

Blood samples should always be labeled with the client's name, the animal's name or number, and the date of collection.

The microfilariae of *D. immitis* are more common in canine blood at certain times of the day than at other times. These microfilariae are found in greater numbers during the evening hours than during the daylight hours.

EXAMINATION OF BLOOD

General observations of blood samples should always be recorded. For example, if the blood appears watery, the animal may be anemic. Clinical pathology tests, such as packed cell volume and white blood cell counts, may aid in the diagnosis of parasitism.

Direct Microscopic Examination

The simplest blood parasite detection procedure is by direct microscopic examination of whole blood, known as the *direct smear* technique. This procedure is aimed primarily at detecting movement of parasites that live outside the red blood cells. In the United States and Canada, direct smear usually is used to demonstrate the microfilariae of the canine heartworm, *Dirofilaria immitis;* trypanosome protozoans also may be observed. The direct smear is quick and easy to perform, but only a small amount of blood is examined; that is, the sample size is very small. This is a major disadvantage to using this technique; unless the parasites are present in very large numbers, they may be easily overlooked.

Trypanosomes are found primarily in the tropical regions of the world; occasionally, however, they may be reported in the United States. Trypanosomes are more easily identified as such on stained blood smears than by direct examination of whole blood.

The microfilariae of primary interest in North America are those found in dogs, *D. immitis* and *Acanthocheilonema reconditum.* It is important that veterinary diagnosticians differentiate between these two filarial parasites, because the treatment for *D. immitis* can be stressful and expensive for the pet owner, whereas treatment for *A. reconditum* is not necessary.

Direct microscopic examination of whole blood is an unsatisfactory method for differentiating microfilariae. There are better methods for diagnosing these parasites. Nevertheless, the microfilariae of *D. immitis* are more numerous than those of *A. reconditum.* It is possible to observe low levels of microfilariae in the peripheral blood. There are also subtle differences in the behavior of these microfilariae in the blood smear. Microfilariae of *D. immitis* tend to remain in one spot on the slide and coil and gyrate in place. If they do move, the movement is sluggish. Microfilariae of *A. reconditum* (on rare occasions) will move rapidly across the microscopic field with a snakelike movement.

Thin Blood Smear

A thin blood smear is prepared in the same manner as a blood smear prepared for a white blood cell differential count (Box 17-14 and Figure 17-16).

The area of the smear farthest from the original drop of blood should be the thinnest part of the smear. This region is known as the *feathered edge* of the smear. Because of the large relative size of microfilariae, they are not carried into the feathered edge. The entire slide is fixed and stained with Diff-Quik.

BOX 17-14 Thin Blood Smear

1. Place a glass microscope slide (the "surface slide") flat on the bench surface, then place a small drop of the whole-blood sample near the short end of the slide.
2. Place the short end of a second slide (the "spreader slide") near the middle of the bench surface slide and hold it at a 35- to 45-degree angle. Holding the spreader slide at that angle, slide the short side of that slide backward across the surface slide until it just contacts the drop of blood (see Figure 17-16). When the drop is contacted, it rapidly spreads along the juncture between the two slides.
3. The spreader slide is then smoothly and rapidly slid forward the length of the surface slide, producing a smear with a feathered edge.
4. Allow the surface slide to air-dry, then stain it. Examine the slide with the 10× objective for microfilariae or trypanosomes; the 100× (or oil-immersion) objective may be used for the intracellular parasites.

A thin blood smear cannot be used for accurate differentiation of the microfilariae of *D. immitis* from those of *A. reconditum.* Trypanosomes can be seen between the red blood cells in the smear. Protozoans such as *Babesia* and *Theileria* species can be seen within the red blood cells. Rickettsiae such as *Anaplasma* species may be seen on the surface of the red blood cells.

This blood examination technique uses minute amounts of whole blood. As with the direct smear, the thin blood smear uses only a small amount of blood. Again, the sample size is very small. This is a major disadvantage to using this technique; unless the parasites are present in very large numbers, they may be easily overlooked. To ensure that mild infections are not missed, several blood concentration techniques using larger volumes of blood have been developed.

Thick Blood Smear

A thick blood smear allows examination of a slightly larger amount of blood than a thin blood

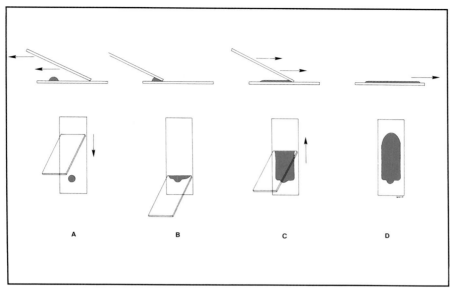

Figure 17-16 Demonstration of correct angle and direction of movement of thin blood smear.

BOX **17-15** Thick Blood Smear

1. Place 3 drops of the blood sample together on a glass slide, and with a wooden applicator stick, spread them out to an area about 2 cm in diameter.
2. Allow the smear to air-dry.
3. Place the glass slide in a slanted position, smear side down, in a glass beaker containing distilled water. Allow the slide to remain in the beaker until the smear loses its red color.
4. Remove and air-dry the slide, then immerse it for 10 minutes in methyl alcohol. Stain with Giemsa stain for 30 minutes. Wash excess stain with tap water.

---

smear (Box 17-15). Microfilariae, protozoa, and rickettsiae may be seen using this method.

Buffy Coat Method

The buffy coat method is a concentration technique for detection of microfilariae in blood samples (Box 17-16). The buffy coat is the layer of white blood cells located between the red blood cells and the clear plasma formed by the centrifugation of whole blood. The specific gravity of microfilariae causes them to gravitate to the upper surface of the buffy coat layer (Figures 17-17 and 17-18). This test is quick and can be performed in conjunction with a packed cell volume determination. It is not possible, however, to determine the species of microfilariae.

Modified Knott's Technique

The modified Knott's technique is a fairly rapid method that detects microfilariae and allows for differentiation between the microfilariae of *Dirofilaria immitis* and *Acanthocheilonema reconditum* (Box 17-17). This technique concentrates the microfilariae from 1 mL of blood and hemolyzes the red blood cells so that the microfilariae may be observed more clearly.

Using the modified Knott's technique, the characteristics in Table 17-1 can be used to distinguish the microfilariae of *D. immitis* from those of *A. reconditum*. Some of these characteristics are unique to the modified Knott's procedure and may not be indicative of other tests that

BOX 17·16   Buffy Coat Method

1. Fill a hematocrit tube with the whole-blood sample and seal one end with hematocrit clay.
2. In the hematocrit centrifuge, centrifuge the hematocrit tube for 5 minutes.
3. If desired, read the packed cell volume to determine if the animal is anemic. Observe the location of the buffy coat layer between the red cell layer and the plasma (Figure 17-17).
4. Place the hematocrit tube on the stage of the compound microscope. Using the 4× objective, examine the zone between the buffy coat layer and the plasma for the presence of microfilarial activity. Use the iris diaphragm to decrease the light, because low light intensity and high contrast increase visualization of the motile microfilariae.

or

Using a small file or glass cutter, deeply scratch the hematocrit tube at the level of the buffy coat. Snap the hematocrit tube by applying thumb pressure opposite the scratch. Immediately take the part of the buffy coat and plasma and tap the buffy coat onto the center of a microscope slide, including some plasma with it. Add a drop of physiologic saline and a drop of methylene blue stain, and cover with a coverslip. Using the 10× objective, examine the slide for the presence of microfilariae.

BOX 17·17   Modified Knott's Technique

1. In a centrifuge tube with a conical end, mix 1 mL of the whole-blood sample and 9 mL of 2% formalin (2 mL of 40% formaldehyde per 98 mL of distilled water). Stopper the tube and rock it back and forth for 1 to 2 minutes until the mixture becomes a clear, red-wine color.
2. Centrifuge the tube at 1500 rpm for 5 minutes.
3. Pour off the liquid supernatant. It is permissible to let the tube stand with open end down for 45 minutes to 1 hour, if time permits. The purpose of this step is to remove as much fluid as possible, leaving sediment only.
4. Add 1 drop of methylene blue stain to the sediment at the bottom of the tube. Transfer a drop of the mixture to a glass slide and apply a coverslip.
5. Examine the slide for the presence of microfilariae using the 10× objective. When microfilariae are found, use a higher-power objective (40×) to observe the fine differences between them (see Table 17-1).
6. The diagnostician may stop this procedure at one of two stopping points: (a) the diagnostician has identified microfilariae as those of *D. immitis* or *A. reconditum,* or (b) the diagnostician runs out of the sediment/stain mixture.

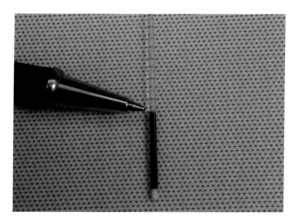

Figure 17-17   Buffy coat in hematocrit tube.

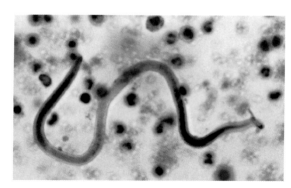

Figure 17-18   Microfilariae in buffy coat smear of canine blood. (560×.)

TABLE **17-1**   Morphologic Characteristics for Differentiation of Microfilariae of *Dirofilaria immitis* and *Acanthocheilonema reconditum*

CHARACTERISTIC	DIROFILARIA IMMITIS	ACANTHOCHEILONEMA RECONDITUM
Body shape	Usually straight	Usually curved
Body length	295-325 µm (average, 310 µm)	250-288 µm (average, 280 µm)
Anterior end	Tapered	Blunt ("broom handle")
Posterior end	Straight	Curved or hooked (artifact of formalin fixation)

depend on observation of morphologic features of the microfilariae. The most accurate features are the total length of the microfilaria, the midbody width, and the shape of the cranial end. Body length and width should be measured using an ocular micrometer (see p. 233). The body length of the microfilaria of *A. immitis* ranges from 295 to 325 µm (average, 310 µm), whereas the body length of the microfilaria of *A. reconditum* ranges from 250 to 288 µm (average, 280 µm). The midbody width of the microfilaria of *D. immitis* ranges from 5 to 7.5 µm, whereas the midbody width of the microfilaria of *A. reconditum* ranges from 4.5 to 5.5 µm. It is important for the differentiation between the morphologic parameters of the parasites on the modified Knott's procedure that veterinary clinics own and calibrate an ocular micrometer within at least one compound microscope. The anterior end of the microfilaria of *D. immitis* tapers gradually from its midbody, whereas the microfilaria of *A. reconditum* has a blunt anterior end, much like the end of a wooden broom handle. Likewise, the posterior end of the microfilaria of *D. immitis* is said to be straight, whereas the microfilaria of *A. reconditum* may have a curved or "button hook" or "shepherd's crook" tail. It is important to remember that the bending, or hooking, of the tail of the microfilaria of *A. reconditum* is an artifact of 2% formalin fixation and may not be observed as a consistent diagnostic feature. Likewise, other microfilarial tests (e.g., commercial filter tests) will not produce this "hooking" characteristic. Veterinary diagnosticians should remember to measure several microfilariae to confirm that the microfilaremia is not a concomitant infection (i.e., both parasites may be present). In some areas of North America

(those with high indigenous populations of both mosquitoes and fleas), infection with both filarial parasites is quite possible.

Commercial Filter Technique

A commercial filter technique, such as the DIFIL-Test, is another means of concentrating microfilariae within blood samples. The materials required are available in a diagnostic kit.*

This kit contains complete directions for use. One mL of the blood sample (no anticoagulant is required if the test is performed immediately) is mixed with 9 mL of a red blood cell lysing solution in a 10- or 12-mL syringe. A new, disposable porous filter (a sieve with tiny holes) is placed in a filter holder. The fluid in the syringe is injected into the filter holder and is then flushed with 10 mL of water. Unlysed cells and microfilariae are retained on the surface of the filter. The filter is then gently transferred with thumb forceps to a glass microscope slide and stained with 2 drops of the stain provided in the commercial kit. The filter is covered with a coverslip and examined with a 10× objective for the presence of microfilariae (Figure 17-19).

The filter technique uses an amount of blood equal to that used in the modified Knott's procedure and can be rapidly performed. This test is best used as an indicator of microfilaremia, the presence of microfilariae in the peripheral blood. It is important to remember that microfilarial species often cannot be identified using a commercial filter technique. If microfilariae are found, additional tests, such as the modified Knott's technique, should be per-

---

*DIFLIL-Test, EVSCO Pharmaceuticals, Buena, NJ.

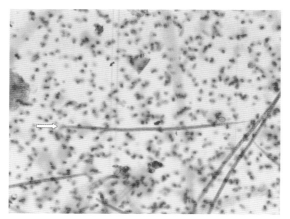

Figure 17-19 Microfilariae of *Dirofilaria immitis* using the DIFIL-Test.

formed to determine if the infection is that of *D. immitis* or *A. reconditum.*

Immunologic Heartworm Tests

About 25% of dogs with adult heartworm infection in the heart and pulmonary vasculature do not have circulating microfilariae in the peripheral blood. These infections may consist of (1) heartworms that are too young to produce microfilariae, (2) a "unisex" or "single sex" infection, (3) an infection in which circulating microfilariae are produced by the adult female heartworms but for some reason are removed by the host, or (4) an infection in which the circulating microfilariae have been killed by a drug, but the adults have not been affected. This type of infection is referred to as an *occult infection.* The hosts are said to be *amicrofilaremic,* without microfilariae. It is important to remember that cats also can be infected with canine heartworms. Because the heartworms are in cats rather than in their natural host (the dog), the adult heartworms produce either low numbers of microfilariae or none at all.

To detect infections, tests have been developed in which antibodies against antigens of adult *D. immitis* react with chemicals to produce a color change when those antigens are in a blood sample. These tests are available commer-

cially and are easy to perform and fairly rapid (15-20 minutes) if the directions are carefully followed and samples are correctly labeled. Older styles of kits detected only canine antibodies in response to heartworm and were unsuitable for use in cats.

Other tests for parasites such as *Toxoplasma gondii* can be performed by diagnostic laboratories. The laboratory will provide information on the nature and amount of specimens they require. Box 17-18 provides a method for collecting serum for these immunologic tests.

Miscellaneous Methods for Microfilarial Identification

Other heartworm diagnostic procedures used in detection and differentiation of microfilariae include staining with brilliant cresyl blue and acid phosphatase. These procedures are often too cumbersome and time-consuming to be used in a veterinary practice. Many of the reagents used in the processing of these specimens are not found in the practice setting. Diagnostic referral

---

BOX 17-18 Serum Collection

1. Using a needle and syringe, dispense 10 mL of blood into a blood collection vacuum tube lacking anticoagulant (tube with red stopper). Slowly dispense the blood from the syringe into the tube to avoid lysis of the red blood cells. Lysis of red blood cells often interferes with the functions of many tests.
2. Keep the blood at room temperature (25° C) for 2 to 3 hours to allow a solid clot to form.
3. Remove the formed blood clot with a wooden applicator stick by gently "rimming" the clot and then sliding it up the side of the tube with the applicator stick. Discard the clot. (Some laboratories request that the clear serum then be transferred to a new tube.)
4. Correctly label each tube of serum with the client's name, animal's name or number, and practitioner's name. Refrigerate the sample until it can be shipped.
5. Ship samples to the laboratory packed in an insulated container with ice or a cool pack. Use the fastest shipper possible, for next-day delivery.

laboratories usually are able to perform both procedures.

DIAGNOSIS OF PARASITISM OF THE RESPIRATORY SYSTEM

FECAL EXAMINATION FOR RESPIRATORY PARASITES

The life cycles of helminth (nematode and trematode) parasites of the lungs are completed through the passage of their eggs or larvae up the airways to the pharyngeal region, from which they are swallowed and passed to the outside environment in the feces. Because of this dependence on fecal transmission, parasitism of the lungs and airways is often diagnosed by microscopic examination of the feces, as described previously. The Baermann technique can be used to recover the larvae of lungworms from feces. Again, this method takes advantage of the fact that warm water stimulates the larvae in a sample to move about. Once the larvae move out of the sample, they relax in the water and sink to the bottom of the container. The Baermann apparatus should be employed when parasitism with lungworms is suspected (see p. 243).

EXAMINATION OF SPUTUM AND TRACHEAL WASHES

The larvae and eggs of respiratory parasites have the same characteristics as those found in the feces. An exception is *Dictyocaulus* species, lungworms of cattle and sheep, which are usually seen in the sputum as eggs containing larvae rather than as free larvae in the feces.

A drop of sputum or nasal discharge on a microscope slide is easily examined. Several slides should be examined. When the sputum is especially viscous, a drop of the material should be placed between two microscope slides and both slides examined microscopically. Larger quantities of fluid obtained from the respiratory tract should be concentrated by centrifugation at 1500 rpm for 5 minutes. A drop of the sediment can then be placed on a slide and examined microscopically.

Dogs may occasionally become infested with the nasal mite, *Pneumonyssoides caninum,* or *Linguatula serrata,* the tongue worm. A cotton swab dipped in mineral oil may be inserted into the nose of a suspect dog and rubbed against the nasal membranes. *Pneumonyssoides* mites have eight legs and are white and hairless and 1 to 1.5 mm long. The eggs of *L. serrata* measure 90 by 70 μm and contain a mitelike larval stage. Tiny hooked feet may be observable in the interior of the egg.

DIAGNOSIS OF PARASITISM OF THE URINARY SYSTEM

Roundworms are common parasites of the kidney and urinary bladder. They complete their life cycle by passing eggs out of the host's body in the urine. These nematodes include *Capillaria* species, which inhabit the walls of portions of the urinary system of both dogs and cats, *Dioctophyma renale,* the giant kidney worm of dogs, and *Stephanurus dentatus,* the swine kidney worm.

COLLECTION OF THE URINE SAMPLE

Urine for parasitologic examination may be collected during normal urination. Catheterization and cystocentesis are usually not necessary unless part of the sample is to be used for bacteriologic or cytologic examination. A waxed paper cup (3-5 mL) with a lid or other clean container may be used for collection. The cup is held in the urine stream and filled. Unless the sample is to be used for other tests, it is not necessary to collect the sample at a certain time during urination. Clients can be instructed to collect a sample at home. Urine samples should be properly labeled with the client's name and the animal's identification and refrigerated until the examination can be conducted.

URINE EXAMINATION FOR PARASITES

The primary method of examining urine for parasites is by microscopic examination of the sediment (Box 17-19). Just as with microscopic examination of feces using the compound microscope, uniform movement and a thorough search

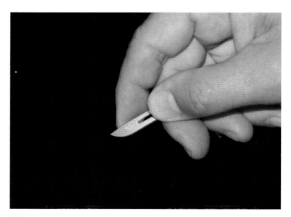

Figure 17-20   Safe method of holding scalpel blade with thumb and second finger for skin scrapings.

of the microscope slide must be performed. Regardless of how the slide is moved, the area under the coverslip must be thoroughly and uniformly searched (see Figure 17-8). When a parasite egg is observed at low magnification, higher-power objectives may be used to examine it more closely.

DIAGNOSIS OF PARASITISM OF THE SKIN

SKIN SCRAPINGS

The skin scraping is one of the most common diagnostic tools used in evaluating animals with dermatologic problems. Equipment required includes an electric clipper with a no. 40 blade, a scalpel or spatula, mineral oil in a small dropper bottle, microscope slide, coverslip, and a compound microscope. Typical lesions or sites likely to harbor the particular parasite should be scraped (e.g., margins of ear for *Sarcoptes scabiei*).

The scraping is performed with a no. 10 scalpel blade, used with or without a handle. A stainless steel spatula is preferred by some clinicians. The scalpel blade should be held between the thumb and the second finger, with the first finger used to help prevent cutting the animal (Figure 17-20). Before the skin is scraped, the blade is dipped in a drop of mineral oil on the slide, or a drop of mineral oil may be placed on the skin.

During the scraping process, the blade must be held perpendicular to the skin. Holding at another angle may result in the animal being incised. The average area scraped should be 6 to 8 cm².

The depth of the scraping varies with the typical location of the parasite in question. When scraping for mites that live in tunnels (e.g., *Sarcoptes* spp.) or hair follicles and sebaceous glands (e.g., *Demodex* spp.), the skin should be scraped until a small amount of capillary blood oozes from the area. Clipping the area with a no. 40 blade before scraping enables better visualization of the lesion and removes excess hair that impedes proper scraping and interferes with collection of epidermal debris. For surface-dwelling mites (e.g., *Chorioptes* spp., *Cheyletiella* spp.), the skin is scraped superficially to collect loose scales and crusts. Clipping before scraping is not always necessary when infestation with surface-dwelling mites is suspected.

All the scraped debris on the forward surface of the blade is then spread in a drop of mineral oil on a glass microscope slide. A glass coverslip is placed on the material, and the slide is ready for microscopic examination using the 4× (scanning) objective. The slide should be examined systematically in rows so that the entire area under the coverslip is evaluated (see Figure 17-8). Low light intensity and high contrast increase visualization of mites and eggs. If necessary, the slide may be evaluated using the 10× (low-power) objective.

Demonstration of a characteristic mite or egg is frequently diagnostic for most diseases. In certain circumstances, more than only identification of the parasite is necessary. For example, determining live/dead ratios and observing immature stages of demodectic mites are important in evaluating a patient with demodecosis. A decrease in the number of live mites and eggs during therapy is a good prognostic sign.

CELLOPHANE TAPE PREPARATION

When attempting to demonstrate the presence of lice or mites that live primarily on the surface of the skin (e.g., *Cheyletiella* spp.), use a cellophane tape preparation instead of a skin scraping. Clear cellophane tape is applied to the skin to pick up epidermal debris. A ribbon of mineral oil is placed on a glass slide, and the adhesive surface of the tape is placed on a glass slide and then placed on the mineral oil. Additional mineral oil and a coverslip may be placed on the tape to prevent the tape from wrinkling, but this is not necessary. The slide is then examined systematically in rows.

GROSS SPECIMENS

Unknown, large *ectoparasites* such as fleas, ticks, chigger mites, biting flies, and myiasis-producing maggots are often collected from the surface of the animal's skin. It is important that these arthropods be placed in a sealed container in either 10% formalin or 95% ethyl alcohol for shipment to a diagnostic laboratory. As many intact specimens as possible should be collected and shipped to a diagnostic laboratory capable of *speciating* these important ectoparasites. Again, containers should be properly labeled with the client's name and the animal's identification.

DIAGNOSIS OF PARASITISM OF MISCELLANEOUS BODY SYSTEMS

PARASITES OF THE EYE

Thelazia species are nematodes that live within the conjunctival sac and on the surface of the eye of several species of domestic animals, including cattle, sheep, goats, horses, dogs, and cats. The adult parasites are milky white, 7 to 17 mm long, and reside in the conjunctival sac, just under the eyelids, particularly the third eyelid. Diagnosis is made by anesthetizing the eye with a local ophthalmologic anesthetic and directly examining the eye for parasites. If observed, these nematodes should be removed while the eye is anesthetized.

Another nematode parasite often associated with the eye is *Dirofilaria immitis*, the canine heartworm. This parasite is often associated with aberrant locations throughout the body of both dogs and cats. A site that may become infected is the anterior chamber of the eye; this is usually noted with alarm by the pet owner. Treatment is by surgical extraction of the wandering ("lost") parasite by a veterinary ophthalmologist.

PARASITES OF THE EAR

Otodectes cynotis, the ear mite, is a common cause of external ear irritation in both dogs and cats. These white mites are frequently observed during otoscopic examination. *O. cynotis* are approximately the size of a grain of salt; they may be seen on a cotton swab after it has been moistened with mineral oil and used to clean the dark, waxy debris from the ears of infested animals. This material may be transferred to a drop of mineral oil on a microscope slide and spread out with the swab. A coverslip is applied to the debris, and the slide is examined microscopically in a systematic manner. This mite has suckers on short stalks at the tips of some of its legs (Box 17-20).

BOX 17-20 Ear Smear Procedure

1. Obtain a sample of debris from the affected ear.
2. Place 2 or 3 drops of mineral on the slide and an equal amount of ear debris.
3. Mix the ear debris and mineral oil with a wooden applicator to form a homogenous solution.
4. Remove large pieces of debris.
5. Place a coverslip over the smear.
6. Examine under the compound microscope and record any parasites or parasite eggs found.

PARASITES OF THE GENITAL TRACT

Tritrichomonas foetus is a protozoan parasite of the reproductive tract of cattle. These parasites reside in the prepuce of infected bulls and in the vagina, cervix, and uterus of infected cows. It may also be found within the stomach contents of aborted fetuses. *T. foetus* is pear shaped and 10 to 25 μm long, with a sail-like, undulating membrane and three rapidly moving, whiplike anterior flagella. In fresh specimens, these protozoans move actively with a jerky motion. Diagnosis is by finding the organisms in washings from its predilection sites or from the stomach of the aborted fetus. Fluid material should be centrifuged at 2000 rpm for 5 minutes. The supernatant is then removed and a drop of sediment transferred to a slide for microscopic examination for the organisms. Several slides should be examined. For more accurate diagnosis, fluid material from the predilection sites can be cultured in a special medium. Laboratories specializing in diagnostic parasitology should be consulted for information on these techniques.

18

Reference to Common Parasite Ova and Forms Seen in Veterinary Medicine

A major part of the veterinary technician's job is identifying parasites in feces and blood. This chapter is a quick reference guide for identifying those parasites often seen in feces and blood of the dog and cat, the horse, the ruminants, and the swine.

COMMON PARASITES OF DOGS AND CATS

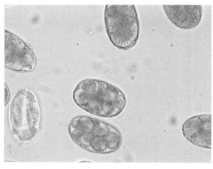

Figure 18-1 *Ancylostoma caninum* ("hookworm").

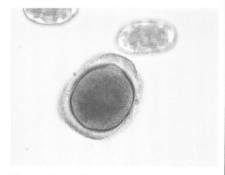

Figure 18-2 *Toxocara canis* ("roundworm").

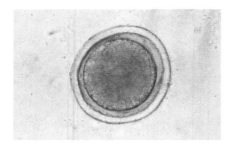

Figure 18-3   *Toxocara cati* ("roundworm").

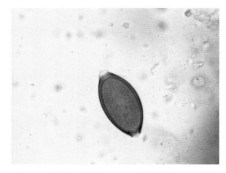

Figure 18-4   *Trichuris vulpis* ("whipworm").

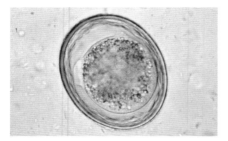

Figure 18-5   *Toxascaris leonina* ("roundworm").

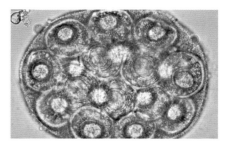

Figure 18-6   *Dipylidium caninum* ("tapeworm").

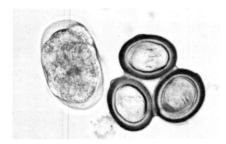

Figure 18-7   *Taenia pisiformis* ("tapeworm").

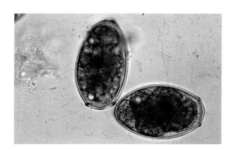

Figure 18-8   *Paragonimus kellicotti* ("lung fluke").

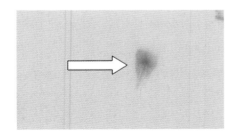

Figure 18-9   *Giardia* species trophozoite.

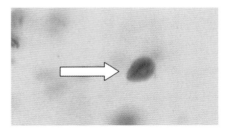

Figure 18-10   *Giardia* species oocyst.

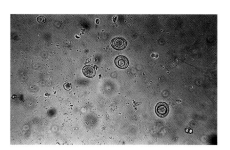

Figure 18-11   *Isospora canis,* large oocysts ("coccidia").

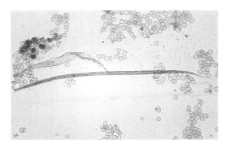

Figure 18-12   *Dirofilaria immitis* microfilariae ("heartworm").

COMMON PARASITES OF HORSES

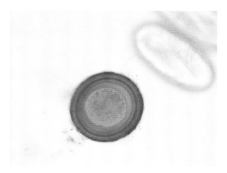

Figure 18-13   *Parascaris equorum* ("equine roundworm").

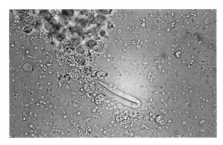

Figure 18-14   *Habronema* species ("equine stomach worm").

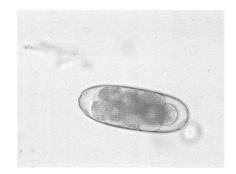

Figure 18-15   *Strongylus vulgaris* ("equine hookworm").

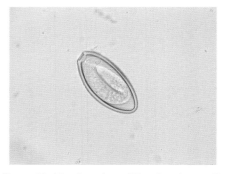

Figure 18-16   *Oxyuris equi* ("equine pinworm").

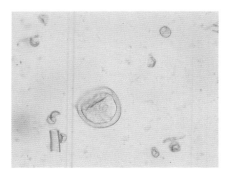

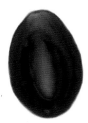

Figure 18-18   *Eimeria leuckarti* ("equine coccidia").

Figure 18-17   *Anoplocephala perfoliata* ("equine tape-worm").

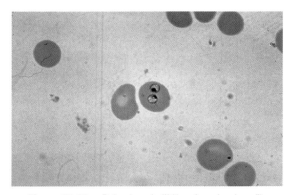

Figure 18-19   *Babesia caballi* ("equine piroplasm").

COMMON PARASITES OF RUMINANTS

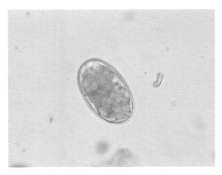

Figure 18-20   *Trichostrongylus* species ("ruminant hookworm").

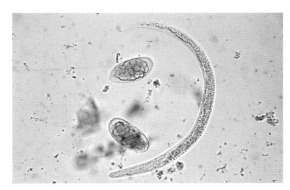

Figure 18-21   *Dictyocaulus viviparus* ("bovine lungworm").

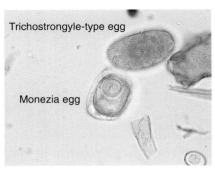

Trichostrongyle-type egg

Monezia egg

Figure 18-22   *Monezia* species, square ("ruminant tapeworm").

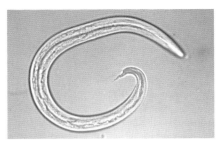

Figure 18-23   *Muellerius capillaris* ("lungworm of sheep and goats").

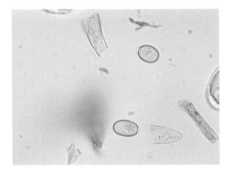

Figure 18-24   *Eimeria* species ("ruminant coccidia").

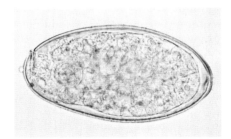

Figure 18-25   *Fasciola hepatica* ("ruminant liver fluke").

COMMON PARASITES OF SWINE

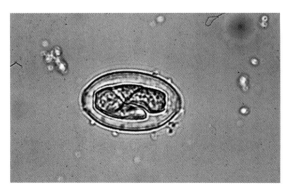

Figure 18-26   *Ascarops strongylina* ("swine stomach worm").

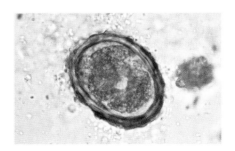

Figure 18-27   *Ascaris suum* ("swine roundworm").

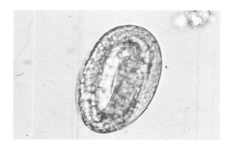

Figure 18-28 *Metastrongylus apri* ("swine lungworm").

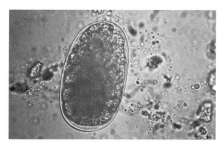

Figure 18-29 *Stephanurus dentatus* ("swine hookworm").

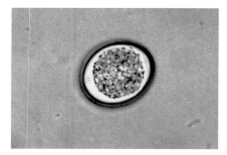

Figure 18-30 *Isospora suis* ("swine coccidia").

Parasite Reference List by Species and Parasite Type

PARASITES OF DOGS AND CATS

NEMATODES

Aelurostrongylus abstrusus, pp. 36, 244
Acanthocheilonema reconditum, pp. 33, 41, 233, 246, 247, 249
Ancylostoma braziliense, pp. 28, 219
Ancylostoma caninum, pp. 28, 219, 220, 255
Ancylostoma tubaeforme, pp. 28, 219
Aonchotheca putorii or *Capillaria putorii*, p. 25
Capillaria feliscati, p. 39, 257
Capillaria plica, pp. 39, 251
Dioctophyma renale, pp. 38, 251
Dirofilaria immitis, pp. 31, 40-42, 223, 233, 245-247, 249, 250, 257
Dracunculus insignis, p. 42
Enterobius vermicularis, p. 31
Eucoleus aerophilus or *Capillaria aerophila*, pp. 25, 38
Eucoleus böehmi, p. 38
Filaroides hirthi, p. 37
Filaroides milksi, p. 37
Filaroides osleri, p. 37
Ollulanus tricuspis, pp. 25, 244, 245
Pelodera strongyloides, pp. 40, 46
Physaloptera species, pp. 23, 245
Spirocerca lupi, p. 23
Strongyloides stercoralis, pp. 29, 244
Strongyloides tumiefaciens, p. 29
Thelazia californiensis, pp. 42, 253
Toxascaris leonina, pp. 25, 244, 256
Toxocara canis, pp. 25, 216, 244, 255
Toxocara cati, pp. 25, 216, 244, 256
Trichuris campanula, p. 30
Trichuris serrata, p. 30
Trichuris vulpis, pp. 30, 233, 256
Uncinaria stenocephala, pp. 28, 219

CESTODES

Diphyllobothrium species, pp. 77, 98, 100, 215
Dipylidium caninum, pp. 73, 86, 214, 230, 256
Echinococcus granulosus, pp. 74, 94, 213
Echinococcus multilocularis, pp. 74, 94, 213
Mesocestoides species, p. 95
Multiceps multiceps, pp. 74, 91
Multiceps serialis, pp. 91, 93
Spirometra species, pp. 77, 99
Taenia hydatigena, p. 88
Taenia ovis, p. 88
Taenia pisiformis, pp. 74, 88, 230, 256
Taenia taeniaeformis or *Hydatigera taeniaeformis*, p. 91

TREMATODES

Alaria species, p. 110
Heterobilharzia americanum, pp. 111, 112
Nanophyetus salmincola, p. 110
Paragonimus kellicotti, pp. 104, 111, 256
Platynosomum fastosum, p. 109

ACANTHOCEPHALANS

Oncicola canis, pp. 115, 118

PROTOZOANS

Babesia canis, pp. 127, 246
Balantidium coli, pp. 125, 239
Cryptosporidium species, pp. 126, 209

Eimeria bovis, pp. 129, 240, 259
Eimeria zuernii, pp. 129, 240, 259
Tritrichomonas foetus, pp. 129, 253
Trypanosoma species, pp. 129, 246

ARTHOPODS

Aedes species, p. 158
Amblyomma americanum, p. 193
Amblyomma maculatum, p. 194
Anopheles species, p. 158
Boophilus annulatus, p. 194
Calliphora species, p. 163
Chorioptes bovis, pp. 177, 252
Chorioptes caprae, pp. 177, 252
Chorioptes ovis, pp. 177, 252
Chrysops species, p. 159
Cochliomyia hominivorax, p. 164
Culex species, p. 158
Culicoides species, p. 158
Damalinia bovis, p. 151
Demodex species, pp. 179, 180, 252
Haematobia irritans, p. 160
Hypoderma bovis, p. 165
Hypoderma lineatum, p. 165
Lucilia species, pp. 162, 163
Lutzomyia species, p. 158
Melophagus ovinus, p. 161
Musca autumnalis, p. 162
Musca domestica, p. 163
Oestrus ovis, p. 167
Otobius megnini, p. 192
Phaenicia species, p. 163
Phormia species, p. 163
Psoroptes bovis, p. 177
Psoroptes ovis, p. 177
Sarcoptes scabei, pp. 173, 175, 252
Simulium species, p. 157
Solenopotes capillatus, p. 151
Stomoxys calcitrans, p. 159
Tabanus species, p. 159
Trombicula species, p. 182

ANNELIDS

Dinobdella species, p. 205
Haemopis terrestris, p. 204
Limnatis species, p. 205

PARASITES OF HORSES

NEMATODES

Dictyocaulus arnfieldi, p. 53
Draschia megastoma, p. 47
Habronema microstoma, pp. 47, 53, 257
Habronema muscae, pp. 47, 53, 257
Onchocerca cervicalis, p. 54
Oxyuris equi, pp. 53, 243, 257
Parascaris equorum, pp. 49, 257
Setaria equina, pp. 55, 242
Strongyloides westeri, p. 53
Strongylus edentatus, p. 51
Strongylus equinus, p. 51
Strongylus vulgaris, pp. 51, 257
Thelazia lacrymalis, pp. 54, 253
Trichostrongylus axei, p. 49

CESTODES

Anoplocephala magna, p. 85
Anoplocephala perfoliata, pp. 85, 258
Paranoplocephala mamillana, p. 85

PROTOZOANS

Babesia caballi, pp. 131, 246, 258
Babesia equi, pp. 131, 246
Eimeria leuckarti, pp. 130, 240, 258
Giardia equi, pp. 130, 239
Klossiella equi, p. 131
Sarcocystis neurona, p. 132

ARTHROPODS

Aedes species, p. 158
Amblyomma americanum, p. 193
Amblyomma maculatum, p. 194
Anopheles species, p. 158
Calliphora species, p. 163
Chorioptes equi, pp. 177, 252
Chrysops species, p. 159
Cochliomyia hominivorax, p. 164
Culex species, p. 158
Culicoides species, p. 158
Demodex equi, pp. 180, 252
Gasterophilus species, pp. 166, 231, 232
Haematobia irritans, p. 160
Lucilia species, p. 163

Menacanthus stramineus, p. 151
Ornithonyssus sylviarum, p. 183

ANNELIDS

Theromyzon tessulatum, p. 205

PARASITES OF RABBITS

NEMATODES

Obeliscoides cuniculi, p. 64
Passalurus ambiguus, p. 63
Trichostrongylus calcaratus, p. 64

PROTOZOANS

Eimeria irresidua, pp. 136, 240
Eimeria magna, pp. 136, 240
Eimeria media, pp. 136, 240
Eimeria perforans, pp. 136, 240
Eimeria stiedai, pp. 136, 240

ARTHROPODS

Cediopsylla simplex, p. 170
Cheyletiella parasitivorax, pp. 184, 252
Cuterebra species, p. 164
Dermacentor variabilis, p. 193
Haemaphysalis leporispalustris, p. 195
Hemodipsus ventricosus, p. 156
Listrophorus gibbus, p. 189
Odontopsylla multispinosus, p. 170
Psoroptes cuniculi, pp. 175, 176
Sarcoptes scabei, pp. 173, 175, 252

PARASITES OF GUINEA PIGS

NEMATODES

Paraspidodera uncinata, p. 63

PROTOZOANS

Cryptosporidium wrairi, pp. 140, 209
Eimeria caviae, pp. 140, 240
Entamoeba caviae, p. 140
Giardia caviae, pp. 139, 239
Giardia muris, pp. 139, 239
Tritrichomonas caviae, p. 140

ARTHROPODS

Chirodiscoides caviae, p. 188
Dermacentor variabilis, p. 193
Gliricola porcelli, p. 155
Gyropus ovalis, p. 155
Notoedres muris, p. 173
Ornithonyssus bacoti, p. 183
Sarcoptes scabei, pp. 173, 175, 176, 252
Trixacarus caviae, pp. 175, 176

PARASITES OF RATS

NEMATODES

Aspiculuris tetraptera, p. 61
Syphacia muris, pp. 59, 61
Syphacia obvelata, p. 61
Trichosomoides crassicauda, p. 61

CESTODES

Hymenolepis diminuta, p. 79
Hymenolepis nana, pp. 79, 215

PROTOZOANS

Eimeria nieschultzi, pp. 139, 240
Giardia muris, pp. 139, 239
Spironucleus muris, p. 139
Tetratrichomonas microti, p. 139
Tritrichomonas muris, p. 139

ARTHROPODS

Cuterebra species, p. 164
Dermacentor variabilis, p. 193
Notoedres muris, p. 173
Ornithonyssus bacoti, p. 183
Polyplax spinulosa, p. 155
Radfordia ensifera, p. 188

PARASITES OF MICE

NEMATODES

Aspiculuris tetraptera, p. 59
Syphacia muris, p. 59
Syphacia obvelata, p. 59

CESTODES

Hymenolepis diminuta, p. 79
Hymenolepis nana, pp. 79, 215

PROTOZOANS

Eimeria falciformis, pp. 138, 240
Eimeria ferrisi, pp. 138, 240
Eimeria hansonorum, pp. 138, 240
Eimeria hansorium, pp. 138, 240
Giardia muris, pp. 137, 239
Klossiella muris, p. 138
Spironucleus muris, p. 137
Tetratrichomonas microti, p. 137
Tritrichomonas muris, p. 137

ARTHROPODS

Cuterebra species, p. 164
Dermacentor variabilis, p. 193
Myobia musculi, p. 185
Myocoptes musculinus, p. 185
Polyplax serrata, p. 153
Ornithonyssus bacoti, p. 183
Radfordia affinis, p. 185
Radfordia ensifera, p. 188

PARASITES OF HAMSTERS

NEMATODES

Syphacia muris, p. 62
Syphacia obvelata, p. 62

CESTODES

Hymenolepis diminuta, p. 79
Hymenolepis nana, pp. 79, 215

PROTOZOANS

Giardia species, pp. 139, 239
Spironucleus muris, p. 139

Tetranucleus microti, p. 139
Tritrichomonas muris (criceti), p. 139

ARTHROPODS

Demodex aurati, p. 180
Demodex criceti, p. 180
Ornithonyssus bacoti, p. 183

PARASITES OF GERBILS

NEMATODES

Dentostomella translucida, p. 62

CESTODES

Hymenolepis diminuta, p. 79
Hymenolepis nana, pp. 79, 215

ARTHROPODS

Demodex aurati, pp. 180, 252
Demodex criceti, pp. 180, 252
Hoplopleura meridionidis, p. 155

PARASITES OF FISH

PROTOZOANS

Chilodonella species, p. 141
Cryptocaryon irritans, p. 141
Ichthyophthirius multifiliis, p. 141
Piscinoodinium species, p. 141
Tetrahymena species, p. 141

PARASITES OF REPTILES

PENTASTOMES

Armillifer species, pp. 198, 225
Porocephalus crotali, pp. 198, 225
Porocephalus species, pp. 198, 225
Kiricephalus species, pp. 198, 225

Glossary

Aberrant parasite Parasite that has wandered from its usual site of infection into an organ or location in which it does not ordinarily live; also called *erratic parasite*.

Acanthella Larval acanthocephalan within the intermediate host, where the acanthella will develop into a juvenile acanthocephalan, the *cystacanth*.

Acanthocephalan A thorny-headed worm.

Acanthor Larval acanthocephalan parasite within an egg.

Acariasis Any infestation or infection by either mites or ticks.

Acaricides Chemical compounds developed to kill mites and ticks.

Acetabulum One of four suckers on anterior end of a true tapeworm *(eucestode)*.

Aliquot Percentage of a solution or sample.

Amicrofilaremic Referring to the absence of immature filarial parasites.

Amphistome Type of digenetic fluke with an oral sucker on one end and a ventral sucker on the other end.

Anthelmintics Chemical compounds developed to kill roundworms, tapeworms, flukes, and thorny-headed worms; also *anthelminthics*.

Antiprotozoals Chemical compounds developed to kill protozoan organisms.

Apicomplexan Banana-, comma-, or boomerang-shaped protozoan found in epithelial cells of intestine, in blood cells, and in cells of reticuloendothelial and nervous systems. Apicomplexans have complex life cycles that are intimately integrated into physiology of host's body. Their locomotory (movement) organelles are internal and are not grossly visible as with other types of protozoans.

Armed tapeworm True tapeworm that possesses a rostellum on its anterior end.

Arthropodology The study of arthropods.

Arthropods The creatures possessing a chitinous exoskeleton and jointed legs.

Ascariasis Infection with ascarids, either larval or adult.

Aseptically Referring to the use of sterile technique.

Baermann technique Type of diagnostic technique in which nematode larvae are collected using gravity (sedimentation).

Bothria Two slitlike holdfast organs on anterior end of a pseudotapeworm.

Buccal cavity Large opening that connects to the mouth of a nematode; connects the mouth to the esophagus.

Bursal rays Fingerlike projections that make up the copulatory bursa of a male nematode.

Calcareous corpuscles Microscopic calcium deposits unique to the tissues of cestodes (tapeworms); also called *calcareous bodies*.

Cantharidin Toxic or blistering compound found in a certain group of beetles; often referred to as "Spanish fly" but has no aphrodisiac effect.

Capitulum Mouthparts of an acarine (mite or tick).

Cercaria Asexual stage within the life cycle of a digenetic trematode. The cercarial stage emerges from the snail, the first intermediate host. Each cercarial stage will produce one metacercarial stage, found in the second intermediate host or on vegetation. Sometimes the cercaria can penetrate the definitive host directly.

Cervical alae   Lateral expansion of the cuticle in anterior end of nematodes.

Cestodes   Tapeworms.

Chelicerae   Two cutting or lacerating organs of the capitulum.

Cilia   Tiny hairs that cover the body surface of one type of protozoans, the ciliates, which move by these beating hairs.

Cloaca   Opening of the intestine of the male nematode to the outside.

Coenurus   Type of metacestode (larval tapeworm) stage characterized by a large, fluid-filled bladder with a number of invaginated (inside-out) scolices attached to the wall of the bladder.

Commensalism   Type of symbiotic relationship in which one symbiont benefits while other neither benefits nor is harmed.

Common name   Name for a living organism in different regions of the world; may refer to different organisms in different places.

Complex metamorphosis   One of two types of metamorphosis by insects; four developmental stages are egg, larva (maggot), pupa, and adult. Each stage is morphologically and structurally different from the other stages.

Copulatory bursa   Flattened, lateral expansion of a nematode's cuticle in posterior region of certain male nematodes; serves to hold onto or grasp the female nematode during the mating process; composed of fingerlike projections called *bursal rays.*

Coracidium   Ciliated hexacanth embryo unique to the pseudotapeworms (cotylodans); when ingested by the first intermediate host (an aquatic crustacean), forms a procercoid within the intermediate host.

Cotylodan   Pseudotapeworm, or "false" tapeworm.

Cutaneous larva migrans   Migration of larval stages of a nematode through the skin of humans, most often seen with *Ancylostoma braziliense.*

Cyst stage   Nonmotile, resistant stage of a protozoan parasite.

Cystacanth   Juvenile acanthocephalan that possesses an inverted proboscis.

Cysticercoid   Type of metacestode (larval tapeworm) stage characterized by a small, fluid-filled bladder containing a single, noninvaginated scolex; usually microscopic.

Cysticercus   Type of metacestode (larval tapeworm) stage characterized by a large, fluid-filled bladder containing a single invaginated (inside-out) scolex.

Definitive host   Host that harbors the adult, sexual, or mature stages of the parasite.

Demodicosis   Infection with demodectic (*Demodex*) species of mites.

Dioecious   Having separate sexes, both male and female; the nematodes and the arthropods are dioecious.

Direct life cycle   Life cycle that does not involve an intermediate host.

Ectoparasite   Parasite that lives *on* the body of the host.

Ectoparasitism   Parasitism by an external parasite; an ectoparasite will produce an *infestation* on the host.

ELISA test   Enzyme-linked immunosorbent assay, an immunodiagnostic technique that detects the presence of antigen.

Embryophore   Tapeworm hexacanth embryo with striated eggshell.

Empodia   Clawlike features on the end of the second pair of legs of *Myobia musculi* and *Radfordia affinis.*

Endoparasite   Parasite that lives *within* the body of the host; an endoparasite will produce an *infection* within that host.

Endoparasitism   Parasitism by an internal parasite.

Erratic parasite   See *Aberrant parasite.*

Eucestode   True tapeworm.

Euryxenous parasite   Parasite with a very broad host range.

Facultative myiasis   Condition resulting from fly larvae, normally free-living, that become parasitic and use a host for their development.

Facultative parasite   Organism that is usually free-living (nonparasitic) in nature that develops a parasitic existence in certain hosts.

Feathered edge   Thinnest part of a blood smear at the edges.

Fistula   Pore or hole within tissue.

Flagellum   Long, whiplike or lashlike appendage that is used by group of protozoans (the flagellates) as a means of moving about in a fluid medium.

Flea dirt   Partially digested blood defecated by fleas; also called *flea feces* and *flea frass.*

Flotation solutions   Liquids used to float parasite ova, cysts, and larvae for identification.

Fly strike   Lesion(s) produced in the tissues of vertebrate hosts by maggots or fly larvae.

Gadding   Action of a vertebrate host marked by running away from irritating flies.

Hermaphroditic   Having complete sets of both male and female reproductive organs; the tapeworms and the flukes (except for the schistosomes) are hermaphroditic.

Hexacanth embryos   Type of tapeworm egg containing a six-toothed embryo (an embryo that contains six hooklets).

Hirudin   Anticoagulant produced in the oral cavity of leeches.

Hirudiniasis   Infestation with leeches.

Holdfast organelle   Scolex or head of the pseudotapeworm.

Homoxenous parasite   Parasite that will infect only one type of host; also called *monoxenous parasite.*

Host   In a parasitic relationship, the member in which or on which the parasite lives.

Hydatid cyst   Large, fluid filled bladder that contains brood capsules, which bud from the internal germinal membrane; each brood capsule contains several protoscolices.

Hydrometer   Tool used for measuring specific gravity of solutions.

Hypodermis   Thin layer beneath the cuticle that secretes the cuticle layer of the nematode.

Hypostome   Penetrating, anchorlike sucking organ of the tick.

Idiosoma   Abdomen of a mite or a tick.

Incidental parasite   Parasite that is found in a host in which it does not usually live.

Indirect life cycle   Life cycle of a parasite that requires an intermediate host.

Insecticides   Chemical compounds developed to kill insects.

Intermediate host   Host that harbors the larval, juvenile, immature, or asexual stages of the parasite. A parasite may have more than one intermediate host.

Invaginated scolices   Tapeworm heads turned inside out within the bladder worm life stage.

Larviparous   Type of female nematode that retains her eggs within the uterus and produces live first-stage larvae.

Leeches   Bloodsucking annelids.

Life cycle   Development of a parasite through its various life stages. Every parasite has its own distinct, individual life cycle with at least one *definitive host* and may have one or more *intermediate hosts.*

Linnaean classification scheme   Classification for all living organisms (animals, plants, fungi, protozoa, and algae) perfected by Linnaeus, an early Swedish biologist. Every living organism can be classified using the following scheme: kingdom, phylum, class, order, family, genus, and species.

Maggots   Fly larvae.

Measly meat   Meat that is infected with the cysticerci (larval stages) of certain human and canine tapeworms; includes measly beef (*Cysticercus bovis*), measly pork (*Cysticercus cellulosae*), and measly mutton (*Cysticercus ovis*).

Metacercaria   Asexual stage within life cycle of a digenetic trematode. The cercarial stage emerges from the snail (first intermediate host) and produces one metacercarial stage. If the cercaria is ingested by the second intermediate host, it will encyst within its tissues. The metacercarial stage may be found encysted on vegetation.

Metacestode Larval tapeworm found within the intermediate host; types of metacestodes include cysticercoid, cysticercus, coenurus, hydatid, tetrathyridium, procercoid, plerocercoid, and sparganum

Metamorphosis To achieve the adult stage, an insect must undergo a series of developmental changes in size, form, or structure called metamorphosis; two types are simple metamorphosis and complex metamorphosis.

Metazoan parasites Multicellular or complex organisms that include trematodes, tape-worms, pseudotapeworms, roundworms, thorny-headed worms, leeches, and arthropods.

Microfilaria Immature stage of filarial parasites.

Microfilaricide Dewormer that kills the immature filarial worm.

Miracidium Developmental stage in the life cycle of a digenetic trematode. This stage emerges from the operculated egg and penetrates the first intermediate host, usually a snail.

Molt Shedding of the outside cuticle.

Monoecious Hermaphroditic; having both sexes in a single organism.

Morula Type of nematode egg that contains an undeveloped grapelike cluster of cells within the eggshell.

Mutualism Type of symbiotic relationship in which both organisms in the symbiotic relationship derive some benefit.

Myiasis Infection or infestation of the tissues or organs of humans or domesticated or wild animals by larval members (maggots) of the Order Diptera (two-winged flies).

Neck Germinal or growth region of a tapeworm that lies just posterior to the scolex.

Nematodes Roundworms.

Nit Egg of a sucking or chewing louse.

Obligatory myiasis Lesions caused by fly larvae that require a vertebrate host for their development.

Obligatory parasite Parasite that must lead a parasitic existence; most parasites of domestic animals are obligatory parasites.

Occult infection Parasitic filarial infection without the presence of microfilaria.

Operculum Tiny "door" at either end (pole) of an egg.

Oviparous Type of nematode egg that contains either a single cell or a morula, a grapelike cluster of cells.

Ovoviviparous Type of nematode egg that contains a first-stage larva.

Papillae Fingerlike or bumplike projections on the cuticle of a nematode.

Parasite In a parasitic relationship, the member that lives on or within the host.

Parasitiasis Type of parasitic relationship in which the parasite is present on or within the host and is potentially pathogenic (harmful); however, the animal does not exhibit outward clinical signs of disease.

Parasiticides Chemical compounds (either very simple or very complex) used to treat specific internal and external parasites (endoparasites and ectoparasites); different types include anthelmintics, acaricides, insecticides, and antiprotozoals.

Parasitism Type of symbiotic relationship between two organisms of different species in which one member (the *parasite*) lives on or within the other member (the *host*) and may cause harm; parasite is metabolically dependent on host for its survival.

Parasitology The study of parasitic relationships.

Parasitosis Type of parasitic relationship in which the parasite is present on or within the host and causes obvious injury or harm to the host animal; host exhibits obvious outward signs of clinical parasitism.

Parthenogenesis Modified form of sexual reproduction characterized by the development of offspring by a female nematode from eggs that have not been fertilized by a male nematode; genus best known for parthenogenesis is *Strongyloides*.

Pediculosis   Infestation by either chewing or sucking lice.

Pedipalps   Two leglike accessory appendages attached to the capitulum that act as sensory support.

Pentastome   Tongue worms, or linguatulids. These annelid-like arthropods have a mitelike larval stage; nymphal stages are found in the visceral organs of many mammalian intermediate hosts; adults usually parasitize snakes and other reptiles. The one pentastome found in domestic animals is *Linguatula serrata*.

Periodic parasite   Parasite that makes frequent short visits to its host to obtain nourishment or other benefits.

Phoresis   Type of symbiotic relationship in which the smaller member in the relationship is mechanically carried by the larger member.

Piroplasmosis   Disease caused by *Babesia canis*.

Plerocercoid   Type of metacestode stage unique to the pseudotapeworms (cotylodans); this solid-bodied metacestode stage with slitlike mouthparts is found within the second intermediate host, usually a fish or an amphibian; also called a *sparganum*.

Predator-prey   Extremely short-term symbiotic relationship in which one symbiont benefits at the expense of the other; for example, a lion (the *predator*) will kill a zebra (the *prey*). The prey ultimately pays with its life and serves as a food source for the predator.

Prepatent period   Time from the point of infection by a nematode until a specific diagnostic stage can be recovered.

Proboscis   Retractable "nose" on anterior end of an acanthocephalan covered with tiny, backward-facing spines and serving to anchor the acanthocephalan to the mucosa of the intestine.

Procercoid   Type of metacestode stage unique to the pseudotapeworms (cotylodans). This metacestode stage is found within the first intermediate host, usually a tiny aquatic crustacean.

Proglottid   Individual boxlike components of the tapeworm strobila; three types are immature, mature, and gravid proglottids.

Protoscolices   Multiple tapeworm heads in a hydatid cyst that will develop into adult tapeworms when ingested by a definitive host.

Protozoan parasites   Unicellular, or single-cell, organisms that may be flagellates, amoebae, sporozoans, apicomplexans, or ciliates.

Pseudoparasites   Living creatures or inanimate objects that are not parasitic but may be mistaken for, or erroneously identified as, parasites.

Pyriform apparatus   The innermost lining (third lining) of the covering of certain types of tapeworm eggs; pear shaped.

Redia   Asexual stage in life cycle of a digenetic trematode. This stage is preceded by the sporocyst stage, which will produce many rediae; each redia will form many cercariae.

Reportable parasites   Parasites that must be reported to both state and federal authorities (e.g., *Cochliomyia hominivorax*, *Psoroptes* species in large animals, *Boophilus annulatus*).

Repugnatorial glands   Areas beneath the legs of millipedes that produce caustic substances.

Reservoir host   Vertebrate host in which a parasite or disease occurs in nature and is a source of infection for humans or other domesticated animals.

Rhabditiform esophagus   Type of nematode esophagus that has a corpus, isthmus, and posterior bulb.

Rostellum   Holdfast organ on anterior end of an armed true tapeworm; has backward-facing hooks used to anchor the tapeworm to wall of the host's gut.

Sarcoptic acariasis   Infection caused by *Sarcoptes* mites.

Schistosome cercarial dermatitis   Swimmer's itch; highly pruritic papular or pustular dermatitis in humans caused by cercarial stages of bird schistosomes.

Scientific name   Name for a living organism that is composed of two Latin words, usually written in italics. The *genus name* (capitalized; e.g., *Felis*) indicates the group to which a particular type of animal or plant belongs;

the *specific epithet* (lowercase; e.g., *catus*) indicates the type of animal itself.

Scolex The "head" of a tapeworm.

Scutum Hard, chitinous plate that covers the body of some ticks.

Simple metamorphosis One of two types of metamorphosis by insects; three developmental stages are egg, nymph, and adult. The nymphal and adult stages are similar in morphology and structure; nymphal stage is smaller than the adult and is not sexually mature.

Siphonapterosis Infestation with fleas.

Sparganosis Infection with the plerocercoid stage within the tissues of the second intermediate host.

Sparganum See *Plerocercoid.*

Spicule pouch Pocket that contains the male reproductive organs used to open the female nematode's vulva.

Spicules Male nematode intromittent organs ("penis") associated with the copulatory bursa.

Sporocyst Asexual stage in life cycle of a digenetic trematode. This miracidium penetrates the snail (first intermediate host) and forms the sporocyst stage.

Stenoxenous parasite Parasite with a narrow host range.

Strobila Body of the tapeworm composed of individual proglottids (immature, mature, and gravid).

Strobilocercus Type of metacestode stage found in the liver of rats; has a scolex that attaches to a long neck, which connects to a fluid-filled bladder.

Stylostome Tube that forms in the host at the attachment site of chiggers.

Symbiont Each living organism in a symbiotic association.

Symbiosis Any association (temporary or permanent) between at least two living organisms of different species.

Tegument Body wall of a helminth.

Tetrathyridium Solid-bodied metacestode stage with a deeply invaginated acetabular scolex. This stage is capable of asexual reproduction and divides by splitting into two stages; two then become four, four become eight, and so on.

Tick paralysis Paralysis seen in animals and humans caused by the toxic saliva in some ticks.

Transport host Special type of intermediate host in which the parasite does not undergo any development, but instead remains arrested, or encysted ("in suspended animation"), within the host's tissues; also called *paratenic host.*

Trematodes The flukes.

Trophozoite stage Motile or moving form of a protozoan.

Unarmed tapeworm True tapeworm that lacks a rostellum on its anterior end.

Urticating The act of stinging.

Vermicide Dewormer that kills the parasite so that it can be broken down by the host's body.

Vermifuge Dewormer that paralyzes (but does not kill) the adult parasite so that it passes in the feces.

Visceral larva migrans Migration of larval stages of a nematode through the organs or tissues of humans (e.g., lungs, liver, eye); most often seen with *Toxocara canis.*

Warbles Larvae of dipteran flies found in the skin of domestic or wild animals, producing cutaneous myiasis.

Wolves See *Warbles.*

Zoonosis Any disease or parasite that is transmissible from animals to humans.

INDEX

Page numbers followed by f indicate figures; b, boxes.